RADIOGRAPHIC ANATOMY OF THE CHEST AND ABDOMEN

In friendship and gratitude to MF who believed that the book was necessary and prevailed in our authorship of it; and to our readers who may prove all of us right.

Radiographic Anatomy of the Chest and Abdomen

D. NOREEN CHESNEY *FSR, TE*
Group Superintendent Radiographer
Coventry Hospitals

MURIEL O. CHESNEY *FSR, TE*
Principal Radiographer, Central
Birmingham School of Radiography

BLACKWELL SCIENTIFIC PUBLICATIONS
OXFORD LONDON EDINBURGH MELBOURNE

Osney Mead, Oxford,
8 John Street, London, WC1
9 Forrest Road, Edinburgh,
P.O. Box 9, North Balwyn, Victoria, Australia.

First published 1976

Chesney, D. Noreen
Radiographic anatomy of the chest and abdomen.
Bibl. – Index.
ISBN 0-632-09440-0
1. Title 2. Chesney, Muriel O.
617'.54'0757 RC941
Chest – Radiography
Abdomen – Radiography

Distributed in the United States of America by
J.B. Lippincott Company, Philadelphia,
and in Canada by
J.B. Lippincott Company of Canada Ltd., Toronto.

Printed and bound in Great Britain by
William Clowes & Sons, Limited
London, Beccles and Colchester

Contents

Preface

Any reader of this book is entitled to know that it is not a textbook of anatomy, a subject of which the authors readily confess to having a smattering of ignorance. However, if we know very little anatomy, there is no doubt that we have had radiographs in front of our eyes on so many occasions, by now uncountable, that we should be able to recognise what we see and appreciate the reasons for the appearances. Because of this, when we were asked if we would write a book on radiographic anatomy we began to think that perhaps we could.

What constitutes such a book? We have interpreted our remit to mean that the book should recognise, describe and in some degree explain the physical realities of the normal human being, which in the radiograph are presented as an esoteric, two-dimensional image.

Radiographs, therefore, have been the raw material of this book and the structures and processes displayed upon them have made the pattern of its fabric; but necessarily the book is only a partial exposition of anatomy and physiology, which must be sought entire in other volumes. To such standard works this is an appropriate companion but it cannot be a substitute for them. Our book is intended to help radiographers understand radiographs, not give them the total knowledge of anatomy which they should have.

If this is not a textbook of anatomy, neither is it an atlas of pathology. There are many radiological textbooks and journals which illustrate the X-ray appearances of the abnormal for any radiographer or other reader who has the wish or need to know them. These necessarily are outside our scope; our purpose refers exclusively to normal radiographic anatomy. This is not to say that the reader of these pages will encounter no single allusion to radiological diagnosis. Here and there we hope to have increased the student's understanding of radiographs by some account—on an appropriately broad level—of the features of an image which may constitute the axis of radiological diagnosis.

We see anatomical nomenclature as an abstruse, elusive subject and might find it difficult to name the one we have used in this book. Our aim has been in general to employ the terms which students may expect to hear from their teachers and encounter in the contemporary anatomical texts which we hope are the companions of their studies. We trust that nowhere have we committed the solecism of an unacceptably mixed terminology or failed to be understood.

Why only the chest and abdomen? We have limited its subject matter mainly in the interests of the book's physical proportions. If there is any need for a work of this kind, we think that the book is likely to be most useful if it is not a massive volume, unable to wander far from the library's shelves. The place for this text is not in a library but wherever its readers are looking at radiographs.

A second consideration dictating the present choice of material is concerned with ease of interpretation. It is evident that newcomers to radiography more readily and more rapidly recognise the skeletal image than they are able to appreciate the significance of other radiographic detail. If limited help is to be given, it is proper to offer it in the more difficult region.

Even within the boundaries determined by X-ray appearances of the chest and abdomen, a claim that this is a complete text would be unjustified. A few pertinent radiological examinations receive no reference here. We have made our selection in the main from radiographs which students are likely fairly often to encounter in the general diagnostic

X-ray departments where they spend the greater part of their time. Highly specialised and infrequently employed procedures we have disregarded. To give space to what is seldom undertaken is almost certainly to ensure that some pages of the book remain unopened.

Finally—if such a word is appropriate in a preface—we owe and gladly give thanks to radiological friends who have read our manuscript and our radiographs and from whose consequent advice the book has benefited. These helpful mentors on the consultant radiological staffs of our several hospitals were Dr D.M. Alexander, Dr J.E. Glasgow, Dr J.F.K. Hutton, Dr M.P. Patel and Dr A.W. Robinson. We are deeply grateful for their interest and willingness to support our project in real terms of time, thought and the supply of apposite radiographs.

We are happy to express appreciation to Dr R. Astley of Birmingham Children's Hospital who obtained for us angiocardiograms from his valuable records and allowed us to use them. We likewise appreciate a similar courtesy from Dr E.H. Mucklow who gave us certain thoracic lymphangiograms. We are grateful also for Dr J.C. Bishop's kind permission to copy radiographs of the chest which were in the radiological library of the Birmingham General Hospital. From the darkroom staff of both these hospitals we acknowledge help received in the duplicating of certain originals.

We sometimes think that writing a book is the easiest part, being aware that once the raw material leaves the author's desk there is much which is critical still to do before a first reader turns the finished pages. It is therefore a pleasure to express appreciation to our publisher, printers and blockmakers for their careful work in creating this book.

1975

D.N.C.
M.O.C.

Prologue

What do the words mean?

'When I use a word' Humpty Dumpty said in a rather scornful tone 'it means just what I choose it to mean, neither more nor less.'

We thought of Lewis Carroll's Humpty Dumpty when we began to write this book and to think about the words used to describe radiographic appearances and denote the varying extent to which different materials absorb X-rays. The words are often confusing and confused.

So we decided to illuminate the matter by explaining at the outset what meanings we have chosen for some of the words we use. There may be other writers and talkers who will disagree with our choice of words and be prepared to argue about the meanings we have assigned to them. Doubtless those who feel strongly in the matter will express themselves on it.

A main objective for writers must be to make themselves understood by their readers, unless they write merely to exercise their minds and their typewriters. We think that this prologue may help to achieve understanding and we hope that it does.

Differences in absorption

The conventional radiograph is produced by passing an X-ray beam through a patient towards a film so that the beam impinges on the film, having emerged from the patient. Different structures of the body absorb X-rays to varying extents; for example, bone absorbs X-rays quite heavily; metal fillings in the teeth absorb X-rays even more; fat does not absorb much X-radiation; air-containing structures such as the lungs absorb X-rays to a smaller extent still. So what emerges from the patient is an X-ray pattern produced by these different absorptive powers of the various tissues and organs of the body.

Through the structures which absorb X-rays heavily comes a low intensity of radiation which in some instances is so slight as to produce no visible effect on the film. Through the structures which absorb hardly any of the X-rays there comes a much higher intensity of radiation which has a very marked effect on the film so that it is very dark on development. Thus a pattern is created.

We needed a word to mean *heavily absorptive of X-rays*; a word to mean *moderately absorptive of X-rays*; a word to mean *hardly absorptive of X-rays*. We chose the following.

Radiopaque	**heavily absorptive of X-rays**
Radiolucent	**moderately absorptive of X-rays**
Radioparent	**hardly absorptive of X-rays**

The student may (and doubtless will) find writers who use these words with other meanings or other words with these same meanings or similar meanings. Practice is not standardised but we can at least control our own use in this book and explain it as we do here.

Radiographic shadows

The structures which absorb X-rays heavily and thus stop them from coming through to reach the film are said to cast a shadow or to give rise to a shadow in the radiograph. This is analogous to the production of a shadow by visible light: it is commonly observed that any structure that does not wholly transmit light casts a shadow to the side away from the one the light reaches. Such shadows are dark in tone. The shadows in radiographs are light in tone.

To understand why they should be light in tone it is necessary to keep two facts in mind:
(i) structures which stop X-rays from reaching the film produce the shadows;
(ii) where X-rays reach the film it becomes dark and where X-rays do not reach the film it is light on development.
From these statements it follows that the shadows produced by structures absorbing X-rays are light areas in the radiograph. In this book we have therefore used the word shadow with the meaning below.

Shadow **a light area in the radiograph**

Radiographic density

In radiographic contexts the words *dense* and *density* can be used with several meanings. Writing about radiographic appearances we assign to the word *density* its meaning of photographic density. This is a numerical expression of the degree of blackening in the film after exposure and development. It indicates the extent to which the black area can transmit light.

Density **photographic density, the logarithm of the ratio**

$$\frac{\textbf{Incident light}}{\textbf{Transmitted light}}$$

Dense area **a dark area on the radiograph**

We have tried to follow the March Harc's injunction to say what we mean and we have also tried like Alice to mean what we say. We hope that we have succeeded in this and in our intention to be clear to the reader.

Chapter 1
The Posteroanterior Radiograph of the Thorax

The radiograph which most fully surveys the thorax is the posteroanterior projection with the patient erect which is taken to show the lung fields and the outlines of the heart and other structures in the mediastinum. In this radiograph some of the structures which comprise the thorax and its contents are well seen. Prominently shown are the skeletal outlines of the thoracic cage; and the soft-tissue organs are also visualised to some extent.

Familiarity with the posteroanterior radiograph of the thorax is essential to anyone who hopes to learn the radiographic anatomy of the region and so we propose here to consider this radiograph fully. We take as a starting point the display of the bony skeleton which it shows.

The bony skeleton of the thorax

Posteroanterior radiographs of the chest are shown in Fig. 1.1 of a male subject and in Figs. 1.2 and 1.3 of female subjects. The bony thorax is of course the same in all three. What usually differentiates the sexes here are the soft tissue outlines of the female breasts; sometimes the radiographs of males show a breast outline if the subject is obese or is being treated with drugs which may develop the breasts as a side effect.

The female breast outlines are seen as curving shadows

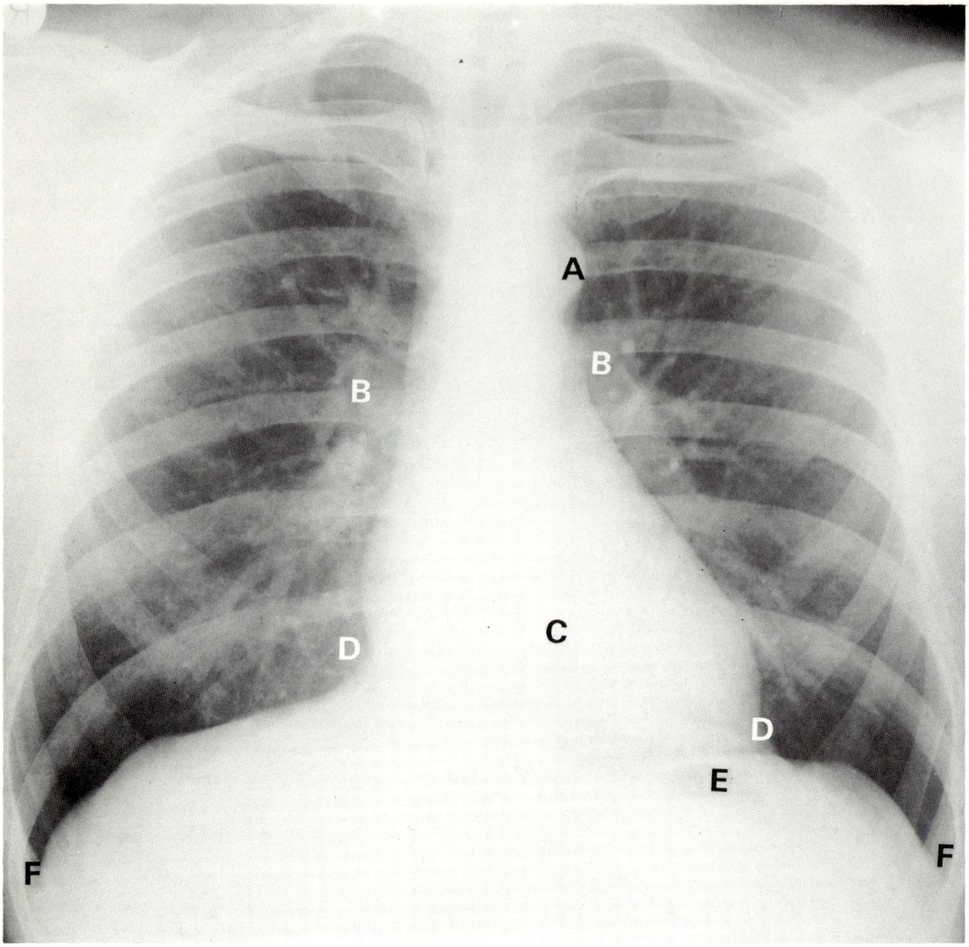

Fig. 1.1. A posteroanterior radiograph of the chest of a male subject.

A Aortic knuckle
B Region of the root of the lung
C Heart shadow
D Cardiophrenic angle
E Gas in the fundus of the stomach
F Costophrenic angle

with the convexity downwards. They may overlie the lung fields towards the basal areas as in Fig. 1.2; they may be higher or lower than this and they may be seen to extend laterally beyond the boundaries of the bony thorax as in Fig. 1.3. Sometimes the nipple can be seen as a circular shadow superimposed on the lung field.

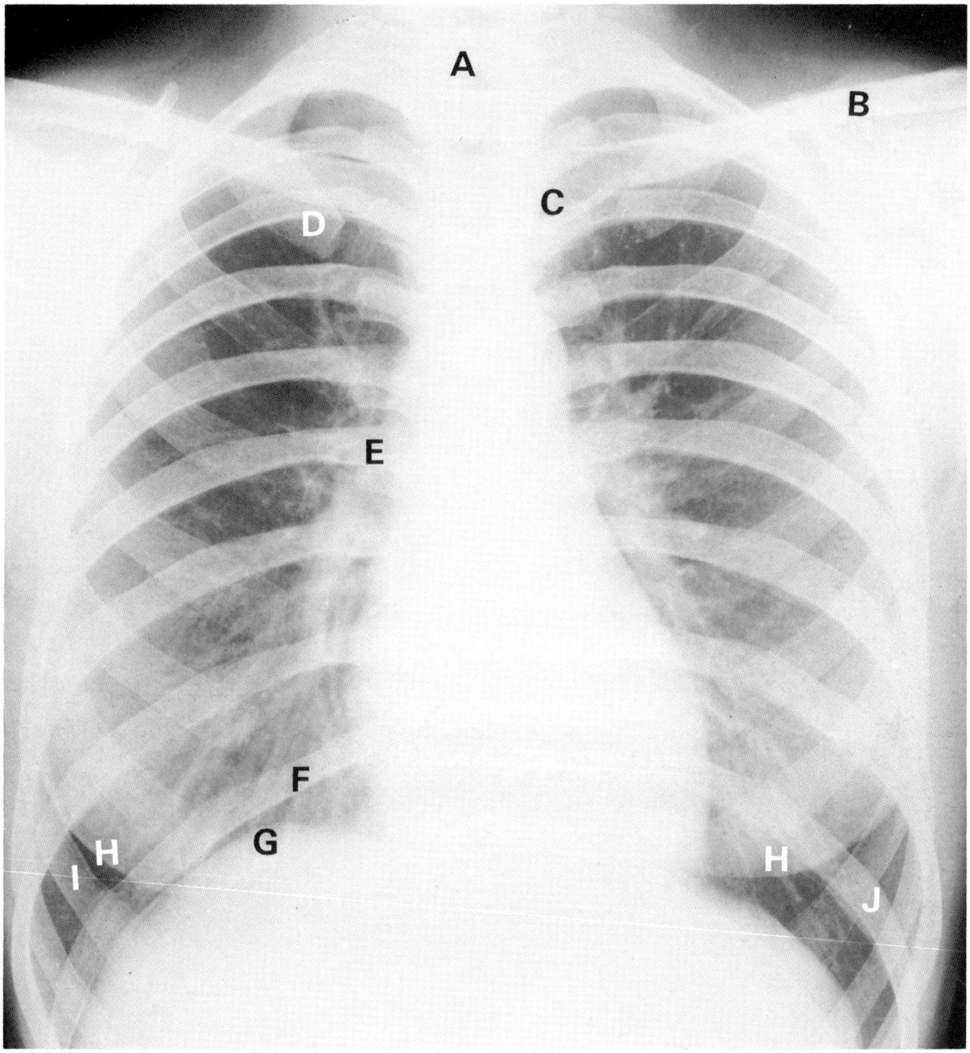

Fig. 1.2. A posteroanterior radiograph of the chest of a female subject with small breasts.

A Thoracic vertebra 1
B Left clavicle
C Inner end of left clavicle
D Right rib 1
E Vertebral end of right rib 7
F Right rib 10
G Right arc of diaphragm
H Breast shadow
I Anterior end of right rib 7
J Left rib 10

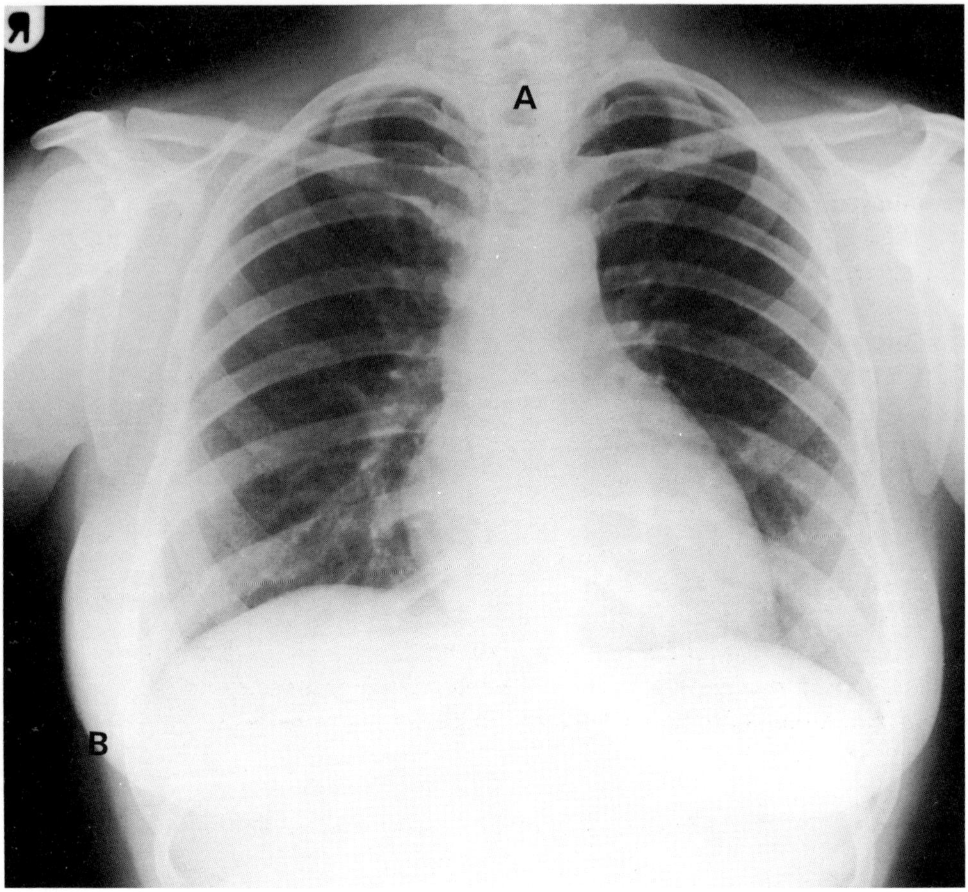

Fig. 1.3. A posteroanterior radiograph of the chest of a female subject (larger breasts than the subject in Fig. 1.2).

A Spinous process of thoracic vertebra 2

B Breast shadow

The variations in the breast outlines are normal features. They arise because nature is diverse in constructing physical interpretations of the fundamental plan. We all of us have more or less the same number of organs functioning for the same purposes; but in detail the individual variations are countless.

SKELETAL ANATOMY

In a medical dictionary the thorax may be found defined as *the chest, the portion of the trunk between the neck and the diaphragm.* Its skeletal boundaries are as follows:

Anteriorly: the sternum, the anterior ends of the ribs, the costal cartilages.

Posteriorly: the 12 thoracic vertebrae, the posterior parts of the ribs.

Laterally: the ribs.

Superiorly at the thoracic inlet: the inlet is bounded by the first thoracic vertebra posteriorly, by the upper edge of the manubrium sterni anteriorly, by the first ribs laterally.

Inferiorly at the thoracic outlet: the outlet is bounded by the twelfth thoracic vertebra posteriorly, by the cartilages of the seventh to tenth ribs laterally. (The thoracic outlet is closed below by the diaphragm. We just note this here because our immediate concern is with skeletal boundaries.)

Not all the bones mentioned above can be well seen on posteroanterior radiographs of the thorax. This is mainly because the radiograph is a two-dimensional representation of a three-dimensional structure and superimpositions occur within the image.

RADIOGRAPHIC APPEARANCES OF THE BONY SKELETON

The region of the thoracic inlet can be identified at the top of the radiograph, the first ribs and the first thoracic vertebra being shown. Of the skeletal boundaries of the thoracic outlet little can be seen. The twelfth dorsal vertebra which is the posterior boundary of the outlet is not shown; the anterior ends of the seventh, eighth, ninth and tenth ribs which indicate the anterior boundary are only partly seen in Fig. 1.2 and their junctions with their respective cartilages (cartilage itself being radioparent) may be presumed. The eleventh and twelfth ribs which are the lateral boundaries of the thoracic outlet are not seen at all.

Prominent thoracic boundaries which dominate the radiograph are the ribs, forming a lattice pattern through which the outlines of organs are seen. In a good radiograph of a suitable subject such as the one illustrated in Fig. 1.2, most of the first ten ribs are to be seen. The rib outlines can be traced from their posterior to anterior ends (although not the whole extent of all of the first ten ribs) and the ribs may be counted from the first downwards.

Counting is most easily done by looking at the posterior parts of the ribs where they are seen to run in towards the vertebrae. Counting the ribs also allows the vertebrae to be located even although they cannot themselves be fully seen. The first dorsal vertebra can be distinguished from the seventh cervical by the directions of the transverse processes: those of the dorsal vertebra are directed in an upwards and a lateral line and those of the cervical vertebra in a downwards and a lateral line. In many cases the first thoracic vertebra is further distinguished by the fact that it has ribs attached to it while the seventh cervical has not but this state of affairs is not invariable: ribs attached to the last cervical vertebra (cervical ribs) are fairly common.

Radiographers should note that the posterior or vertebral ends of the ribs are higher than the anterior ends as the ribs slope downwards; and that the ribs are not all at the same angle of slope. Radiographic projection tends to exaggerate the slope of the ribs so that in the image it can seem to be more than it is in fact. In general the upper ribs are more oblique than the lower ones; obliquity diminishes from the ninth rib to the twelfth. The ribs increase in length from the first down to the seventh. After that they become progressively shorter and the twelfth rib is much shorter than the eleventh and may be shorter than the first.

In the radiograph the anterior ends of the ribs appear to hang in space, not joined to anything. In fact they are attached to the costal cartilages. These are bars of hyaline cartilage extending from the anterior ends of the ribs and they are not seen on the radiograph because cartilage is radioparent. In old age the costal cartilages tend to become calcified or even ossified and it is then possible to visualise on a radiograph the outlines of calcified parts; Figs. 1.13 and 1.14 show examples.

Prominently shown across the upper part of the thorax are the two clavicles lying almost horizontally at the root of the neck. Anatomically the clavicle is part of the shoulder girdle and it functions to brace back the shoulders and to assist in supporting the weight of the upper limb. The medial ends of the clavicles articulate with the upper end of the sternum at the sterno-clavicular joints.

Sometimes the skin and subcutaneous tissues which cover the clavicles and the sternomastoid muscles in the neck can be seen in the posteroanterior radiograph of the chest; for example, in Fig. 1.6. These tissues show as lines which first come down from the neck and can then be seen running along the upper borders of the clavicles from their inner ends laterally.

Figs. 1.1, 1.2 and 1.3 demonstrate that in the posteroanterior radiograph of the chest the sternoclavicular joints are not well seen, although the inner ends of the clavicles can just be distinguished. The sternoclavicular joints are lost through superimposition of the images of other structures: the third to fourth dorsal vertebrae, the vertebral ends of their attached ribs and the structures of the upper mediastinum. Radiographers checking the correctness of radiographic projection and of the positioning of the patient look at the inner ends of the clavicles. They should appear equidistant from the midline. The midline may be represented by a vertical line drawn through the shadows of the spinous processes of the upper dorsal vertebrae and prolonged down the radiograph; these spinous processes form roughly triangular shadows, apex upwards, on the outlines of the vertebral bodies seen in the upper dorsal region.

If the patient is positioned facing the film and is rotated in respect to the film, the appearance of the inner ends of the clavicles is as shown in Fig. 1.4. On the side of the patient which is rotated away from the film, the inner end of the clavicle appears to move further laterally from the vertebral outlines and the viewer can distinguish the sternoclavicular joint and the manubrium sterni. On the side of the patient which is nearer the film, the inner end of the clavicle appears to move medially towards the vertebral outlines. So for the radiograph shown in Fig. 1.4 the patient was rotated with her left side further from the film. (In the particular case of Fig. 1.4 there is some degree of scoliosis or abnormal lateral curvature of the spine and this may have misled the radiographer who positioned the patient.) This appearance of the

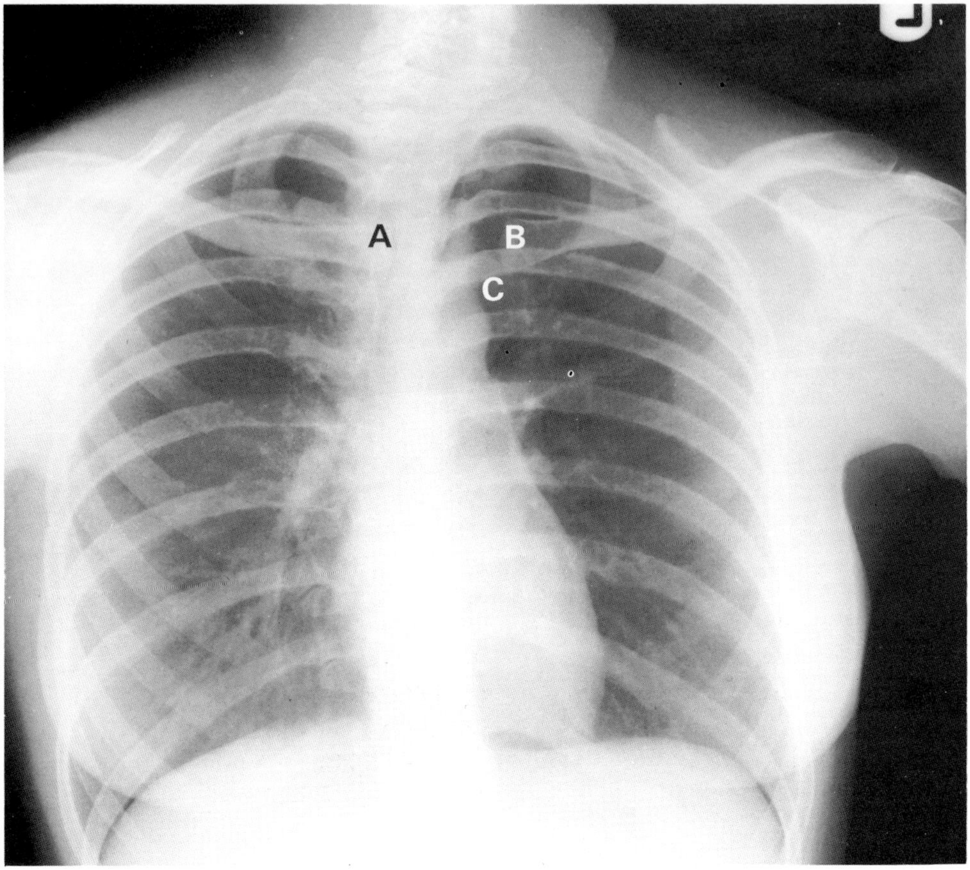

Fig. 1.4. A posteroanterior radiograph of the chest with the patient slightly rotated in position.
A Inner end of right clavicle
B Inner end of left clavicle
C Manubrium sterni

inner end of the clavicles in respect to the spine which is given by the positioning of the patient *could* result also from a very oblique alignment of the X-ray beam; malpositioning of the patient is a much more likely cause of such an appearance in the general run of radiographs produced in an X-ray department.

The diaphragm

The diaphragm is a fibromuscular structure which separates the thoracic and abdominal cavities. It forms a dome with the convexity upwards. On a posteroanterior radiograph of the thorax the diaphragm shows prominently as two curving lines, one on the right side of the thorax and one on the left, both being convex upwards.

These two lines which radiographically represent the diaphragm are not truthful. They make the diaphragm look simpler in structure than it is. Furthermore, in the postero-anterior projection they do not reveal the extent to which from its anterior attachments to sternum and costal cartilages the domed structure slopes up to its highest peak and then down posteriorly to the attachments of its lumbar fibres eventually to the upper lumbar vertebrae. In the radiograph we see an outline which corresponds only to the highest part of the dome.

The two arcs of this radiographic outline run medially towards the midline but are not seen to meet each other because they become lost in the heart shadow. The angles formed where the two arcs of the diaphragm meet the heart are called the cardiophrenic angles. Laterally the two arcs meet the thoracic wall on the right and left sides and the angles thus formed are called the costophrenic angles.

The diaphragm shows thus prominently because it closes the thoracic cavity and is therefore a boundary between two regions which are different in their abilities to absorb X-radiation. Above the diaphragm are the air-containing lungs and the air makes them radioparent. Below the diaphragm is the abdomen packed with viscera and the only air normally present is a certain amount in the gastrointestinal tract. The abdomen relative to the thorax is more radiopaque and hence in the posteroanterior radiograph exposed for the thoracic contents the subdiaphragmatic regions appear as an empty white space; through these parts of the body no radiation has reached the film to blacken it. The arcs of the diaphragm represent radiographically its upper surface shown against the air-filled lungs. The lower surface of the diaphragm is not seen unless there is air beneath it to outline the lower surface, as the air in the lungs does for the upper surface.

AIR BENEATH THE DIAPHRAGM

The only air which can be beneath the diaphragm must be in one or more of the following situations:

(i) air which is normally present in the gastrointestinal tract;

(ii) air which has entered the peritoneal cavity because a hollow air-containing viscus has perforated (for example, a gastric ulcer has eroded the wall of the stomach and the resultant opening allows air within the organ to escape into the peritoneal cavity);

(iii) air which has entered because the abdomen has been

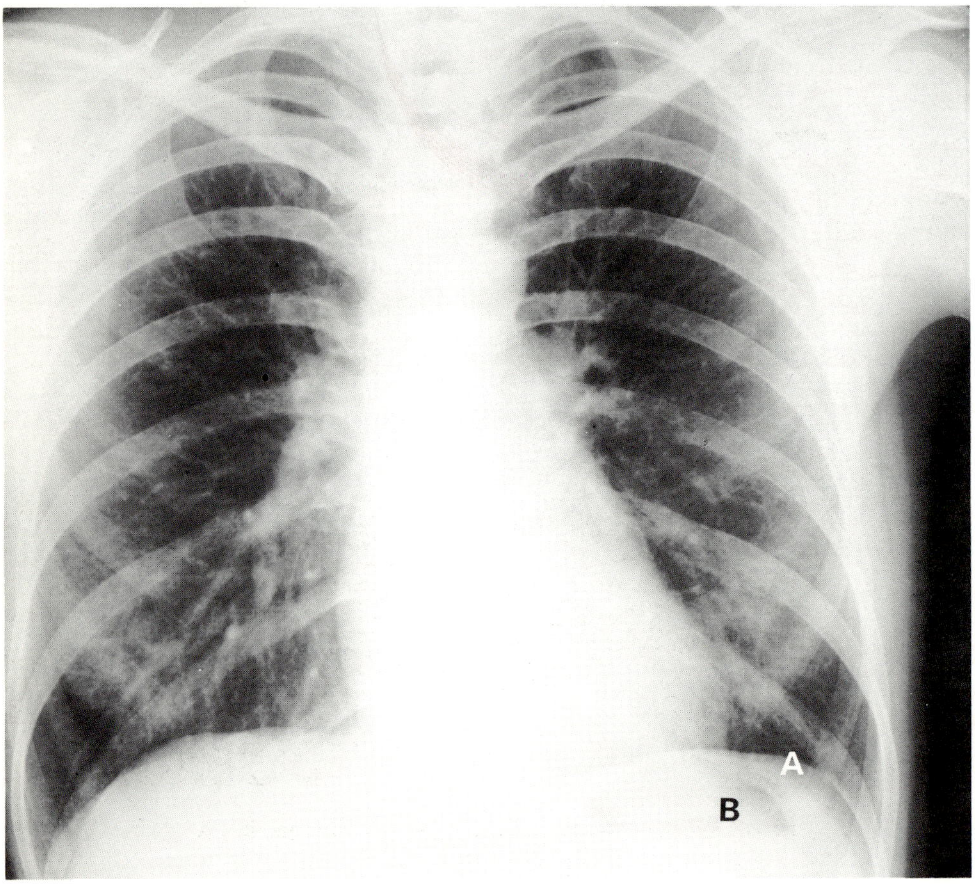

Fig. 1.5. A posteroanterior radiograph of the chest showing gas in the fundus of the stomach beneath the diaphragm.

A Left arc of diaphragm B Gas in the fundus of the stomach

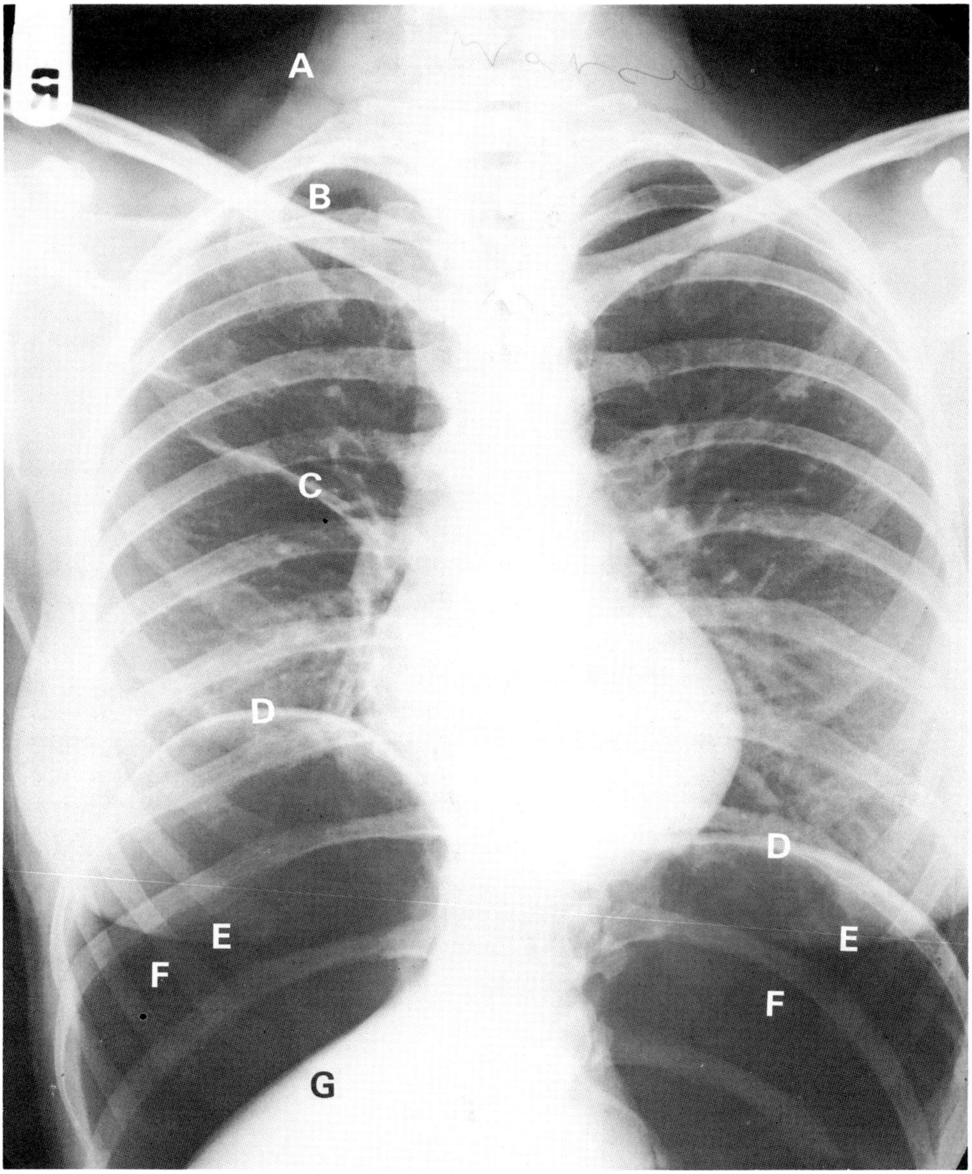

Fig. 1.6. A posteroanterior radiograph of the chest showing gas in the peritoneal cavity beneath the diaphragm.

A Sternomastoid muscle
B Soft tissue covering the clavicle
C Horizontal fissure of right lung
D Diaphragm
E Breast shadow
F Free air beneath the diaphragm
G Liver

opened recently, either deliberately in a surgical operation or traumatically through a penetrating wound (this air is absorbed in due course and by a few days after an operation it has disappeared);
(iv) air which has been deliberately introduced as a part of diagnostic investigations.
The air, whether contained within the gastrointestinal tract or free in the abdominal cavity, rises to the highest level it can achieve for a given posture of the patient. When the patient is erect, the highest level within the abdomen is the undersurface of the diaphragm and air which can reach there will do so. The diaphragm is then radiographically outlined on its undersurface by the contrast of the air.

Hence on a posteroanterior radiograph of the thorax taken with the patient erect, the left arc of the diaphragm may be seen to have beneath it a 'gas bubble' of air in the stomach. It is present on the left side only because the air is contained within the stomach and the location of the stomach is immediately beneath the left dome of the diaphragm. This is the situation in Fig. 1.5 which shows a quantity of air in the fundus of the stomach and the diaphragm is seen outlined above this air. A smaller gas bubble in the stomach is seen in Fig. 1.1. Where the air is not held within the stomach and is in the peritoneal cavity, it will outline the under-surface of the diaphragm on both sides because it is free to rise on both sides. This is the situation in Fig. 1.6 where free air in the peritoneal cavity shows the diaphragm in contrast above it on both sides. The presence of the air has depressed the abdominal organs so that they have been pushed downwards from close contact with the diaphragm. The under-surface of the diaphragm is thus very clearly seen.

THE LEVEL OF THE DIAPHRAGM

The level or height of the diaphragm within the thorax varies considerably with different conditions.

Factors which alter its level are as follows.
(i) The phase of respiration. During inspiration muscular fibres in the diaphragm contract and its central portion is drawn downwards and forwards. If the costal margin is not

much raised in the act of inspiration, the curvature of the diaphragmatic arcs is little altered, the whole dome moving downwards so that it stays parallel to its original line with the abdominal organs being pushed downwards as it goes. If the rib movements are great on inspiration, the diaphragmatic arcs are flattened in outline as well as being lower in level. In expiration there is elastic recoil of the chest wall from its expansion and the action of the abdominal muscles puts upwards pressure on the diaphragm through the abdominal organs. The level of the diaphragm is thus lower in the phase of inspiration and higher in the phase of expiration.

It has been stated that the difference in level between deep inspiration and full expiration averages 30 mm on the right and 28 mm on the left; in quiet respiration the average movement is 12 mm on the right and 12·5 mm on the left.

Fig. 1.7 shows radiographs of a child taken within a few minutes of each other. At (a) the child had not taken the deep inspiration required; at (b) is the repeat radiograph taken when the patient had inspired fully. Figs. 1.8 and 1.9 show an adult. The radiograph in Fig. 1.8 was taken on full inspiration; that in Fig. 1.9 is of the same patient taken on expiration. A difference in the level of the diaphragm between inspiration and expiration can be seen both for the child and the adult.

In general with an average subject, the domes of the diaphragm move between full inspiration and full expiration a distance equivalent to two dorsal vertebrae. The right dome moves between the levels of the eleventh and the ninth dorsal vertebrae and the left dome moves between the levels of the twelfth and the tenth dorsal vertebrae.

(ii) The size of the liver and the amount of space occupied by the stomach and intestines, depending on their degree of distension. As can be seen in the radiographs of Figs. 1.1 to 1.5, on the right the diaphragmatic arc is higher in level than on the left. Some difference is maintained whether the general level is the lower one in the phase of inspiration or the raised one of expiration.

Immediately beneath the right side of the diaphragm is the right lobe of the liver and over this convexity and over the right kidney and suprarenal gland the diaphragm is closely moulded. On the left side the diaphragm is shaped over the

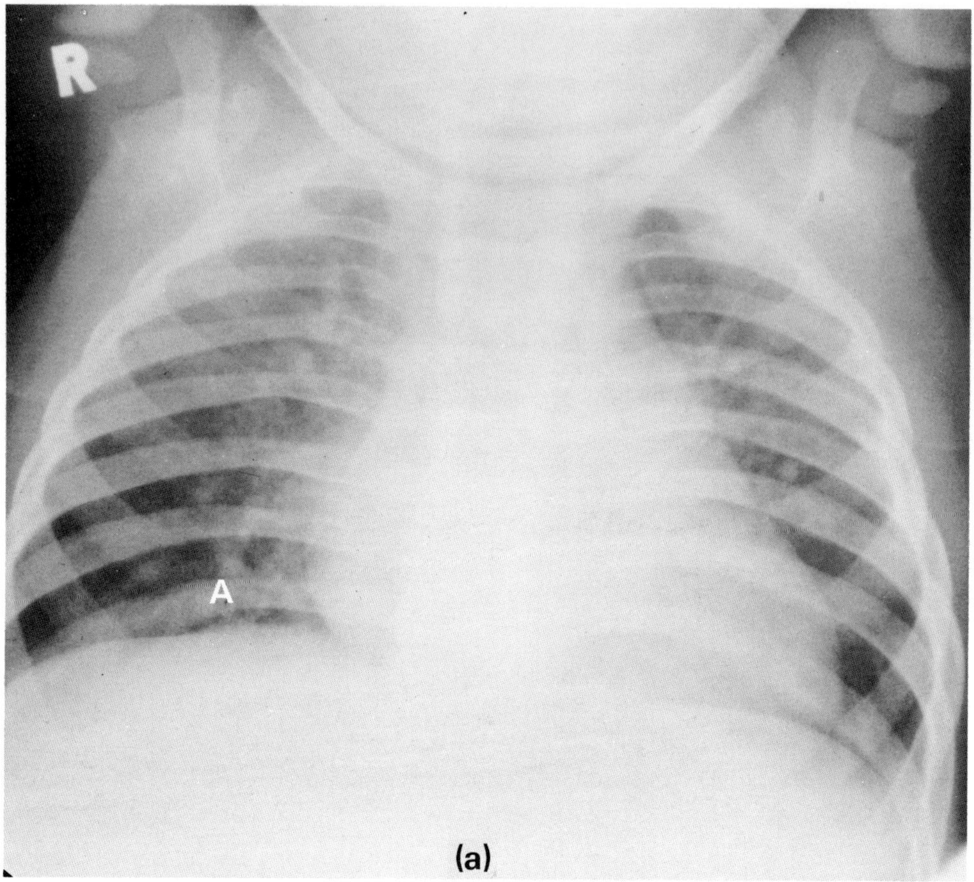

Fig. 1.7a. Posteroanterior radiograph of the chest of a child taken on expiration.
A Right rib 9

much smaller left lobe of the liver, the fundus of the stomach (which is a hollow organ), the spleen and the left kidney and its suprarenal gland. It is differences in the viscera related to the undersurface of the diaphragm which account for the dissimilarity between the right and left sides.

(iii) The body-build of the subject. The level of the diaphragm is not the same for all subjects and shows variation between people of different body-build and of different weights. Some people have 'high diaphragms' and some people have 'low diaphragms' and most people have what might be described as an average diaphragm situated at an expected intermediate

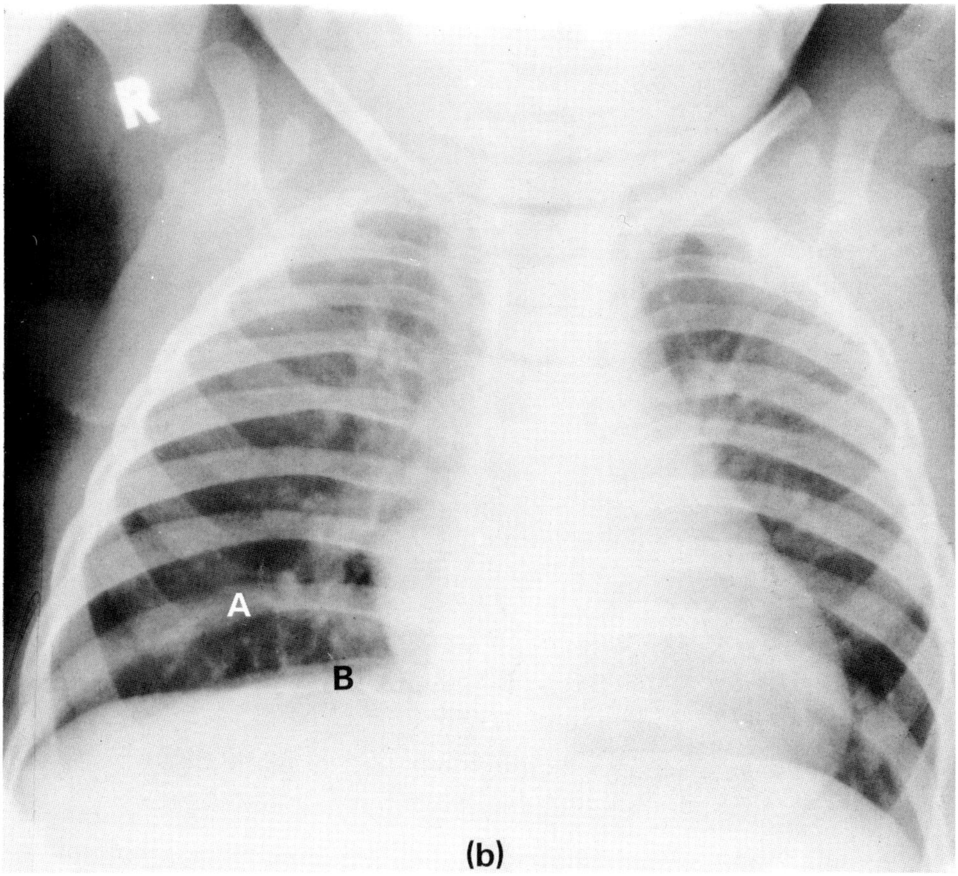

Fig. 1.7b. Posteroanterior radiograph of the chest of a child taken on inspiration.

A Right rib 9 B Right rib 10

level between the high and the low. This intermediate level relates the right dome of the diaphragm posteriorly to the level of the tenth to eleventh thoracic vertebrae and anteriorly to the fifth costal cartilage; and the left dome to the level of the eleventh to twelfth thoracic vertebrae posteriorly and to the sixth costal cartilage anteriorly. The high diaphragm is about one vertebra higher (and the low similarly one vertebra lower) than these levels. If the subject is short and broad in the trunk, the diaphragm is more likely to be high, while long slender people probably have lower diaphragms.

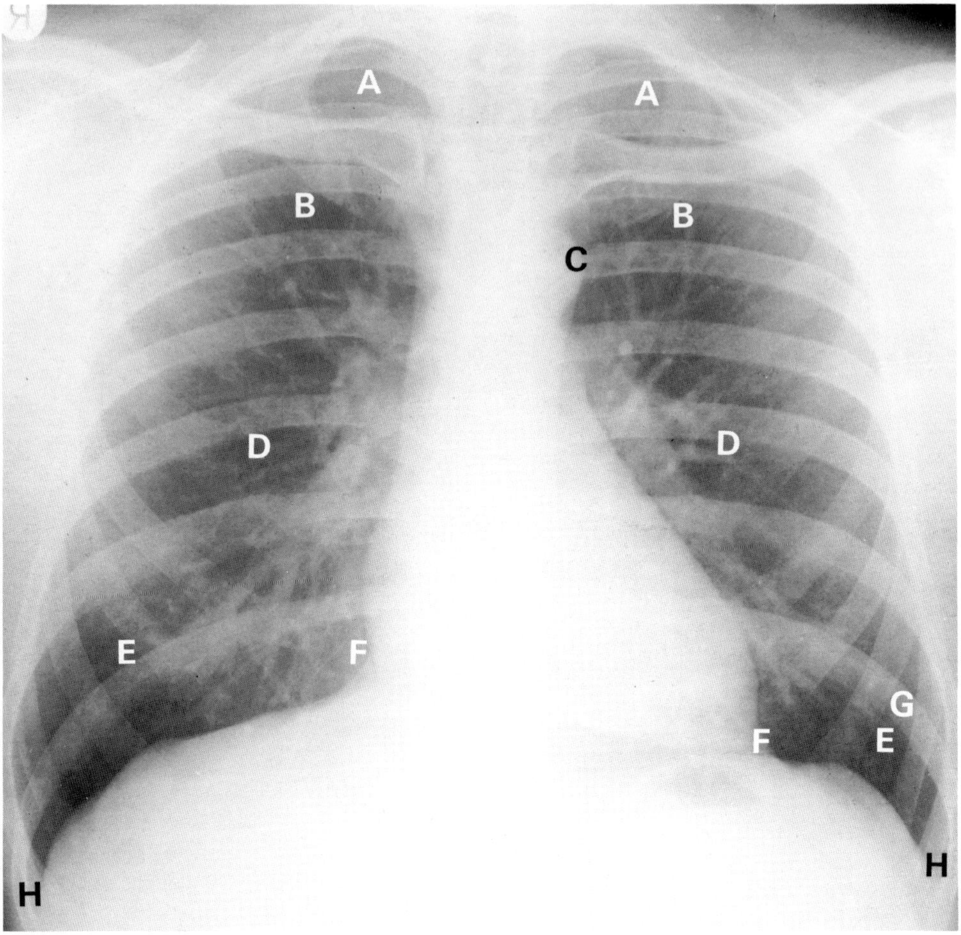

Fig. 1.8. Posteroanterior radiograph of the chest of an adult taken on inspiration.

A	Apical region	E	Basal region
B	Infraclavicular region	F	Cardiophrenic angle
C	Aortic knuckle	G	Left rib 10
D	Hilar region	H	Costophrenic angle

(iv) The posture of the subject. The level of the diaphragm changes in any subject with the position of the body. Comparisons may be made between these positions: lying supine, standing erect, sitting, lying down on one side. The diaphragm is at nearly its highest when the subject is lying flat on his back and when it is highest its range of movement with normal

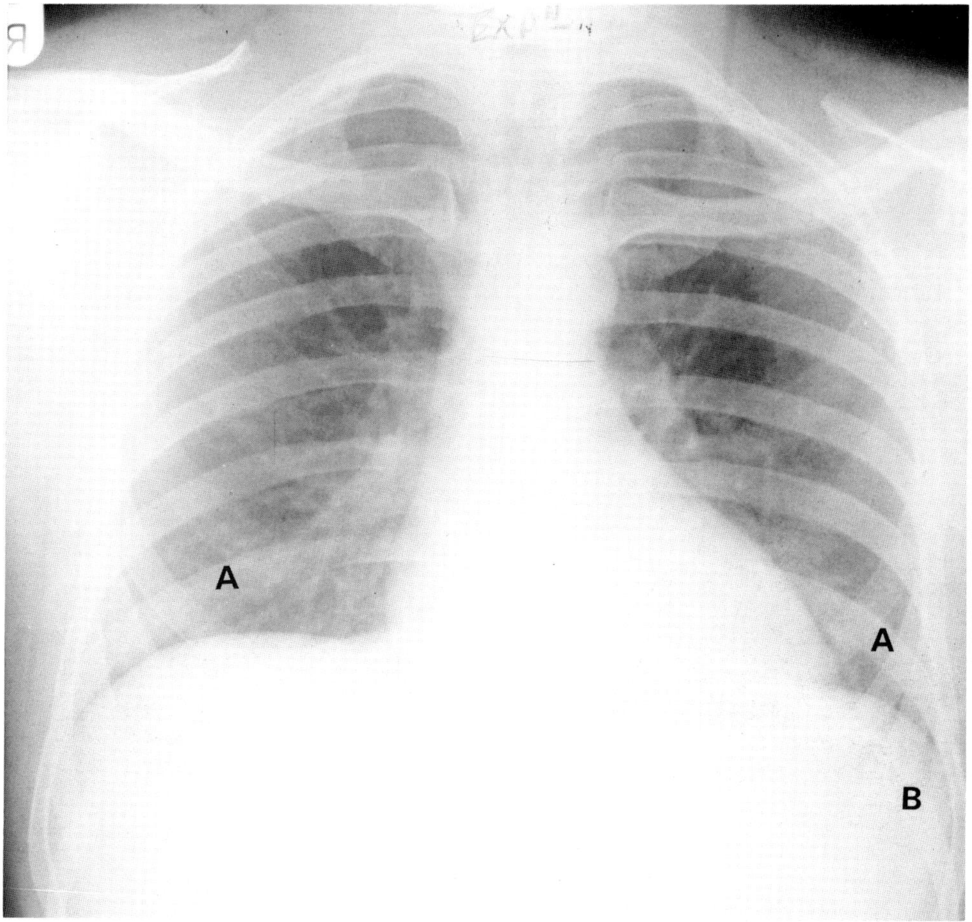

Fig. 1.9. Posteroanterior radiograph of the chest of an adult taken on inspiration.

A Right and left ribs 9 B Left rib 10

respiration is greatest. With the subject standing erect, the level of the diaphragm is lower in the trunk because it has fallen, the extent of movement with respiration then being smaller than previously.

Because when the subject is standing the abdominal muscles are in a state of contraction but are not so when he sits down, it is in the sitting posture that the diaphragm is found at nearly its lowest level with nearly the smallest excursion from expiration to inspiration. When the subject lies down on one side, the two halves of the diaphragm react separately: the half which is to the side on which he is lying achieves the highest level and an increased degree of movement with respiration; the half which is to the uppermost side reaches its lowest level and shows only slight movement with the phase of breathing.

(v) Pregnancy. During the last months of pregnancy the diaphragm is high. This is not surprising in view of the fact that the gravid uterus, expanding upwards into the abdominal cavity, occupies much more space than usual and pushes movable abdominal organs upwards as it grows.

The trachea

The trachea is almost wholly a midline structure that begins in the neck at the lower border of the cricoid cartilage. At the level of the fourth or fifth dorsal vertebra the trachea ends by dividing into the right and left main bronchi; at the point of bifurcation it lies slightly to the right of the midline. On the standard posteroanterior radiograph of the chest, the trachea is seen in the midline as a shadow which is radioparent because it contains air. The spinous processes of the dorsal vertebrae which we noticed previously are visible in the midline through the air-containing trachea. At about the level of the sternoclavicular joints or the third dorsal vertebra (whichever of the two bony landmarks you fancy) the radioparency of the trachea becomes lost behind the medisatinal shadow at which we shall be looking in more detail later (page 35).

Thus the end of the trachea and its bifurcation into the right and left main bronchi are not seen. These features can, however, be demonstrated on a posteroanterior view of the thorax if the radiographic exposure factors and technique are selected to give a result in which the mediastinal region is penetrated; see Fig. 1.10.

The cartilaginous rings which make up the trachea are seen when they are calcified. This happens often in very old people and on a radiograph the rings then show as horizontal light lines. In Chapter 4 we have more to say about the trachea and the bronchi for in that chapter we discuss the use of

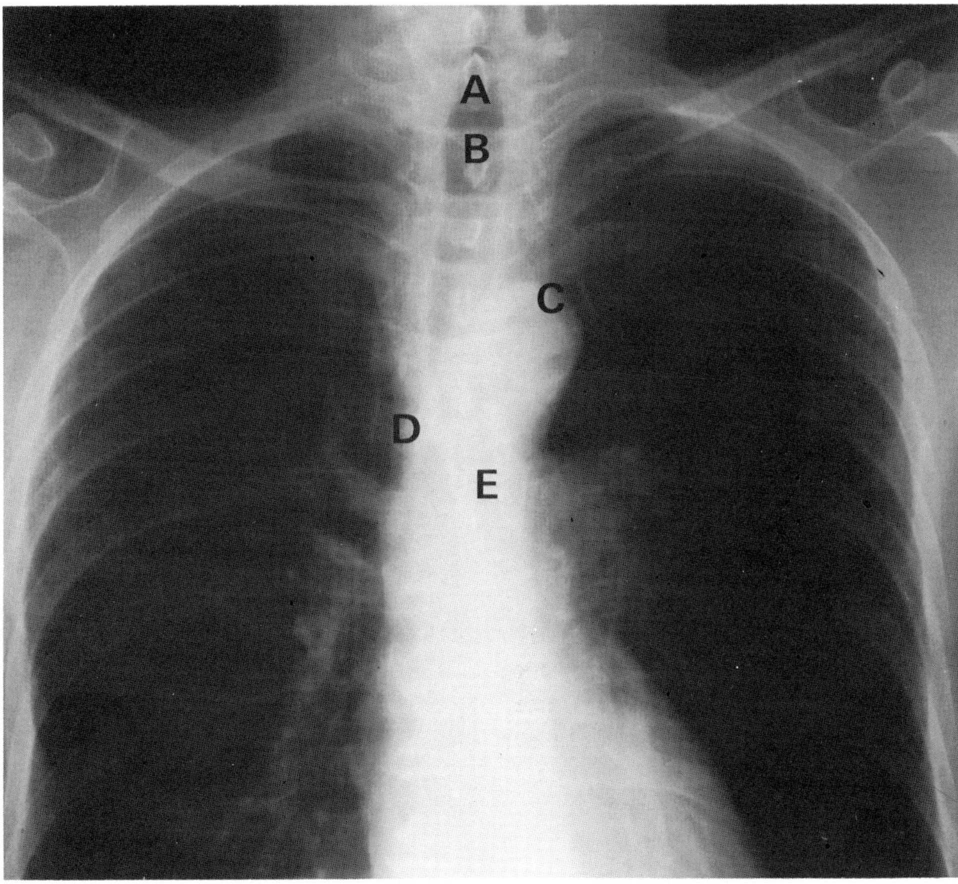

Fig. 1.10. Posteroanterior radiograph of the thorax with the lung fields overexposed, demonstrating the air-filled trachea.

A Spinous process of thoracic vertebra 1 behind the trachea
B Air-filled trachea
C Aortic knuckle
D Right edge of ascending aorta
E Bifurcation of trachea

contrast agents: when positive contrast agents have been introduced the trachea and bronchi are well demonstrated on radiographs.

The lungs

The right and left lungs lie on either side of the mediastinum within the thorax. Radiographs of the thorax show them as dark areas (their content of air making them radioparent) over which the shadows of the ribs are superimposed. These areas on a radiograph are usually called *the lung fields*. The lung fields are divided roughly into six separate parts. These parts are described in relation to the shadow of the clavicle, lying across the uppermost portion of each lung field, and to the hilum of the lung.

The hilum of each lung is a roughly triangular depression on its medial surface above and behind the deep concavity called the cardiac impression which accommodates the pericardium and the heart. The hilum is the place where the structures which form the root of the lung enter and leave the organ. For each lung, these structures are the main bronchus, the pulmonary artery and veins, the bronchial arteries and veins, nerves, lymph vessels and glands. Fig. 1.11 shows calcified left hilar lymph nodes, indicating the location of these structures in the hilum of the lung.

The descriptive areas for each lung are as follows (see Fig. 1.8):
(i) the apical region lying above the clavicle;
(ii) the infraclavicular region lying between the clavicle and the upper part of the hilum of the lung;
(iii) the middle region of the lung field which is below the infraclavicular part and is the region of the hilum of the lung (hilar region);
(iv) the basal region which is below the middle one and reaches from the lower part of the hilum down to the diaphragm;
(v) the cardiophrenic angle where the outline of the heart meets the arc of the diaphragm;
(vi) the costophrenic angle where the arc of the diaphragm runs into the thoracic wall at the side of the thorax.
By the use of these terms the location of any particular lesion, shadow or appearance in the posteroanterior view of the chest can be described in words.

The radiograph does not reveal the whole truth concerning the lungs for the radiographic lung fields do not include all parts of the lung. The anatomist recognises that the anterior border of each lung overlies the front of the pericardium and that the posterior and inferior part of each lower lobe is at a lower level than the anterior and inferior portion of each lung.

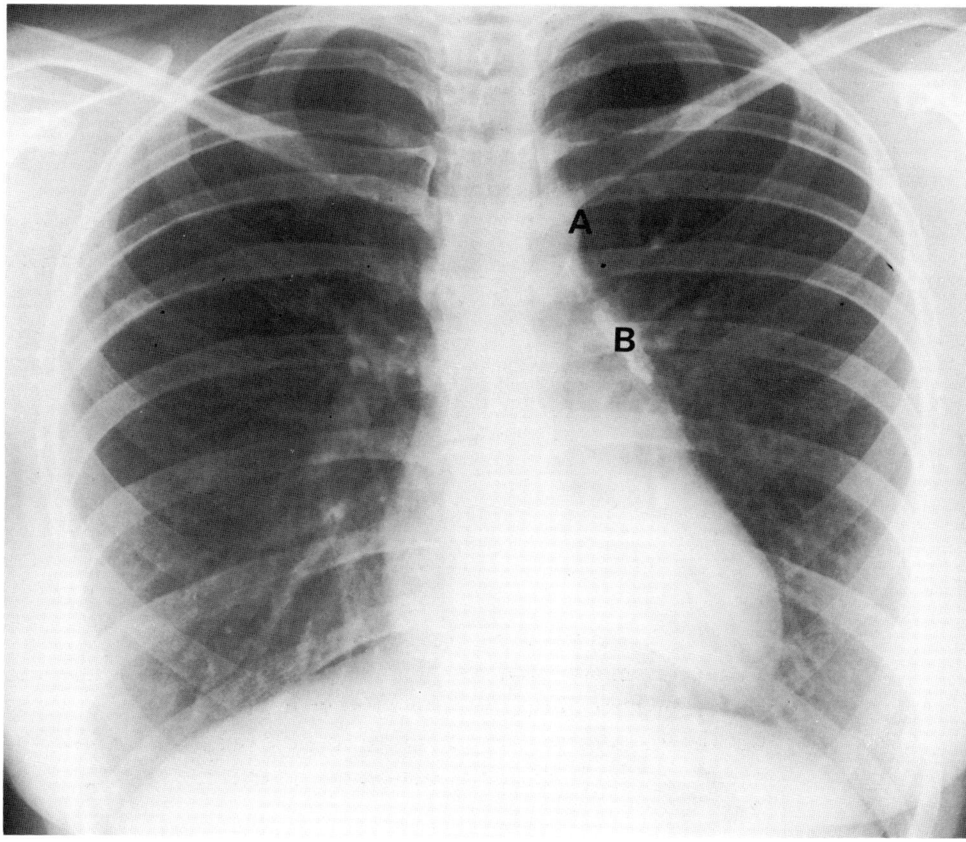

Fig. 1.11. Posteroanterior radiograph of the chest showing calcified hilar lymph nodes.

A Aortic knuckle

B Calcified hilar lymph nodes on left

The posteroanterior radiograph reveals none of this and shows as the lung fields only those regions which are projected clearly above the highest part of the diaphragm and are lateral to the mediastinum and the cardiac outline (see Fig. 1.12).

In the posteroanterior radiograph of the chest the lung fields show a pattern of fine lines (grey-white shadows against the darker background of the air-filled lung substance) which radiate fanwise from the hilum of each lung. These lines are formed not by the pulmonary substance itself which is almost completely radioparent when air-filled but by the vessels which pass through it; these are arteries, veins and lymph vessels. Sometimes in a radiograph a vessel is projected axially so that it is viewed end-on and appears as a white circular shadow. In Fig. 1.1, one such shadow is very prominent on the left side just above the letter B which is used to mark the region of the lung root. There is another white

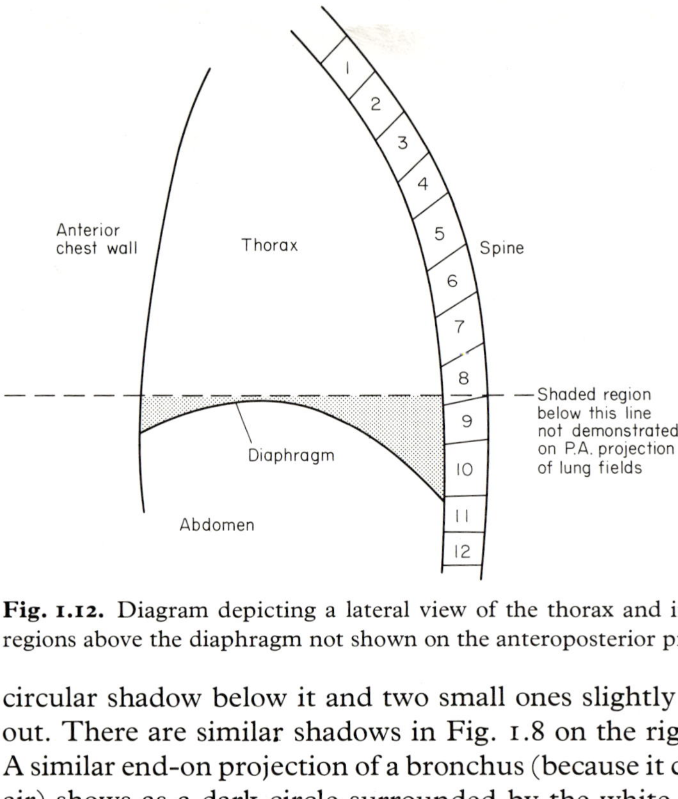

Fig. 1.12. Diagram depicting a lateral view of the thorax and indicating regions above the diaphragm not shown on the anteroposterior projection.

circular shadow below it and two small ones slightly further out. There are similar shadows in Fig. 1.8 on the right side. A similar end-on projection of a bronchus (because it contains air) shows as a dark circle surrounded by the white shadow of the bronchial wall. On a good radiograph of the chest, the pattern of ramifying vessels should be clearly seen throughout from the hilum to the periphery of the lung.

As we have said, the lung substance when air-filled is radioparent and on a radiograph of the chest taken at full inspiration the lung fields are dark. Not unexpectedly, when the lungs have less air in them the lung fields are not so dark. This relative loss of radioparency in the chest radiograph taken on expiration is shown by the comparison of Fig. 1.8 with Fig. 1.9 and of the two sections of Fig. 1.7.

In certain pathological conditions the normal pattern of radioparent lung tissue with the network of vessels displayed against it alters. Radiological diagnosis is based on these alterations. It is no part of our task here to detail what occurs but we felt that we should mention two prominent changes, one leading to an appearance of greater radioparency and one resulting in an appearance of radiopacity. The conditions are respectively a pneumothorax and a pleural effusion. Determined and interested readers should turn to pages 32–35 to read more about them.

THE FISSURES OF THE LUNGS

The lungs are divided into separate lobes by deep fissures which extend inwards from the external surfaces nearly to the roots of the lungs. The arrangement of the fissures differs between the lungs. The right lung has three lobes, two fissures dividing it, one oblique and one transverse; the three lobes are the upper lobe, the middle lobe and the lower lobe. The left lung has one oblique fissure dividing it into an upper and a lower lobe.

On a posteroanterior radiograph of the chest, the transverse or horizontal fissure on the right side may show as a thin curving white line which runs from the hilum of the lung at the level of the fourth costal cartilage out towards the periphery. In Fig. 1.6 this shadow can be seen. In this instance as it goes outwards from the hilum of the lung the upward direction of the fissure is not normal; it has been raised by the presence of air beneath the diaphragm which elevates the domes and pushes upwards the thoracic contents.

When, as a result of disease or any other conditions, the lung fissures are filled with material which is more absorptive of X-rays than is the surrounding tissue, then shadows of the fissures appear clearly in the radiograph. The oblique fissures are seen only in a lateral projection of the thorax. (See Fig. 2.4, p. 59)

ACCESSORY FISSURES OF THE LUNGS

In addition to the fissures which have just been described and are found as a standard feature of the lungs, extra or accessory fissures are often present. These are deviations from the common order and are said to be anomalous but not abnormal.

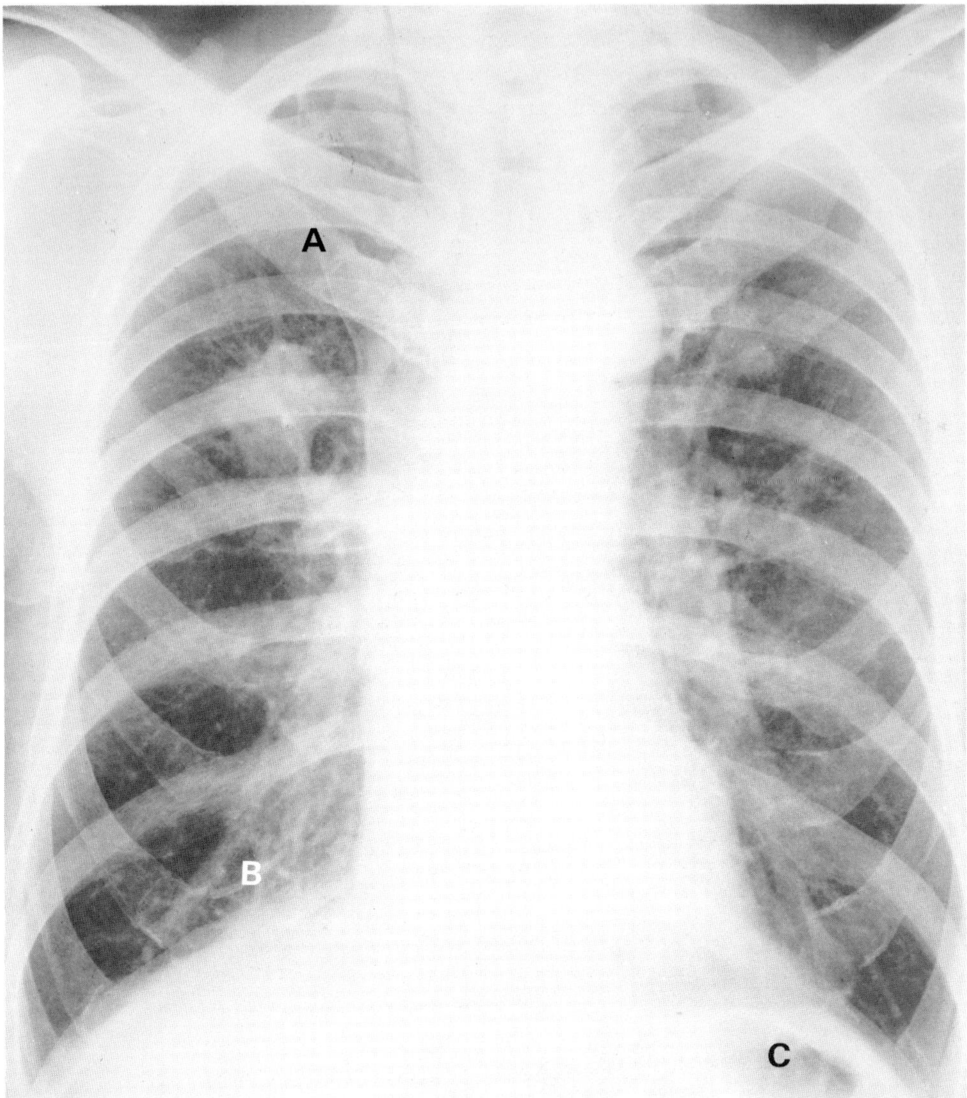

Fig. 1.13. Posteroanterior radiograph of the chest showing on the right the accessory fissure of the azygos lobe.

A Fissure of the azygos lobe
B Calcified costal cartilage.
C Gas in the fundus of the stomach

Pathological lesions are present on this radiograph in both lungs.

Several different accessory fissures are recognised and known but we need not enumerate them all here. It will meet the need of student radiographers if we acquaint them with the two most commonly encountered accessory fissures. These are both on the right side and are (i) the fissure of the azygos lobe and (ii) the right medial basal fissure or inferior fissure.

The fissure of the azygos lobe

The fissure of the azygos lobe may be seen as a curving line in the upper parts of the right lung field, extending through the apical area down into the infraclavicular region towards the mediastinum. When present, the azygos fissure does not follow an unvarying line. Figs. 1.13 and 1.14 show two examples, in one of which the course of the fissure is much closer to the shadows of the spine and mediastinal structures than it is in the other.

The azygos vein ascends in the thorax in the posterior mediastinum and usually arches forward over the root of the right lung. When it develops on an aberrant course it may be very deeply sunk in the pulmonary substance, giving rise to this accessory fissure in the right lung and marking off the azygos lobe.

The right medial basal fissure

An accessory fissure may be found in the right lung dividing off from the right lower lobe a medial basal segment or cardiac lobe of the lung. This fissure is called the right medial basal fissure or inferior fissure and on a posteroanterior radiograph of the chest it may be seen as a curving linear shadow. Situated in the basal region of the lung fields, the line runs out on the right side from the edge of the cardiac shadow, curving downwards towards the diaphragm at an angle which is not constant in all cases. It may be more or less steeply angled and more or less close to the right edge of the cardiac shadow. Fig. 1.15 shows an example.

THE HILAR REGION AND THE ROOT OF THE LUNG

The medial aspect of each lung in its lower part is concave because the lungs must accommodate the heart. This con-

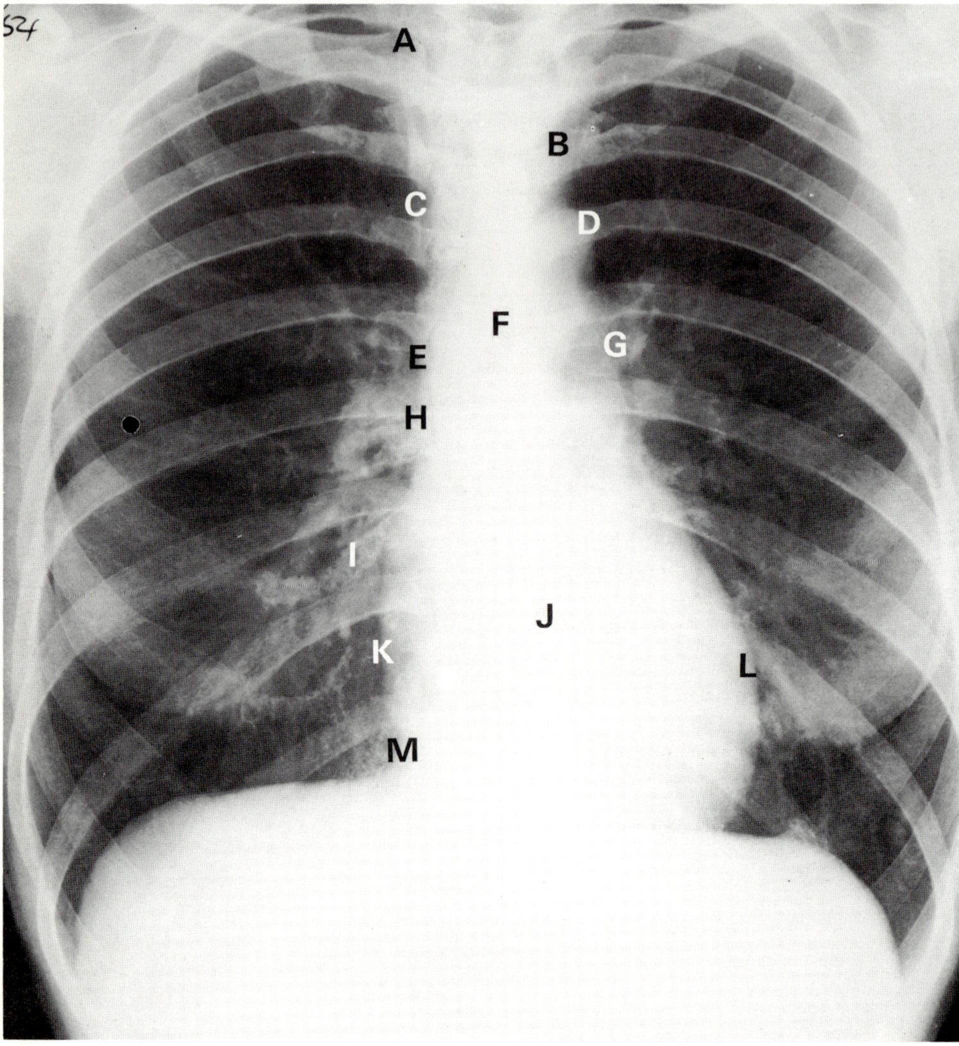

Fig. 1.14. Posteroanterior radiograph of the chest showing on the right the accessory fissure of the azygos lobe.

A Fissure of the azygos lobe
B Left subclavian artery
C Right innominate vein
D Aortic knuckle
E Superior vena cava
F Vascular part of the mediastinal shadow
G Pulmonary trunk and root of left lung
H Root of right lung
I Calcified right costal cartilage
J Right ventricle (cardiac shadow)
K Right atrium (cardiac shadow)
L Left ventricle (cardiac shadow)
M Inferior vena cava

cavity in each lung is called the cardiac impression. In the right lung it is related to the right atrium and part of the right ventricle of the heart; in the left lung it is more deeply concave and is related to the left atrium and the left ventricle. Above and behind the cardiac impression in each lung there is a triangular area called the hilum and it is here that the vessels which form the root of the lung enter and leave the organ. For each lung the vessels are: the main bronchus; the

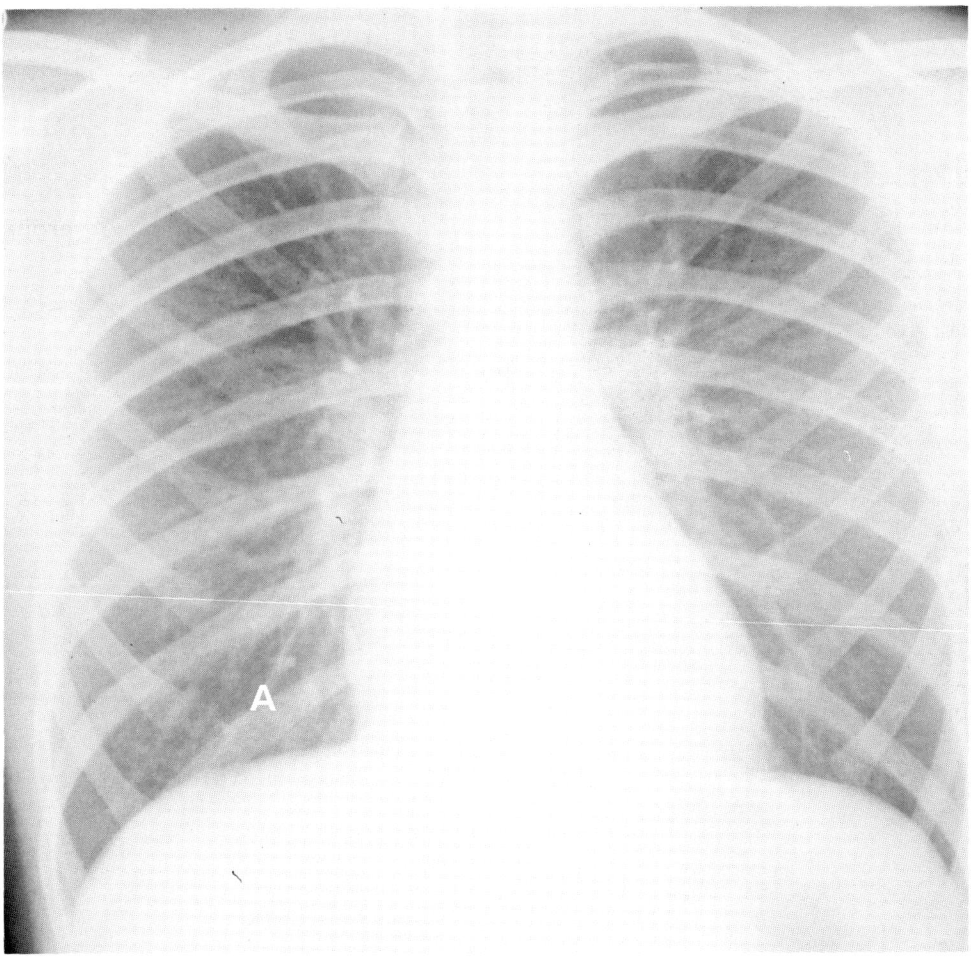

Fig. 1.15. Posteroanterior radiograph of the chest showing on the right the accessory inferior fissure.
A Inferior fissure

pulmonary artery; two pulmonary veins; the bronchial arteries and veins; pulmonary nerves; lymph vessels and broncho-pulmonary glands.

In the posteroanterior radiograph these vessels are not individually delineated but shadows radiating from the root of the lung can be seen; they are marked in Fig. 1.1. The most prominent of these hilar shadows in each lung is formed by the main artery and vein passing downwards and laterally. They are best seen on a radiograph taken on full inspiration and they are nearly at the same level on both sides; the shadow of the pulmonary vessels is only a little higher on the left side in comparison with the right.

PNEUMOTHORAX

The lungs each have a covering which is a closed sac of serous membrane called the pleura or pleural sac. This closed sac has its inner layer closely applied to the surface of the lung, extending into the fissures, and its outer layer attached to the chest wall. The inner layer is called the visceral pleura and the outer layer is called the parietal pleura. Separated only by a film of serous fluid, the two layers are in close contact with each other; they are held together by suction and the space between them is a potential one.

The term pneumothorax means that air is present between the two layers of pleura. The air may be introduced deliberately. For example, an induced pneumothorax used to be a therapeutic measure to rest the lung in cases of pulmonary tuberculosis before modern antibiotic drugs were discovered. Or the air may enter as a result of an injury such as a blow or a penetrating wound on the chest wall. Sometimes a spontaneous pneumothorax happens with no apparent reason for its occurrence.

Whatever its cause, the effect of a pneumothorax is to raise the intrapleural pressure. The space between the two layers becomes a real space and the lung collapses because of the changed pressure, retracting towards the hilum. On the posteroanterior chest radiograph, the side on which the air is present looks abnormally radioparent over an area which is larger or smaller depending on the extent to which the lung is more or less retracted. The extent of the retraction of the lung is in its turn dependent on the intrapleural pressure, higher pressure leading to increased retraction.

Fig. 1.16 shows a pneumothorax on the left side. The edge of the retracted lung can be seen and to one side of the edge is

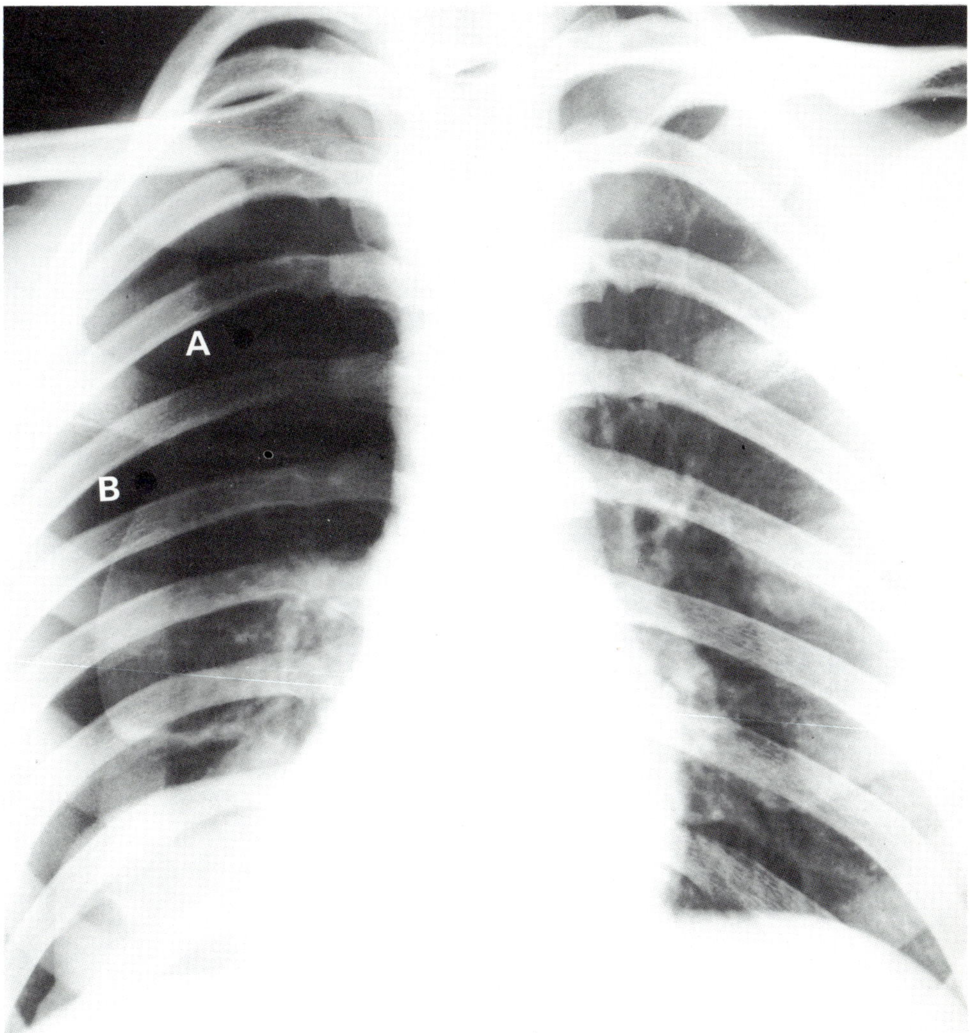

Fig. 1.16. Posteroanterior radiograph of the chest showing a pneumothorax on the right side.

A Pneumothorax B Edge of retracted lung

the pattern of vessels noted as features of the normal lung fields. Beyond the edge to the other side is the large dark area without vascular pattern and of increased radioparency which indicates that air is present in the pleural sac.

It is easy to demonstrate a total pneumothorax radiographically. A partial or localised pneumothorax may not be so readily shown and in such a case a posteroanterior radiograph taken on expiration (that is, with reduced air in the lung) may be of help.

PLEURAL EFFUSION

In medical use the word effusion describes the escape of fluid into a part or tissue and the term pleural effusion indicates that the pleural space has filled abnormally with fluid. The fluid may be an exudate arising from a pathological process or it may be blood following trauma to the chest. If it is blood, the word haemothorax may be used, meaning a collection of blood in the thoracic cavity. A collection of pus in the pleural cavity is called an empyema.

Whatever the nature of the fluid, it constitutes material which is more absorptive of X-rays than is the normal air-containing lung tissue. The region occupied by the fluid appears radiographically as an area of radiopacity, a white shadow covering the lung. The normal vascular pattern against air is lost in this part. For radiographers there are certain points which are important relating to the radiographic appearances produced by fluid.

(i) Fluid in the pleural cavity may give rise to a curving parabolic shadow, concave upwards. A small effusion at the base of the thorax may show itself as a curving shadow of such a type in the costophrenic angle on one side (see Fig. 1.21). In this case the two costophrenic angles do not match in appearance, the one retaining its normal acute angle while in the other the angle is replaced by a gentle concavity. Seeing this, a good radiographer takes a lateral view of the affected side. An appearance somewhat similar to the concave line of an effusion at the base of the lung may be produced in a radiograph taken with a circular cone used as a beam-limiting device if malpositioning of the beam leads to the costophrenic

angle being 'coned off'. Radiographers checking radiographs should look carefully at the costophrenic angles.
(ii) A small amount of fluid may not be apparent on the posteroanterior radiograph taken when the patient is standing erect. This is because the fluid is lying posteriorly in the base of the thorax. It is then lower than the highest part of the diaphragm and is thus not seen in the posteroanterior projection. It can be made to appear if the patient lies down on the affected side and an anteroposterior or posteroanterior projection is taken with a horizontal beam. The fluid then forms a line running along the side of the thorax. This line is a vertical one when the radiograph is viewed in the usual way as if the patient were standing erect before the viewer.

The mediastinal shadow

Very prominent (see Fig. 1.14) on the posteroanterior radiograph of the chest is the white shadow formed by the heart, the pericardium and the great vessels along which blood is carried from the heart and returns to it. The heart and its vessels form what is called the mediastinal shadow on the radiograph. The mediastinum is that anatomical region which is the central part of the thorax, the thorax being considered to have three main parts: these are the right and left pleural cavities containing the lungs and between them the mediastinum extending from the sternum in front to the spine behind and from the thoracic inlet above to the diaphragm below.

For ease of description, the mediastinum is divided into certain regions. These are as follows (see Fig. 1.17):
(i) the superior mediastinum above a line drawn between the manubrium sterni and the fourth thoracic vertebra;
(ii) the anterior mediastinum which is below this line and in front of the heart;
(iii) the middle mediastinum which is below the same line, is behind the anterior mediastinum and contains the heart, the great vessels and other structures;
(iv) the posterior mediastinum which is below the same line and is immediately behind the middle mediastinum and thus behind the heart.

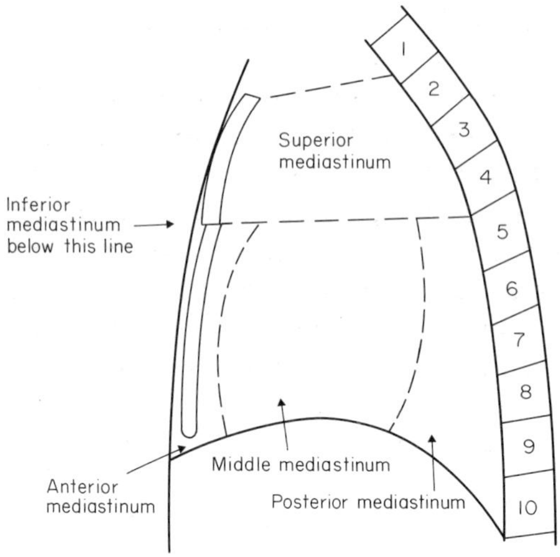

Fig. 1.17. Diagram to show the regions of the mediastinum.

On a posteroanterior radiograph the mediastinal shadow is homogeneous because the structures in it absorb X-rays and, with an exposure technique selected to record the relatively radiolucent lung fields, areas of the film which are beneath these absorbing structures remain unaffected by radiation. The mediastinal shadow looks in fact like an empty space but it is of course nothing of the sort. Radiographers need some understanding of the mediastinal shadow and we propose to elucidate it in the following pages.

In its upper part the mediastinal shadow is formed by the great vessels. In its lower part, where the shadow is expanded and is more or less pear-shaped, it is made by the heart enclosed in the pericardial sac. This part of the mediastinal region on the radiograph is called the cardiac shadow.

THE CARDIAC SHADOW

The heart is a hollow muscular organ enclosed in a fibro-serous sac which is called the pericardium. Normally the heart itself cannot be differentiated from the enclosing pericardium and the two together form one homogeneous white shadow on the radiograph. If calcifications are present in the pericardium they may be seen in some cases, more readily in oblique projections than in the posteroanterior view of the thorax which we are considering now.

The heart lies in the middle mediastinum resting on the diaphragm and placed obliquely so that it lies more towards the left than towards the right. It is divided into right and left sides and each side has two hollow chambers, the atrium above and the ventricle below. The four chambers of the heart are thus: the right atrium above with the right ventricle below and the left atrium above with the left ventricle below. The right atrium communicates with the right ventricle through the tricuspid valve; and the left atrium with the left ventricle through the mitral valve. During foetal life there is an opening between the two atria but normally this opening closes at birth and subsequently there should be no direct communication between the right and left sides of the heart. On a radiograph the white 'empty space' which is the heart shadow does not have the four chambers individually delineated within it. But the locations of the four chambers within this shadow can be identified through knowledge of the anatomy of the heart and its placing in the thorax. As a result of its oblique position in the middle mediastinum (see Fig. 1.18) the heart may be divided into (i) a left and posterior

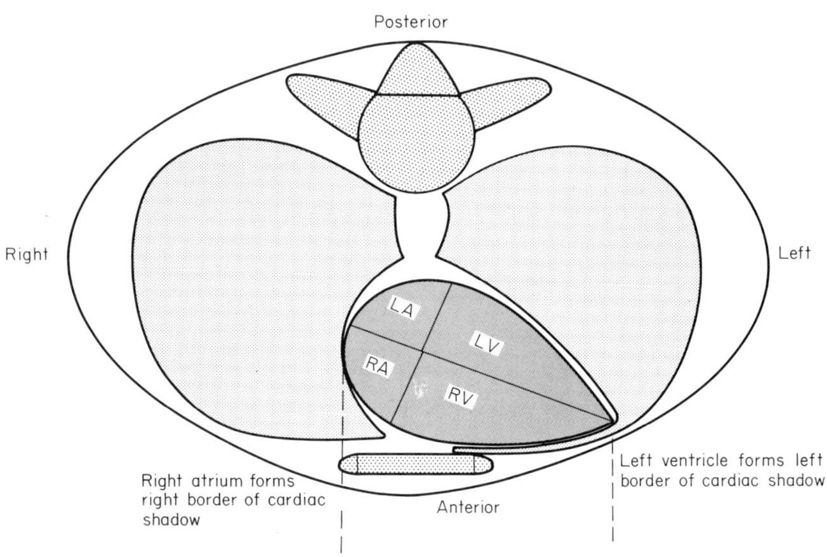

Fig. 1.18. Diagram to show the placing of the heart in the thorax.

part and (ii) a right and anterior part; it may then be further divided with the atrium marked off from the ventricle on each side.

If the diagram in Fig. 1.18 is studied, it can be appreciated that when the heart is viewed from the front (as it is in a posteroanterior view of the thorax) the outline of the cardiac shadow is formed on the one hand by the right atrium and on the other by the left ventricle. The contour of the right atrium is the arc which is the right border of the heart shadow, curving upwards from the diaphragm and overlapping to some extent the shadows of the spine. If the heart is not in its normal position but is displaced to the right, this arc further overlaps the spine and moves to the right; if the heart is displaced to the left, this arc tends to disappear into the shadows of the vertebrae.

On the left, the outline of the heart shadow curving up from the diaphragm is contoured by the left ventricle. The right and left ventricles together form one ventricular mass which is the major part of the heart shadow as seen in the posteroanterior radiograph. As can be appreciated from the diagram in Fig. 1.18, the right ventricle is towards the front and the left ventricle is towards the back as the heart is placed in the thorax. The right ventricle normally does not reach the cardiac margin on the left and it is thus the left ventricle that forms most of the outline of the heart shadow on that side. The right ventricle is located so as to form no outlines of the heart shadow and it occupies most of the central region of the white space when the heart is viewed radiographically from the front.

The left atrium, as can be seen in Fig. 1.18, is posterior in its situation. A small conical part called the auricle projects forwards from the upper left hand corner of the atrium. This may be visible theoretically when the heart is viewed from the front but in the posteroanterior radiograph the shadow of this appendage cannot be distinguished on the left edge of the cardiac outline from the left ventricle below and the pulmonary artery and root of the left lung above. So the left atrium forms no part of the cardiac outline which can be recognised, except when it is abnormally enlarged.

THE VASCULAR PART OF THE MEDIASTINAL SHADOW

Above the atrial and ventricular parts of the cardiac outline, the mediastinal shadow is seen to narrow as it is followed in an upwards direction through the thorax. Eventually, in the region of the sternoclavicular joints, it becomes lost in the shadows of the upper dorsal vertebrae. Between the cardiac outline and the sternoclavicular joints, the mediastinal shadow is formed by the great vessels which carry blood to and from the heart.

Within the single white shadow the vessels are not delineated separately. Different vessels can be recognised as forming the right and left edges of the shadow and these vessels are thus identifiable in outline to some extent.

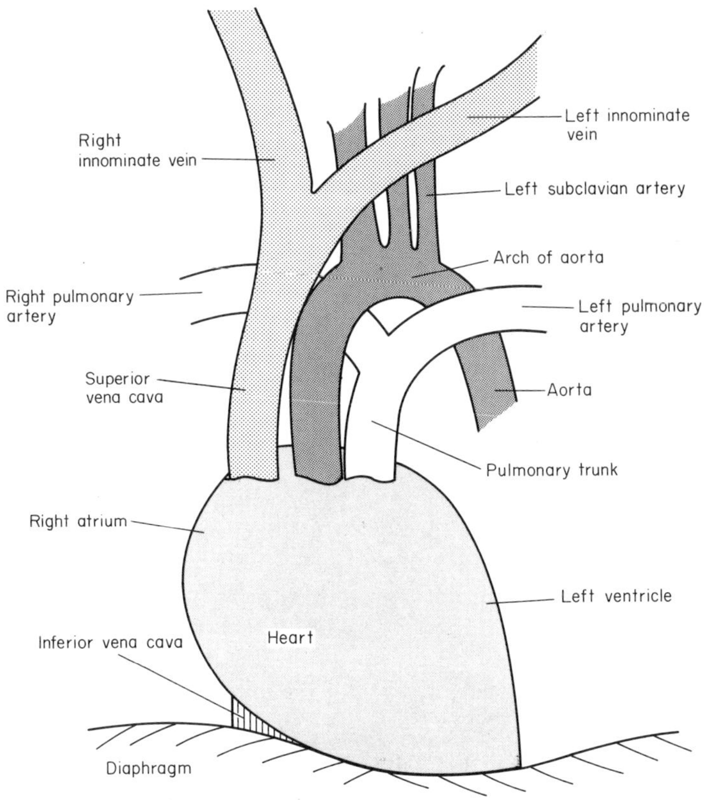

Fig. 1.19. Diagram to show the heart and great vessels forming the mediastinal shadow.

Normally this part of the mediastinal shadow on the right overlaps the vertebrae only a little, the extent to which it does so being different for individuals of different build; a slender subject with a long thorax has less overlap than a stocky subject with a short thorax.

On the left, the mediastinal shadow begins to overlap the vertebrae where the posterior part of the arch of the aorta forms an arc seen at about the level of the vertebral ends of the fifth or sixth rib. Fig. 1.19 shows a diagram of the heart and great vessels and this should be compared with the labelled radiograph shown in Fig. 1.14. Fig. 1.19 shows that the ascending aorta is within the mediastinal shadow and it indicates vessels which form outlines at the edges of the shadow.

On the right (passing from above downwards) the edge of the mediastinal shadow above the cardiac outline is formed by the right innominate vein; the superior vena cava; the root of the right lung with its pulmonary vessels spreading fanwise; the edge of the shadow then becomes formed by the right atrium as the cardiac outline is reached. Just where the curve of the right atrium runs to meet the diaphragm, the inferior vena cava may be glimpsed and forms a small curve concave to the right.

On the left similarly the edge of the mediastinal shadow is formed by the left subclavian artery; the arch of the aorta which makes a small but prominent and easily recognisable arc (the aortic knuckle); the main pulmonary trunk which, under the concavity of the aortic arch, divides into the right and left pulmonary arteries and forms a shallower arc which is less immediately noticeable; the root of the left lung with its fan of pulmonary vessels; the edge of the shadow then becomes left ventricle as the cardiac outline is reached.

VARIATIONS IN THE MEDIASTINAL SHADOW

Both in its cardiac and its vascular parts, the mediastinal shadow does not look exactly the same in all individuals or at different times in the same individual. It shows certain variations which are not indicative of abnormality in the heart and the great vessels themselves and are entirely separate from the changes which abnormal states of these structures produce.

Individual variations occur through the following:
(i) the body-build of the subject;
(ii) the curves of the spine and of the sternum;
(iii) the age of the subject;
(iv) the phase of respiration;
(v) the posture of the subject;
(vi) the condition of pregnancy.

The body-build of the subject

We can all recognise that people have different general body-forms and anatomists perceive associations between the build of the subject and the lie of certain organs within the body. People can be assigned to three general categories of body-build: those with short broad trunks; those with long narrow trunks; those who do not suit either of the previous categories and may be classified as average in build. With these three types of subject three sorts of heart outline can be recognised. People with short broad chests and of square build have hearts which lie with a more horizontal inclination; such hearts are also described as transverse or horizontal hearts. Those with long narrow chests and slender build have hearts which are more vertically inclined. The heart which is most commonly encountered is the one which is described as oblique and is found in people who in their body-build are neither very short and broad nor very long and narrow. Readers may like to look at Figs. 1.3 and 1.5 as examples of horizontal hearts; at Figs. 1.14 and 1.15 as examples of vertical hearts; and Figs. 1.1 and 1.11 as examples of the oblique heart most commonly encountered.

These variations in the cardiac part of the mediastinal shadow are accompanied also by differences in its vascular part. The horizontal heart goes with a vascular mediastinal shadow which is short and wide and overlaps the vertebrae; the vertical heart has a narrow elongated vascular mediastinal shadow with less overlapping of the outline of the dorsal spine.

The level of the heart within the thorax is determined mainly by the level of the diaphragm. People of short square build have higher diaphragms than do people of long narrow build and hence they also have hearts at a higher level. Since the level of the diaphragm in any person changes with the phase of respiration, the position of the heart and the appearance of the mediastinal shadow change too. This is further considered on page 46.

The curves of the spine and of the sternum

Scoliosis. The dorsal spine has normally a kyphotic curve (its curvature is concave anteriorly) and no lateral curve, forming a straight line when viewed directly from the front or the back. The thoracic aorta descending through the thorax follows the spine and deviations of the spine produce changes in the vascular and cardiac parts of the mediastinal shadow. If quite slight spinal aberrations have not been noticed, these changes may be wrongly attributed to abnormalities of the heart and great vessels.

If the spine has abnormal lateral curvature (scoliosis) the heart may be rotated and this alters the radiographic outline of the heart and aorta. If the heart is rotated to the right, more of the left ventricle shows from the front and the heart may seem enlarged. If the heart is rotated to the left, less of the left ventricle can be seen from the front. If the scoliosis is convex to the right, there will be less than the usual overlapping of the vertebral shadows by the outline of the right edge of the cardiac shadow; that is, the heart can look shifted to the left if the spinal curvature is unseen. If the scoliotic curve is convex to the left, there is more than the usual overlap of the vertebral shadows by the heart outline, corresponding to an impression that the heart has shifted to the right.

Kyphosis. Abnormal degrees of kyphotic curvature can make it extremely difficult, if not impossible, to obtain a postero-anterior projection of the chest which approaches the standard view. The mediastinal shadow presents an altered appearance, its degree of difference from the usual being dependent on the extent of the deformity present in the bony thorax.

Depressed sternum. The sternum is a long flat bone which normally is slightly convex anteriorly and concave posteriorly.

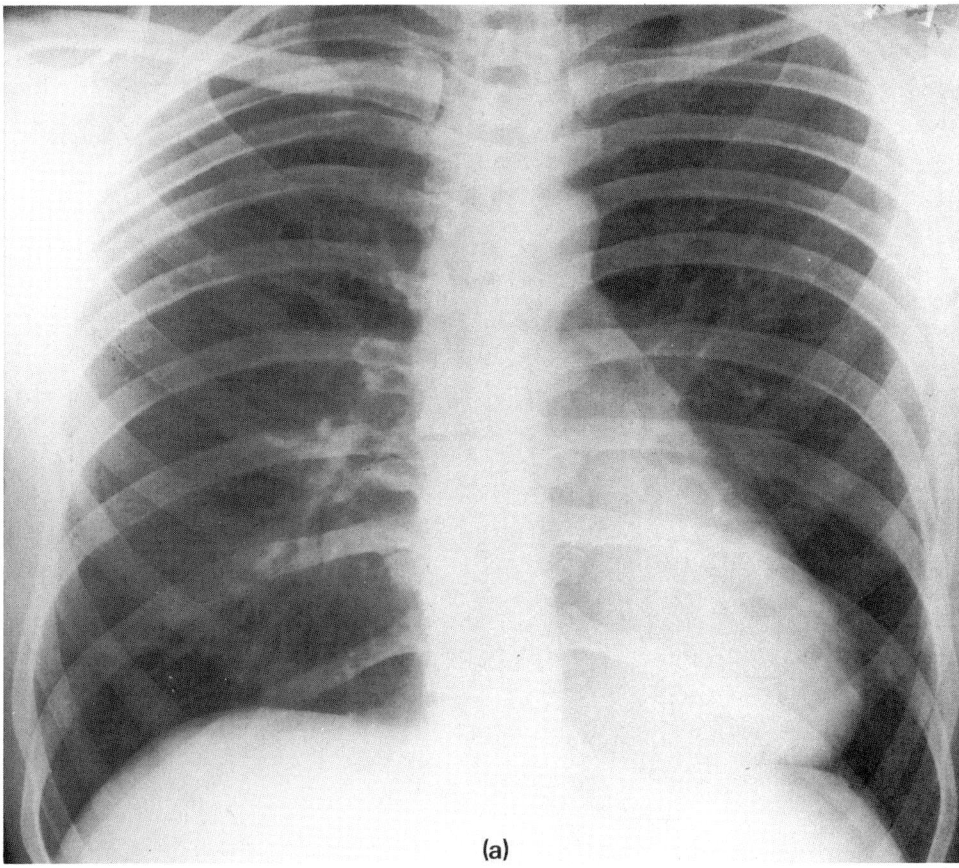

Fig. 1.20a. Posteroanterior radiograph of the chest of a subject who has a depressed sternum.

It is situated in the midline of the anterior chest wall. There is an anomaly called a funnel chest in which there is a funnel-shaped depression in the middle of the anterior chest wall, the deepest part of the hollow being occupied by the sternum. When the sternum is thus depressed backwards from its normal position, it decreases the anteroposterior dimensions of the thorax in the region which is immediately retrosternal. The heart then has less than its normal allocation of room within the mediastinum and can be flattened anteroposteriorly. This sometimes causes it to appear wider than usual when seen from the front in a posteroanterior radiograph of the

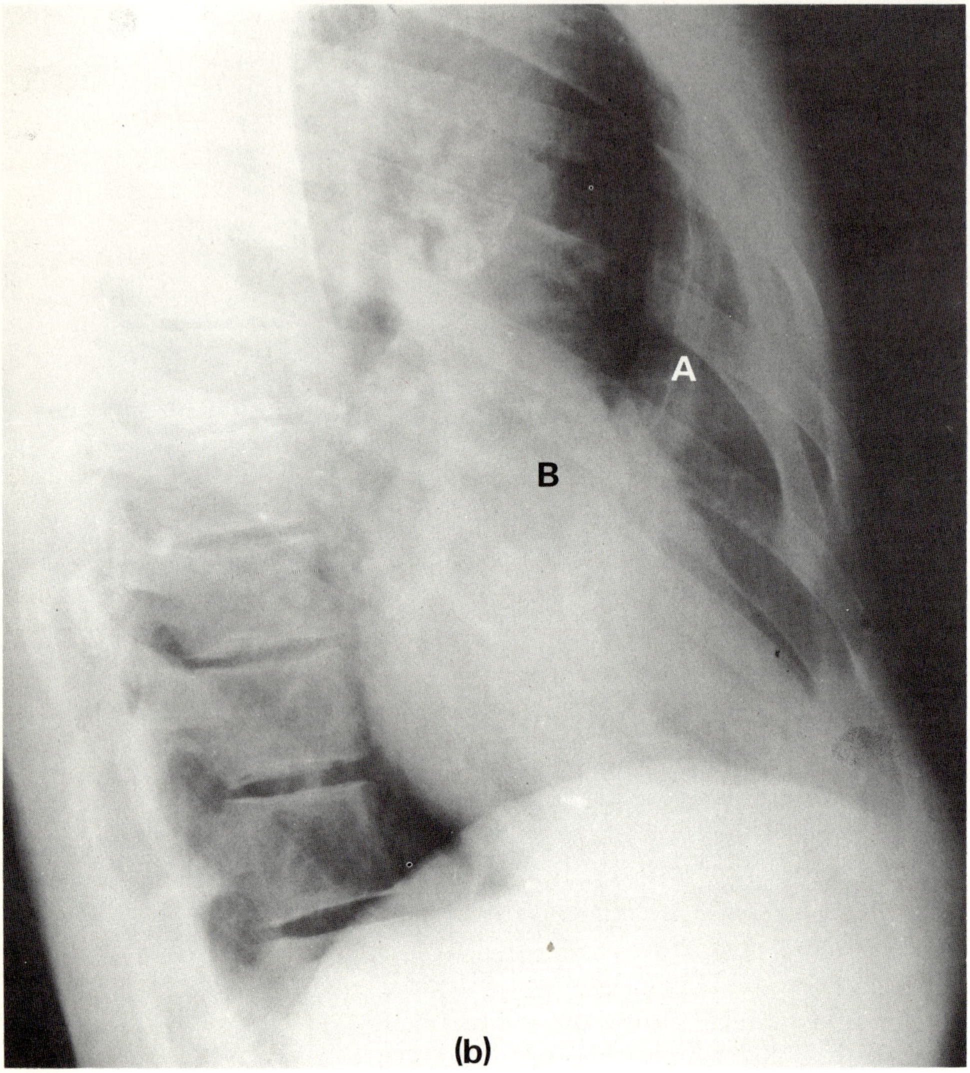

Fig. 1.20b. Lateral radiograph of the chest of the same subject.

A Depressed sternum B Cardiac shadow

chest and it may also appear as shifted to the left in position. Fig. 1.20 shows at (a) the posteroanterior radiograph of the chest of a patient who has a slight scoliosis in the upper dorsal spine and at (b) the lateral radiograph which reveals that he also has a sternum markedly depressed backwards from its usual position. The cardiac shadow on the posteroanterior view looks shifted to the patient's left, there being no overlap of the outline of the right atrium on the vertebrae. On the right side the second to sixth ribs have less space between them than do their opposite numbers in the left thorax. This follows from the scoliosis of the spine which spreads the ribs on the side to which it is convex, narrowing their interspaces on the side to its concavity.

This chest is an example of the way in which skeletal oddities alter the appearance of the mediastinal shadow. A radiographer who sees any deviation from the normal in a patient's thorax should make sure that the radiologist reporting on the chest radiographs is informed about the anomalies present.

The age of the subject

Cardiothoracic ratio. The term cardiothoracic ratio refers to the relationship between the width of the heart and the width of the thorax (see Fig. 1.21). As a guide to the normal size of the heart, in an adult the ratio width of heart/width of thorax should be within the range 1/3 to 1/2. In the child the heart is relatively larger in respect of the thorax and the ratio width of heart/width of thorax exceeds 1/2.

The aorta. As shown earlier, the ascending aorta rising from the heart in front of the vertebral column is within the vascular part of the mediastinal shadow and does not form one of the outlines in this region on the radiograph. As the aorta turns to the left and backwards at the arch of the aorta and then continues down through the thorax as the descending aorta, the posterior part of the arch produces to the left of the vertebral column the rounded outline or arc known as the aortic knuckle (labelled in Figs. 1.1, 1.8, 1.11 and 1.14). It varies in prominence not only with certain pathological states but also in the normal condition.

In young normal people this arc on the left is not prominent; on the right edge of the mediastinal shadow no outline of the aorta is to be seen. By middle age the aorta may have changed somewhat in its course and become distorted so that it forms a curving outline to the right of the spine and on the

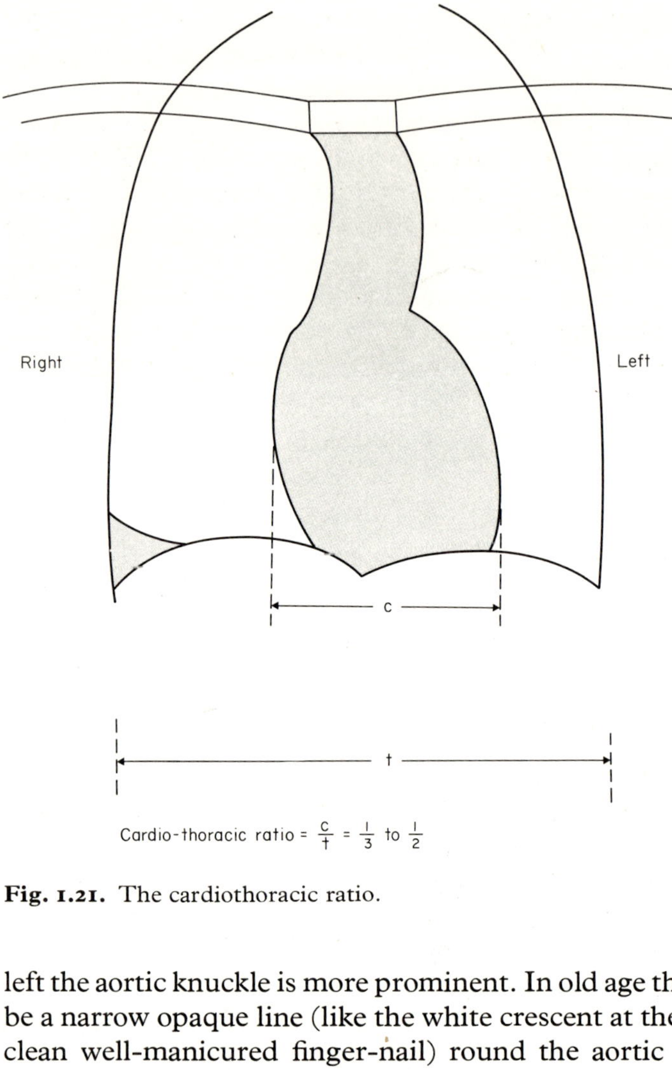

Fig. 1.21. The cardiothoracic ratio.

left the aortic knuckle is more prominent. In old age there may be a narrow opaque line (like the white crescent at the tip of a clean well-manicured finger-nail) round the aortic knuckle because calcification is present.

The phase of respiration

In an earlier section of this chapter the movement of the diaphragm with respiration was described. It has also been said earlier that the level of the heart within the thorax is related to the level of the diaphragm. Hence it follows that when a radiograph is exposed at full inspiration with the diaphragm depressed, the heart is at a lower level in the thorax than for the same patient after a movement of expiration. Figs. 1.8 and 1.9 should be compared.

There is a change not only in level. The mediastinal shadow shows some change in size and shape. When the heart descends with the diaphragm, the cardiac shadow appears narrower, the heart having a more vertical lie, and the vascular part of the shadow is longer and less wide. When the heart is at a higher level in the phase of expiration, its vertical diameter becomes shorter, its lie is more transverse and it looks wider. Correspondingly the vascular part of the shadow is shorter and broader. A study of Figs. 1.8 and 1.9 confirms these statements.

The posture of the patient

In thinking about the posture of the patient and its effect on the mediastinal shadow in a posteroanterior radiograph of the chest, we can consider a patient in the following situations:
(i) standing erect;
(ii) lying supine;
(iii) lying on the right side;
(iv) lying on the left side.
Movement of the diaphragm with posture and the relationship between the diaphragmatic level and the cardiac shadow in its situation and apparent size and shape have already been discussed. Attentive readers, recalling the movements of the diaphragm from pages 20–22, will not be surprised to be told that when the patient is standing erect the heart shadow is more vertical, is narrower and is at a lower level in the thorax in comparison with the transverse lie, the wider cardiac shadow and its higher level when the subject is radiographed lying supine. Correspondingly, because of the higher level of the heart in a supine subject, the vascular part of the mediastinal shadow is wider.

When the patient lies on one side, the heart shadow shifts to the side on which he is lying. If it is the right side, the right edge of the cardiac outline appears further to the right of the vertebral column. If the subject is lying on his left side when the posteroanterior radiograph is taken, the left edge of the cardiac shadow at its widest part extends nearly to the ribs.

The standard technique for a posteroanterior radiograph of the chest requires the patient to be standing erect. Radiologists and others interpreting radiographs recognise a normal mediastinal shadow on the basis of a standard appearance which results from this technique. Should the technique vary from the usual because a patient cannot stand erect, the radiographer should make sure that the radiologist is informed about the posture of the patient when the radiograph was taken.

The condition of pregnancy

It has already been stated that in the later months of pregnancy the diaphragm is high; and that the level of the heart within the thorax is determined mainly by the height of the diaphragm. Hence in the later months of pregnancy the vascular part of the mediastinal shadow looks shorter and wider and the heart is higher in the thorax with a less vertical lie.

THE THYMUS GLAND AND THE MEDIASTINAL SHADOW

The thymus gland is situated in the anterior and superior mediastinum. No definite function has been attributed to it. Its size is variable at different stages in life, the gland being fairly large at birth. It continues to grow during infancy and childhood until about the eighth year of life and after that time the process begins to reverse, the gland dwindling in size until, in the adult, it becomes small and atrophied.

When it is large and actively growing, the thymus gland is situated partly in the neck and partly in the thorax. Its thoracic portion is behind the sternum and in front of the heart and the great vessels. Below, the thymus gland rests on the pericardium and it extends up the thorax from about the level of the fourth costal cartilage, reaching as high in the neck as the level of the thyroid gland.

At its largest the thymus is relatively big for the amount of space available to it in the anterior mediastinum of an infant or a small child. It therefore makes the mediastinal shadow

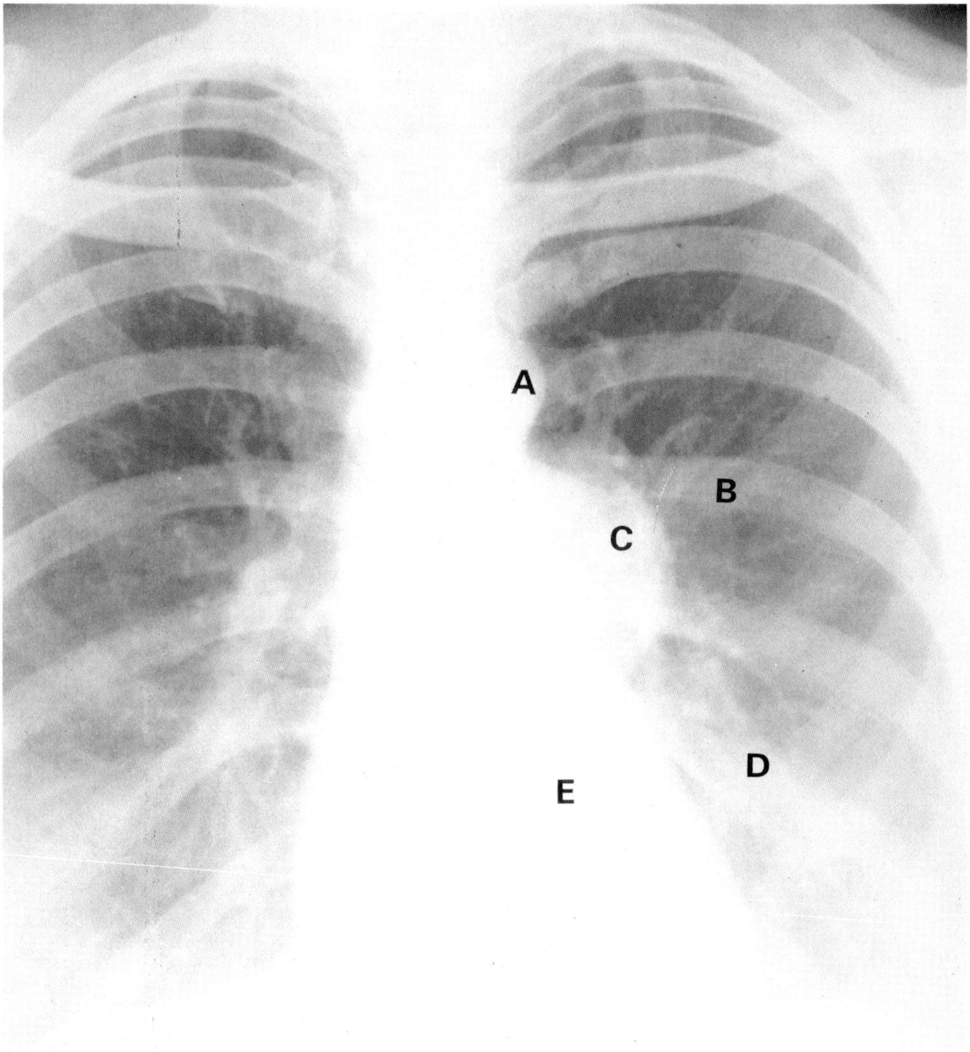

Fig. 1.22. Posteroanterior radiograph of the chest showing a thymic enlargement.

A Aortic knuckle
B Left rib 8
C Thymic shadow
D Left rib 10
E Cardiac shadow

wider and gives rise to a variety of appearances on posteroanterior radiographs of the chest. These appearances vary with the phase of respiration and with slight degrees of obliquity of the subject. Thymic shadows look larger on inspiration than on expiration and they appear exaggerated when the subject is turned slightly oblique from the frontal position.

The classic effect of the thymus on the mediastinal shadow is to produce a triangular projection (described as being like the sail of a boat) from the right edge of the mediastinal shadow above the cardiac outline. Variations on this are for the thymic shadow (a) to extend down to the diaphragm; (b) to be entirely on the left and not at all on the right; (c) to show as a bilateral widening of the mediastinal shadow.

Fig. 1.22 shows a thymic shadow in an adult, the thymus being enlarged beyond what would be considered to be normal in a subject of this age. The thymic shadow is on the left and projects as a curving outline which starts just below the aortic knuckle and just above the shadow of the posterior end of the eighth rib. The curve is convex to the left and lower down it joins the edge of the cardiac outline just above the shadow of the tenth rib.

Chapter 2
The Lateral Radiograph of the Thorax

A lateral radiograph is taken with the X-ray beam passing through the trunk from side to side; that is, in a direction at right angles to the one used for the posteroanterior radiograph considered previously. Examples of the resultant lateral view are seen in Fig. 2.1 of a female subject and in Fig. 2.2 of a male subject. We will consider their main features with reference to the following structures:

(i) the bony skeleton of the thorax;
(ii) the diaphragm;
(iii) the trachea;
(iv) the heart and great vessels;
(v) the lungs.

The bony skeleton of the thorax

In a lateral radiograph prominent features of the bony thorax are its anterior and posterior midline boundaries: the sternum in front and the thoracic spine behind. In Fig. 2.2 the sternum is well displayed. The manubrium, its articulation with the body of the sternum, the sternal angle at this articulation and the body itself of the sternum are all well seen. Posteriorly the outlines of the thoracic vertebrae show clearly both in Fig. 2.1 and in Fig. 2.2. The upper four or five vertebrae are not seen so well as are those below for the shadows of the scapulae and

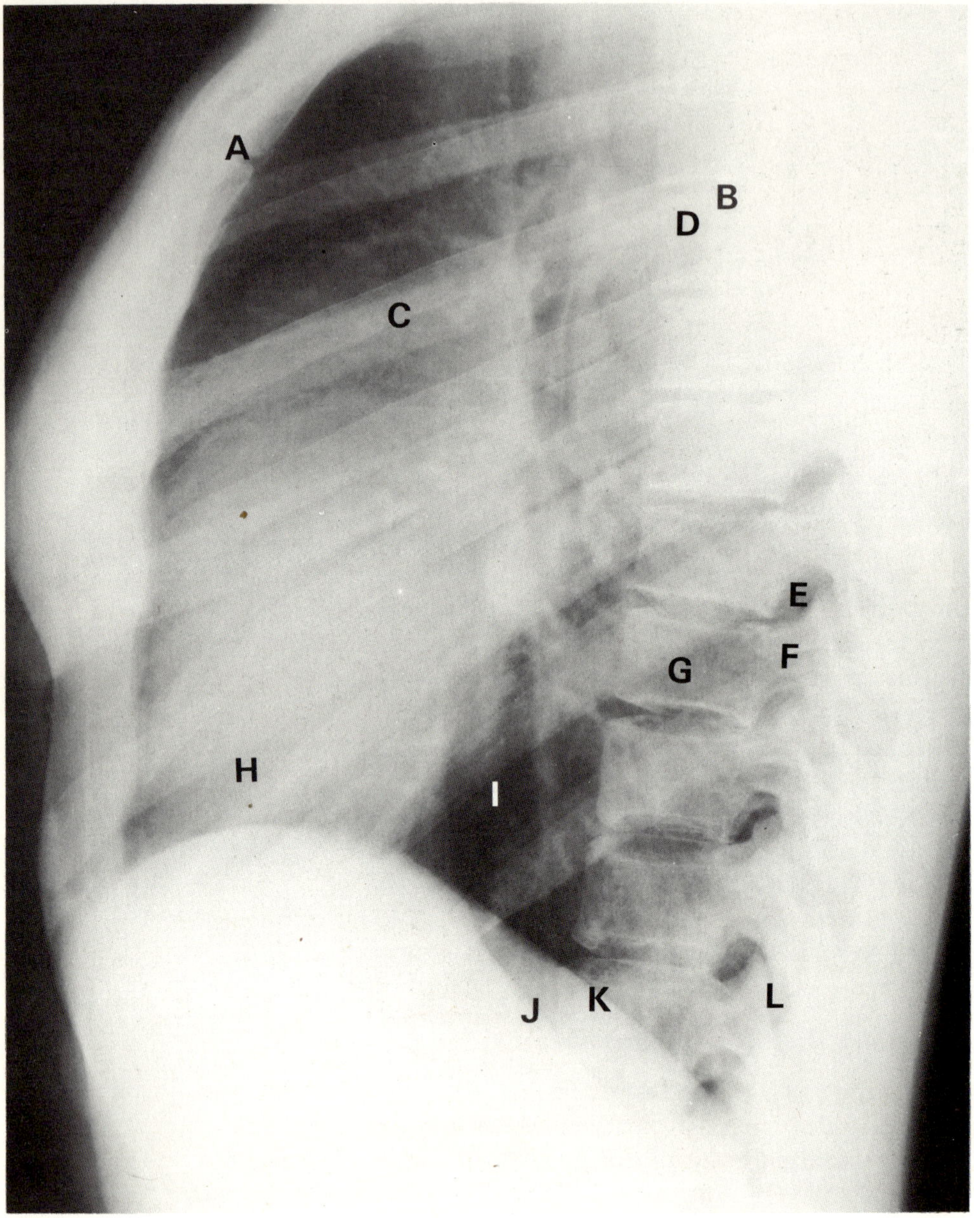

Fig. 2.1. Lateral radiograph of the chest of a female subject.

A Sternal angle
B Border of scapula
C Rib outlines (right and left ribs 4)
D Thoracic vertebra 5
E Intervertebral foramen
F Pedicle of vertebra
G Body of vertebra
H Cardiac shadow
I Retrocardiac space
J Left arc of diaphragm
K Right arc of diaphragm
L Intervertebral articulation

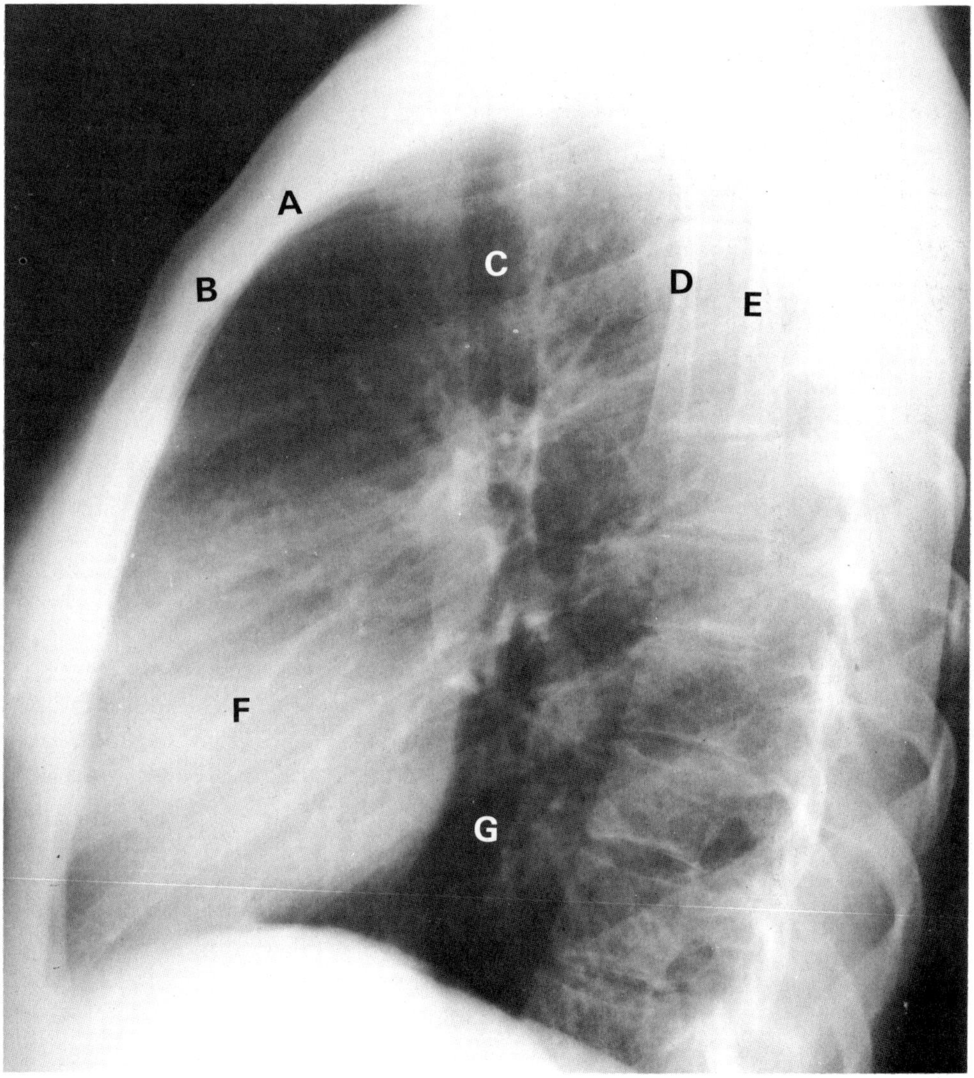

Fig. 2.2 Lateral radiograph of the chest of a male subject.

A Manubrium sterni
B Sternal angle
C Air-filled trachea
D Edge of left scapula
E Edge of right scapula
F Cardiac shadow
G Retrocardiac space

the tissues in the region of the shoulder girdle are superimposed upon them. However, some vertebral bodies can be distinguished readily enough in the upper regions. In those parts of the lateral view where dorsal vertebrae are well shown, the pedicles are seen projecting posteriorly from the vertebral bodies with the concavities of the vertebral notches above and below the pedicles forming the intervertebral foramina. Some intervertebral articulations are distinguishable.

It is not possible to number the individual vertebrae with absolute sureness on lateral radiographs of the chest but some identification can be attempted. It may be assumed that the articulation between the manubrium and the body of the sternum lies about opposite to the lower border of the fourth thoracic vertebra and the upper border of the fifth. With this established, other vertebrae may be counted upwards and downwards from the two identified. The vertebral outlines eventually become lost at the top in the region of the thoracic inlet and the shoulders and at the bottom in the radiographically underpenetrated parts below the diaphragm.

The only remaining structures of the bony thorax to which attention may be drawn on the lateral radiograph are the outlines of the ribs. They can be seen very prominently in Fig. 2.1, nearly superimposed from side to side and slanting downwards and forwards from their posterior articulations (not clearly shown) with the thoracic vertebrae. In Fig. 2.2 the ribs show much less intrusively over the thoracic contents. This difference in representation occurs through variations principally in exposure-technique. Choice of higher kilovoltage produces a radiograph in which the ribs are less prominently displayed.

The diaphragm

The diaphragm closes the thoracic cavity inferiorly. In a lateral radiograph of the thorax it shows prominently as the boundary line between the thoracic region and its contents (relatively radiolucent to the abdomen) and the abdominal region and its organs (relatively radiopaque to the thorax). The sternal fibres of the diaphragm arise from the back of the xiphisternum and the lumbar fibres arise from the upper lumbar vertebrae, which are at a lower level than the xiphisternum. The outline of the diaphragm on a lateral radiograph is seen to arch upwards and backwards from its anterior boundary at the xiphisternum and then follow a downwards and backwards course to disappear posteriorly at about the level of the eleventh or the twelfth dorsal vertebra.

As on the posteroanterior projection, this outline of the diaphragm represents its upper surface shown against the air-containing lungs. Taken on full inspiration with the subjects erect, the lateral radiographs in Figs. 2.1 and 2.2 show the diaphragm at a low level in the trunk.

It was noted in Chapter 1 that the right and left halves of the diaphragm are not at the same level, the right arc being higher than the left arc. This difference in level means that the two arcs are not always superimposed from side to side when seen in the lateral projection of the thorax.

The trachea

The trachea passes down the thorax through the superior mediastinum. Behind it is the vertebral column, from which it is separated by the oesophagus. The oesophagus does not appear on a lateral radiograph of the thorax unless there is a contrast agent present to fill and outline it. The trachea does show because normally it is air-containing and thus is revealed on the radiograph (see Figs. 2.1 and 2.2) as a dark band in front of the spine running from the thoracic inlet to about the level of the sixth dorsal vertebra or the one below it.

The trachea ends by dividing into the right and left main bronchi, the level of this bifurcation being usually given as the fifth thoracic vertebra. However, when a living subject stands erect and takes a deep inspiration, the bifurcation descends within the thorax and is at a lower level corresponding to the thoracic vertebrae which are numbered six and seven.

From the point of bifurcation of the trachea, the two main bronchi run outwards and downwards (the right bronchus rather more vertically than the left) to enter the lung on each side; the right bronchus is said to enter the right lung at the lung root on a level about opposite to the fifth thoracic vertebra while the left bronchus has assigned to it the level of the sixth thoracic vertebra for its point of entry at the root of the left lung. Again, if we think of a living person standing erect and taking in a deep breath (and such are the subjects usually for lateral radiographs of the chest) these levels for the entry points into the lung roots will be lower than those given by traditional anatomists.

Each main bronchus runs outwards from the mediastinum and in a lateral radiograph the direction of the X-ray beam (and hence the line of sight for a viewer) is more or less along the same plane as the direction of travel of the main bronchi and along the main axis of the lumen of each. These air-containing structures become lost on the radiograph and without the introduction of a positive contrast agent it is not possible to follow the divisions and subdivisions into smaller and smaller bronchi within the lung substance.

The heart and great vessels

THE HEART

In a lateral radiograph of the thorax the heart is seen in its situation in the middle mediastinum. As a relatively dense muscular organ, it forms a white shadow behind the sternum, set broadly on the diaphragm and separated from the spine at the rear by a darker space which represents the posterior mediastinum. This darker space on the radiograph may be called the retrocardiac space.

Seen from the side in a plain lateral radiograph the cardiac shadow, as in the posteroanterior projection, is homogeneous and the chambers of the heart are undifferentiated. However, the edges of the shadow may be recognised as being formed by particular parts. If Fig. 1.18 is studied it will be appreciated that the anterior and sternal edge of the cardiac shadow on the lateral radiograph is formed by the right ventricle. For the posterior and vertebral edge, the lower part is formed by the left ventricle and the upper part is formed by the left atrium.

THE GREAT VESSELS

The great vessels which carry blood from and to the heart and

have openings directly out of or into the heart chambers are as follows (see Fig. 1.19):
(i) The ascending aorta. This springs from the base of the left ventricle and passes upwards, forwards and to the right to become the arch of the aorta. Here the vessel continues to run upwards but it takes a backwards direction and the arch is towards the back and passes to the left side of the trachea and of the body of the fourth dorsal vertebra. Then it turns downwards to become continuous with the descending aorta.

The thoracic part of the descending aorta passes down in the posterior mediastinum immediately in front of the vertebral column and behind the left atrium. At about the level of the twelfth thoracic vertebra the descending aorta passes through the aortic opening in the diaphragm and the thoracic part becomes continuous with the abdominal part of the vessel.

In the radiograph shown in Fig. 2.3 the ascending aorta, the arch of the aorta and the descending aorta as far as about the level of the thoracic vertebrae ninth to tenth are well seen.
(ii) The pulmonary artery. This springs from the anterior and upper left angle of the right ventricle and runs upwards and backwards towards the arch of the aorta. Within the concavity of the arch above it, the pulmonary artery divides into right and left branches about opposite to the sixth dorsal vertebra. The right and left branches of the pulmonary artery pass outwards; each goes to the hilum of the appropriate lung and eventually enters the lung substance. In Fig. 2.3 the pulmonary artery is well shown beneath the arch of the aorta.
(iii) The pulmonary veins. These open into the upper posterior part of the left atrium and there are four of them, two right pulmonary veins and two left pulmonary veins.
(iv) The inferior vena cava. This passes upwards through the abdominal cavity on the right side of the aorta, penetrates the central tendon of the diaphragm through an opening and enters the inferior part of the right atrium. It is very clearly seen in Fig. 2.3.
(v) The superior vena cava. This vessel is formed by the junction of the right and left innominate veins and it opens into the upper part of the right atrium. The superior vena cava drains blood from the head and neck and the upper limbs.

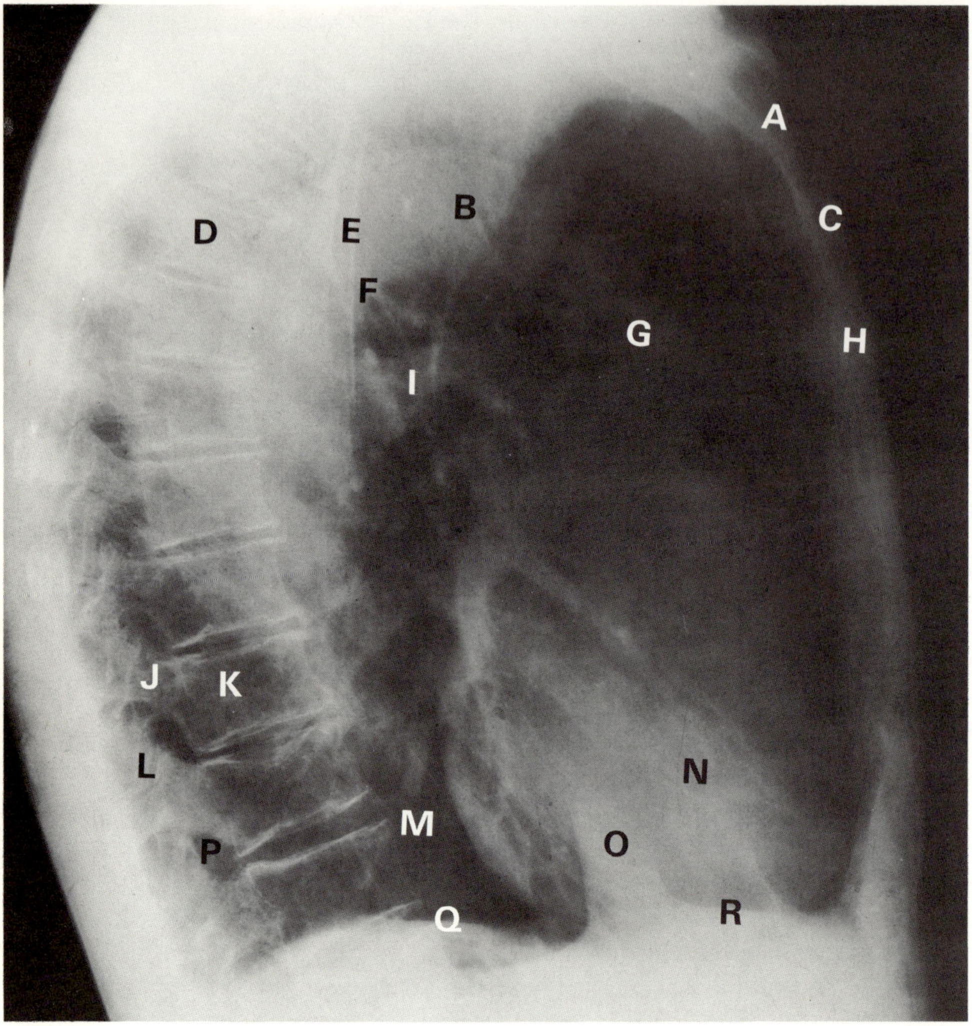

Fig. 2.3. Lateral radiograph of the chest with a good display of the great vessels.

A Manubrium sterni
B Arch of aorta
C Sternal angle
D Thoracic vertebra 5
E Edge of scapula
F Descending aorta
G Ascending aorta
H Body of sternum
I Pulmonary artery
J Pedicle of vertebra
K Body of vertebra
L Intervertebral articulation
M Retrocardiac space
N Cardiac shadow
O Inferior vena cava
P Intervertebral foramen
Q Right arc of diaphragm
R Left arc of diaphragm

If comparison is made between Fig. 2.1 and Fig. 2.3 it will be noticed that the vessels which are prominently shown in Fig. 2.3 are not so displayed in Fig. 2.1. Fig. 2.3 is a radiograph where a fortunate combination of subject and technique of exposure have combined to show the vessels with particular clarity. However, it is usually possible in a lateral radiograph of the thorax to distinguish the shadows of the aorta and of the main pulmonary trunk beneath the arch.

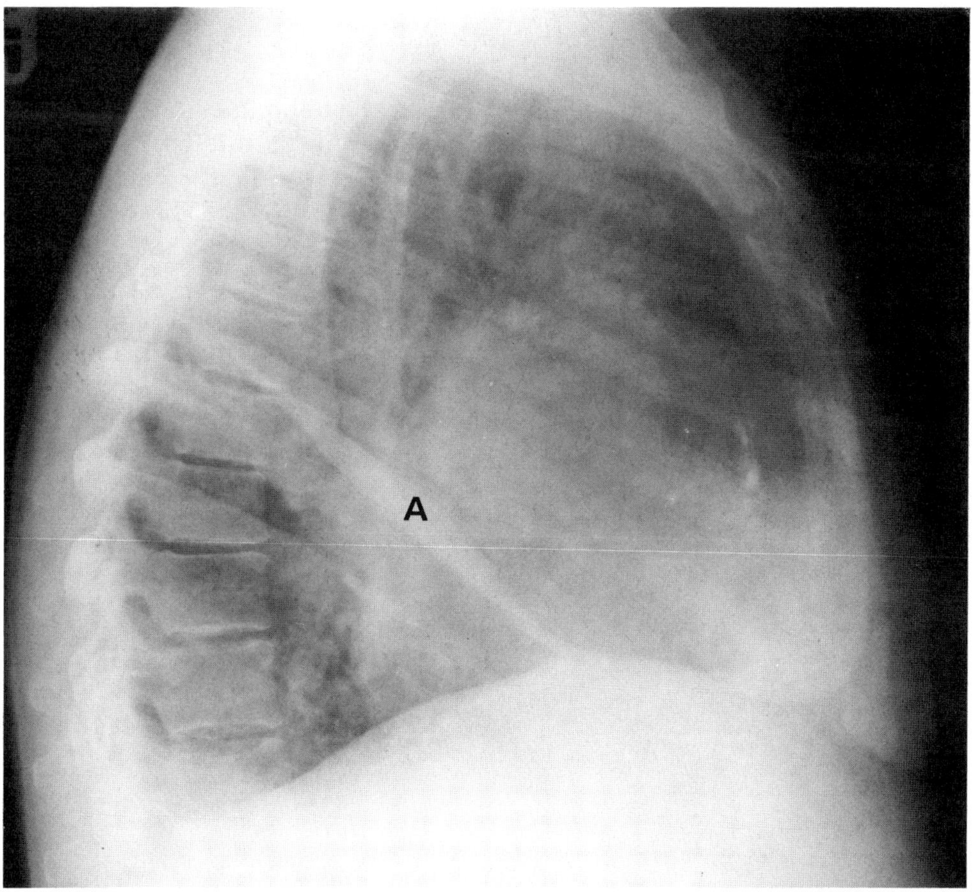

Fig. 2.4. Lateral radiograph of the chest showing an opacified oblique fissure in the right lung (interlobar effusion).
A Opacified oblique fissure

The lungs

In a lateral projection of the thorax the right and left lung fields become superimposed from side to side. The direction of the X-ray beam as it passes through the thorax from one side to the other is more or less along planes in which lie the fissures of the lungs. If they are normal, the fissures are seen as very thin white lines. If they are filled with an abnormal material by a process of disease, this can be detected (see Fig. 2.4). The line of the oblique fissure on each side rises from the diaphragm about 4 cm behind the anterior chest wall and curves upwards to about the level of the fourth dorsal vertebra. The level of the horizontal fissure in the right lung is the fourth costal cartilage and its line runs more or less horizontally backwards to join the oblique fissure.

In Chapter 1 it was pointed out that the posteroanterior radiograph displays only these areas of the lung fields which are projected above the highest part of the diaphragm. In Fig. 2.1 the level of this highest part is seen to be the top of the body of the eleventh thoracic vertebra. The lateral radiograph shows what is not visible on the posteroanterior view: firstly the posterior region in the thorax where the diaphragm dips from its highest point of curvature down to the level (in the case of Fig. 2.1) approximately of the lower edge of the body of the twelfth thoracic vertebra; and secondly the anterior region where the diaphragm dips from its highest level at the upper edge of the eleventh thoracic vertebra to a point corresponding to the lower edge of the same vertebral body.

Chapter 3 Oblique Radiographs of the Thorax

This chapter concerns itself with radiographic anatomy demonstrated by oblique projections of the thorax used in radiographic technique. In these views the X-ray beam is directed neither anteroposteriorly nor laterally from side to side but along angled lines through the thorax that come between these two directions.

The oblique projections are:

(i) the right anterior oblique;
(ii) the left posterior oblique; } very similar anatomically

(iii) the left anterior oblique;
(iv) the right posterior oblique. } very similar anatomically

Fig. 3.1 indicates the direction of the beam, the placing of the patient and the situation of the film for all four oblique views. It can be seen that in the right anterior and the left posterior oblique projections the X-ray beam follows parallel courses; hence the two are essentially similar views. The same is true for the left anterior and the right posterior oblique projections.

We are concerned here with radiographs taken in oblique positions to demonstrate features of the cardiac outline and to examine structures in the mediastinum. For these purposes the patient is usually placed with his anterior chest wall nearer to the film and his back towards the X-ray tube. So we deal here with the two opposite anterior oblique views and disregard their posterior equivalents. This chapter considers the

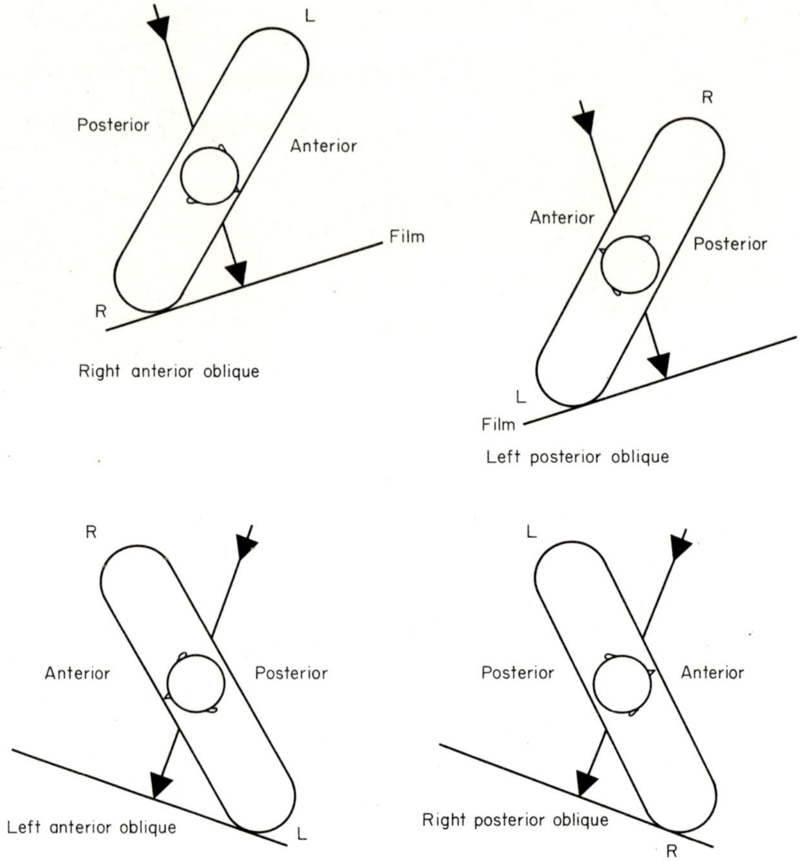

Fig. 3.1. The relative positions of the film, the patient and the X-ray beam in oblique projections of the thorax.

appearances shown in (i) the right anterior oblique projection, disregarding its equivalent left posterior oblique view; and (ii) the left anterior oblique projection, disregarding its equivalent right posterior oblique.

The right anterior oblique projection

Fig. 3.2 shows a radiograph of the chest taken with the patient erect in the right anterior oblique position.

THE BONY SKELETON

In this radiograph prominent bony landmarks, useful for

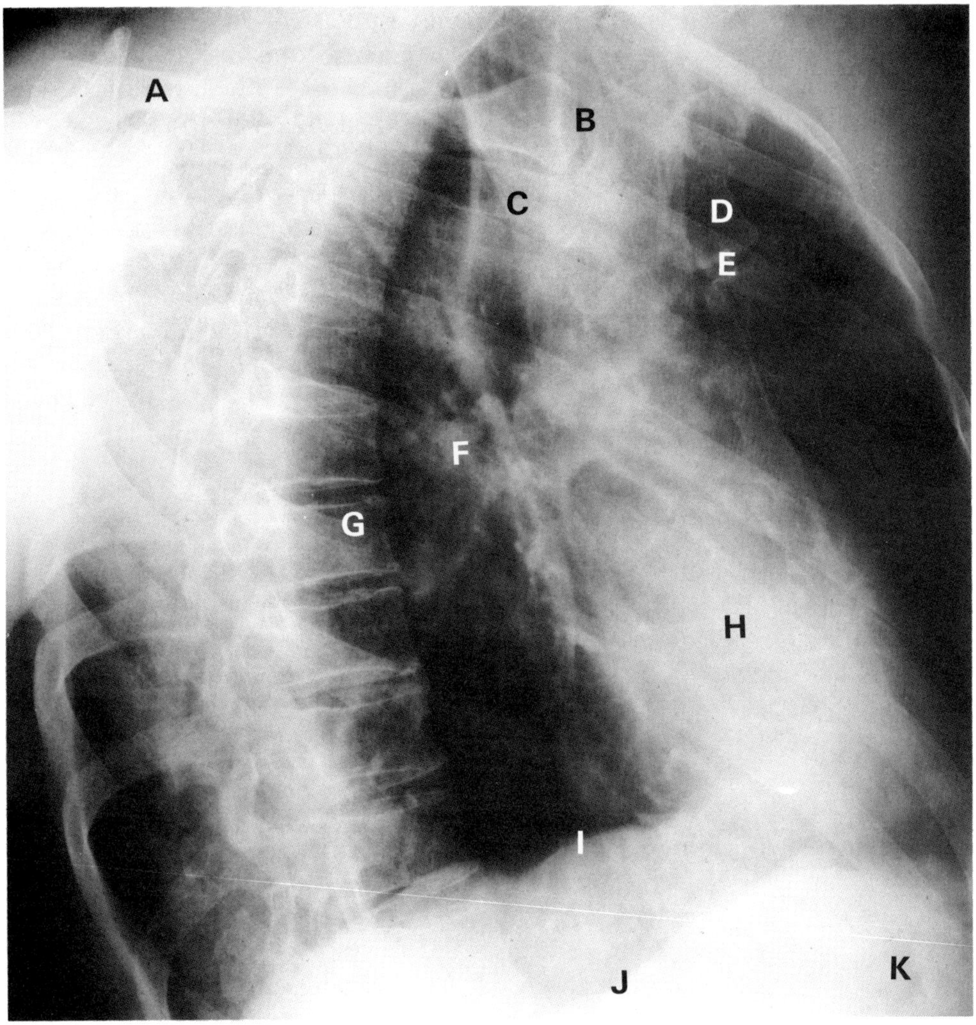

Fig. 3.2. A right anterior oblique radiograph of the chest.

A Right clavicle
B Right sternoclavicular joint
C Arch of aorta
D Manubrium sterni
E Sternal angle
F Region of hilum of right lung
G Body of thoracic vertebra
H Cardiac shadow
I Right arc of diaphragm
J Left arc of diaphragm
K Gas in the fundus of the stomach

orientation and recognition, are the thoracic vertebrae seen in a curve to the viewer's left hand and the sternum seen towards the viewer's right hand. Well shown are the manubrium of the sternum, the patient's right sternoclavicular joint and the articulation between the manubrium and the body of the sternum which marks the sternal angle. The lower part of the sternum is to some extent overshadowed by the heart.

Such a projection may be used to demonstrate the sternum when it is the required subject of examination, other features of the technique being adjusted to show its full extent more clearly than in Fig. 3.2. Our main concern with the projection here is its demonstration of the anatomy of certain of the mediastinal contents so we will not describe in further detail features of the bony skeleton as they happen to be shown. Readers who began with Chapter 1 will be able to recognise in Fig. 3.2 the various parts of the bony thorax.

THE DIAPHRAGM

In Fig. 3.2 the diaphragm is seen as the lower boundary of the thorax, with the radiographically underpenetrated region of the abdomen below it and the relatively less radiopaque thoracic structures above it. In this projection the two domes of the diaphragm are shown as two separate curves: the line of one is above that of the other and they can both be clearly seen in the region on the radiograph which is immediately to the viewer's right of the spine. From this part, the higher of the two lines is seen in the radiograph to run towards the viewer's left, reaching the spine and then curving down towards the costrophrenic angle on the extreme left of the radiograph; this is the right dome of the diaphragm and the costophrenic angle mentioned above is on the subject's right side. The lower of the two lines is seen to run from the spine towards the viewer's right, forming a little below the heart shadow a curve which is convex upwards; this is the left dome of the diaphragm.

In Fig. 3.2 at the extreme edge of the radiograph on the viewer's right where this curve of the left dome of the diaphragm disappears, there can be seen below the diaphragm a faint round dark area. This is gas in the fundus of the stomach.

THE LUNGS

Oblique projections of the chest carried out as plain radiographs without the introduction of any contrast agent are not particularly useful for demonstration of the lung fields. The matter is discussed further in Chapter 4 and readers who wish to pursue it are referred to page 87.

THE MEDIASTINUM

The right anterior oblique projection demonstrates structures within the mediastinum and on a plain radiograph the following can be seen at least in part:
(i) the trachea;
(ii) the ascending aorta, the arch of the aorta and the descending aorta;
(iii) structures in the hilum of the right lung;
(iv) the heart.

The trachea

In a right anterior oblique projection of the thorax the trachea is seen as a dark band in the upper mediastinum running from above downwards, more or less centrally situated between the spine on the viewer's left hand and the sternum on the viewer's right. The band crosses the inner end of the subject's right clavicle and at about the level of the sixth thoracic vertebra it disappears.

In Fig. 3.2 the sternal angle is well seen and is marked. It may be taken to be opposite to the thoracic vertebrae 4 and 5 and from this the sixth thoracic vertebra can be approximately located. At a point to the viewer's right of it the tracheal band ends. This point of disappearance is where the trachea bifurcates into the right and left main bronchi.

The aorta

In a right anterior oblique projection the arch of the aorta with parts of the ascending and descending aorta can be seen, although the line of sight is not such as to open up fully the arch and best display the full extent of the descending aorta.

In Fig. 3.2 the upper border of the highest part of the arch of the aorta shows below the inner third of the subject's right clavicle with the dark band of the trachea superimposed upon it. With the upper border of the arch located it is not difficult to distinguish the lower border; the arch and the first part of the descending aorta which is continuous with it then seem to spring into view. The arch curves upwards and backwards in the thorax, running from the viewer's right to left in this radiograph. The descending aorta can be distinguished passing down through the thorax close to the spine.

In Fig. 3.1 at a point somewhat below the bifurcation of the trachea, the shadow of the descending aorta seems to disappear into a darkish space between the shadow of the heart on the viewer's right hand and the shadow of the spine on the viewer's left. This dark space is the retrocardiac space. The aorta occupies it, behind the unseen oesophagus and in front of the spine, but may not be clearly visualised on a plain radiograph.

The hilum of the right lung

The hilum of each lung is the region where various structures which form the root of the lung pass into and from the lung. For each lung these structures are: the main bronchus; the pulmonary artery; the pulmonary veins; the bronchial arteries and veins; lymph vessels; nerves.

In the right anterior oblique projection the region of the hilum of the right lung is viewed beneath the arch of the aorta. Some of the mentioned structures form shadows which can be appreciated as a composite mass behind the heart, beneath the arch of the aorta and appearing to bridge the retrocardiac space between the heart and the spine. Normal lymph glands do not show as separately recognisable on a plain radiograph and the nerves are unseen.

For the others, if a vessel happens to be visualised from a line of sight which is along its lumen a blood vessel can be distinguished from a bronchus. The vascular structure is a circular radiopacity while the air-containing bronchus has a radioparent centre to the circle and thus appears as a ring and not a disc.

The part of the composite shadow which is just beneath the arch of the aorta is formed principally by the pulmonary trunk which arises from the upper left hand part of the right ventricle and runs upwards and backwards, dividing into the right and the left pulmonary arteries beneath the concavity of the aortic arch.

The heart

The heart shadow is readily recognised because of its radio-pacity, its size and its situation, resting on the diaphragm in front of the thoracic spine with the dark retrocardiac space between it and the vertebral bodies. In the right anterior oblique projection, the border of the heart shadow which is towards the spine and is on the left hand of the viewer is formed by the left atrium in its upper part and by the right atrium in its lower part as the curve runs down towards the diaphragm. Just above the diaphragm the inferior vena cava makes an appearance at the back of the heart shadow.

This projection can be of value to show enlargement of the left atrium for if the condition is gross the line bulges towards the spine; readers are referred to page 102 if they wish to read of the use of this projection when the oesophagus is outlined by means of barium sulphate.

The border of the heart shadow which is towards the sternum and on the right of the viewer in the right anterior oblique projection is formed by the right ventricle throughout most of its length from above downwards. One small part of the outline, anterior and close to the diaphragm, is formed by the left ventricle.

The left anterior oblique projection

Fig. 3.3 shows a radiograph of the chest taken with the patient erect in the left anterior oblique position.

THE BONY SKELETON

The prominent bony landmarks of the spine and the sternum are shown in the left anterior oblique projection similarly to

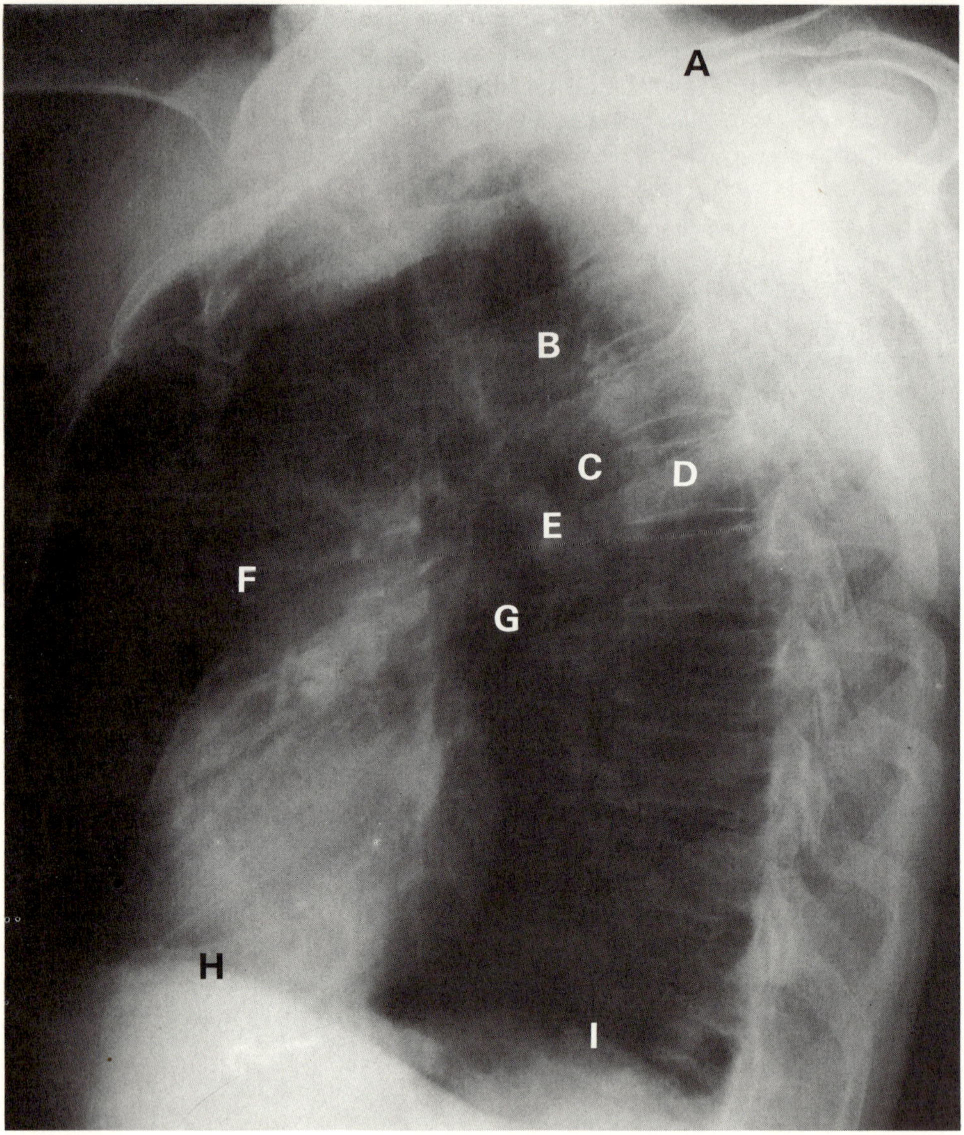

Fig. 3.3. A left anterior oblique radiograph of the chest.

A Left clavicle
B Arch of aorta
C Descending aorta
D Thoracic vertebra 6
E Right pulmonary artery
F Ascending aorta
G Left pulmonary artery
H Right arc of diaphragm
I Left arc of diaphragm

their display in the right anterior oblique radiograph but reversed left to right for the viewer. Thus the subject's spine appears to the viewer's right in the radiograph and the sternum to the viewer's left.

THE DIAPHRAGM

The left anterior oblique projection shows the diaphragm again with its right and left domes separately distinguishable. In Fig. 3.3 running from the spine on the viewer's right towards the heart on the viewer's left, two lines are seen, one above the other. This higher one is the left dome of the subject's diaphragm. The lower one can be followed further across the radiograph towards the viewer's left, passing beneath the heart shadow and running into the costophrenic angle shown to the viewer's left of the heart shadow. This is the right dome of the diaphragm and the costophrenic angle mentioned is on the subject's right side.

THE LUNGS

The reader is referred to page 65 in regard to appearances within the lungs displayed in oblique projections of the thorax.

THE MEDIASTINUM

The mediastinal organs which are to be seen in the left anterior oblique projection not surprisingly differ little from those seen in the right anterior oblique radiograph. The differences are (a) that the hilar region shown is the hilum of the left lung in place of the right; and (b) that the opposite projection of the central ray (from back right to left front in place of from back left to right front) gives another view of the heart and great vessels as they are placed within the thorax.

The structures to be considered are:

(i) the trachea;

(ii) the ascending aorta, the arch of the aorta and the descending aorta;

(iii) structures in the hilum of the left lung;

(iv) the heart.

The trachea

The trachea is again glimpsed as a dark band in the mediastinum, situated between the spine on the viewer's right hand and the sternum on the viewer's left. In Fig. 3.3 the upper part of the trachea is seen faintly, crossing the medial third of the subject's left clavicle. Opposite the sixth thoracic vertebra it is more clearly shown at its point of bifurcation into the right and the left main bronchi.

The aorta

The arch of the aorta is continuous with the ascending aorta. From the point where the arch begins behind the manubrium sterni, it runs upwards, backwards and to the left. At first in front of the trachea, the arch is on the left as it turns downwards and becomes continuous with the descending aorta. The descending aorta thus begins on the left of the vertical column. As it goes down through the thorax, the aorta approaches the midline and at its end where it passes through the diaphragm it lies in front of the spine.

Because of the direction and the position of the descending aorta within the mediastinum, if it follows a course undistorted by age or pathological change the left anterior oblique projection of the thorax can sometimes provide a full-length view of it. For this purpose the left anterior oblique is not necessarily better than the left lateral projection (compare Figs. 2.2 and 3.3).

In Fig. 3.3 the top of the arch of the aorta can be discerned a little in front of the spine, just above a line drawn from the sternal angle on the viewer's left to the upper border of the fifth thoracic vertebra on the viewer's right. The aorta can be seen to turn downwards in front of the fourth and fifth thoracic vertebrae at the point where the arch becomes continuous with the descending aorta. The descending aorta can be followed moderately easily down to about the eighth or ninth dorsal vertebra, close to and in this case partially obscured by the spine. After that it seems to disappear in the dark space (the retrocardiac space) between the heart and the vertebral column which is its situation.

The hilum of the left lung

In the left anterior oblique projection (as in the right anterior oblique) the region of the hilum of the lung occupies on the radiograph an area which is beneath the arch of the aorta and above the dark retrocardiac space. In Fig. 3.3 the letter C which identifies the descending aorta can be seen to have immediately to the viewer's right of it a little dark space shaped more or less like an inverted U. The lower boundary of this inverted U is formed by the right pulmonary artery.

Below the right pulmonary artery is another little dark space which (while we are alphabetically inclined) may be likened to a tilted *D*. Beneath this *D* is the left pulmonary artery. In the left anterior oblique projection the pulmonary trunk and then the left pulmonary artery, after it branches from the trunk beneath the aortic arch, run more or less parallel to the film on the way to the root of the left lung.

The heart

In the left anterior oblique radiograph shown in Fig. 3.3 the heart shadow is clearly seen, resting on the diaphragm between the sternum on the viewer's left and the spine on the viewer's right. This projection makes the right ventricle form the lower part of the edge of the heart shadow which is towards the sternum; the upper part just below the ascending aorta is formed by the right atrium. The left ventricle forms most of the edge of the cardiac shadow which is towards the spine; a small part of the outline at the top and just below the left pulmonary artery is formed by the left atrium.

Thus the viewer sees the right heart on his left hand and the left heart on his right hand. This makes the projection of use in angiography and the reader is referred to the appropriate part of Chapter 4 for more on this topic. The left anterior oblique projection helps also in plain radiographic examinations when enlarged hearts are being studied since it provides separation of the right and left ventricular shadows.

Chapter 4
Appearances on Contrast-Studies in the Thorax

So far this book has considered the radiographic anatomy shown on plain radiographs of the thorax and the reader knows by now that such radiographs present an incomplete account of the structures depicted. By different methods of examination for which contrast agents are used, more information may be gained about the particular structures which a contrast agent fills and about neighbouring organs. The present chapter is given to the anatomical appearances on contrast studies within the thorax. The survey does not claim to be comprehensive and detailed. It is intended to help student radiographers to understand radiographs and to enable them to identify the anatomical parts which are displayed.

The following will be considered:
(i) angiographic appearances;
(ii) bronchographic appearances;
(iii) appearances when the oesophagus is outlined with barium sulphate;
(iv) lymphangiographic appearances.

Angiographic appearances

Angiography is the radiographic examination of the cardiovascular system which circulates the blood. It is achieved by introducing a suitable contrast agent into the blood and then exposing a series of radiographs which demonstrate the region being examined. We are to consider here some radiographic anatomy to be displayed within the thorax by such a method and in particular we explain the appearances of the heart and the great vessels on normal angiocardiograms.

In order to be able to understand the radiographic anatomy which appears on angiocardiograms, the student needs to keep in mind the following: (a) the sequence of blood flow and hence of the contrast agent through the heart and the great vessels and (b) the situation of the heart in the thorax and the views obtained of it by the projections used.

Contrast agent and blood filling the superior vena cava pass from there into the right atrium and thence to the right ventricle. From the right ventricle the blood is pumped to the pulmonary artery and its branches and thus it reaches the lungs. The return route to the heart brings opacified blood along the pulmonary veins to the left atrium, which fills. Next the left ventricle fills and finally the blood is pumped out to the general circulation via the aorta. So the sequence is:

right heart to lungs to left heart to general circulation.

In an unselective angiocardiographic examination (that is, one in which the contrast agent has not been selectively placed by catheterizing a particular chamber of the heart) a viewer of the radiographs sees the whole series of events: the opacification first of the right heart, then of the pulmonary trunk and the right and left pulmonary arteries as the blood leaves the heart; then on the return of blood from the lungs, the left heart and finally the aorta are opacified and visualised.

On plain radiographs the cardiac shadow presents as a homogeneous radiopacity with the separate heart chambers undifferentiated. Angiocardiograms are different pictures because in them the right and the left sides of the heart are separately filled and demonstrated in isolation from each other. Thus it becomes possible to identify within the mediastinal shadow the four chambers of the heart and the several great vessels in turn displayed. We consider below the appearances of (i) the right heart and its associated vessels and (ii) the left heart and its associated vessels.

The right heart and the left heart, each separately filled in turn, can be seen in the frontal view of a posteroanterior or anteroposterior projection. The location of the heart within the thorax places its right half towards the front and its left half towards the back. Thus from the front there is some superimposition of the two sides and the vessels associated with them. Normally in contrast studies the two sides fill separately and thus can be studied in turn on a frontal view, the superimposition ceasing to matter as the two sides are not together filled.

When the patient is turned into the left anterior oblique position (or the equivalent right posterior oblique position) the left heart is seen on the one side towards the spine and the right heart is seen on the other towards the sternum. These projections thus give a clear view of the right heart and the left heart separated on the radiograph. In contrast studies this is of value in elucidating such variations as abnormal shunts of blood between the two sides of the heart.

THE RIGHT HEART AND ITS VESSELS

Fig. 4.1 is a diagrammatic presentation to remind the reader of anatomical arrangements with which we are concerned as

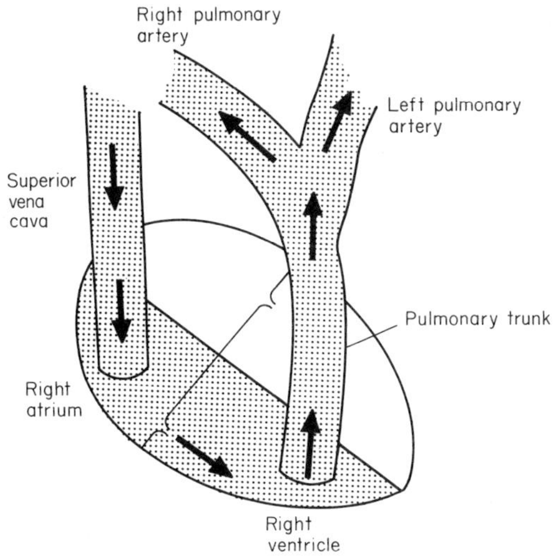

Fig. 4.1. Diagram of the filled right heart during angiocardiography.

they would appear when seen from the front. The shaded areas indicate the following structures opacified: the superior vena cava; the right atrium; the right ventricle; the pulmonary trunk and its branches which are the right and the left pulmonary arteries. The arrows point in the direction of blood flow.

To be compared with Fig. 4.1 are Figs. 4.2 and 4.3. These are radiographs which show the right heart and its associated

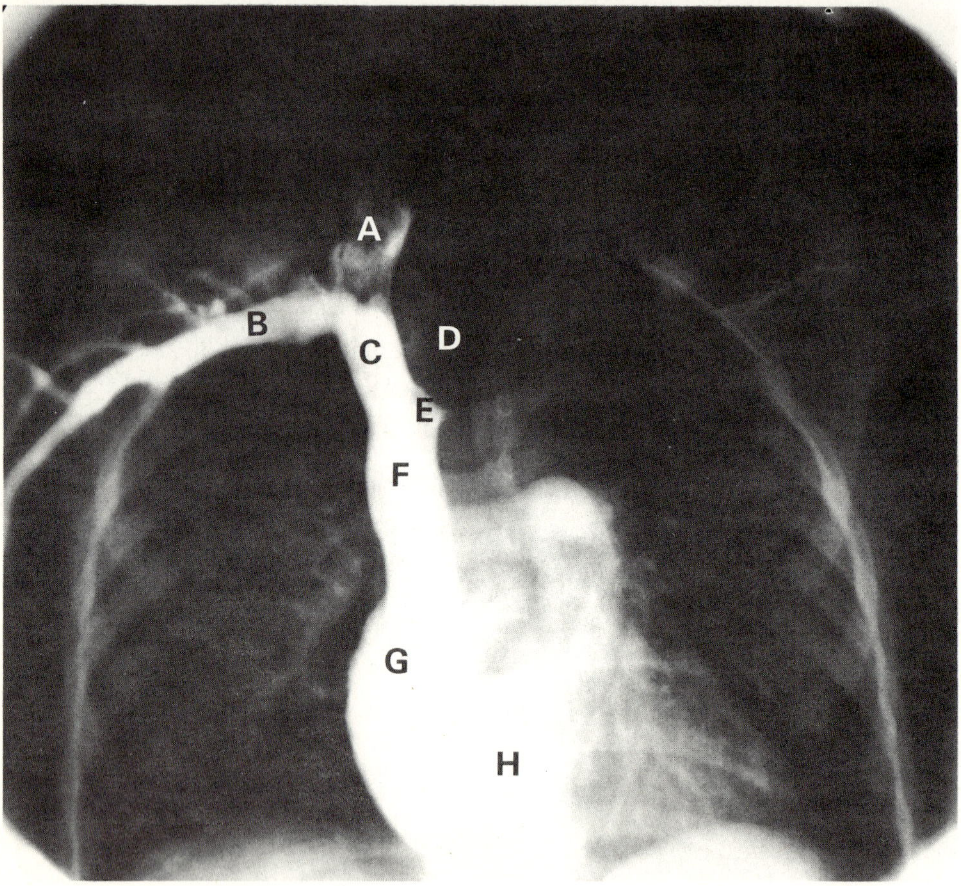

Fig. 4.2. Angiocardiogram of the normal right heart early in the series (frontal projection).

A Right internal jugular vein
B Right subclavian vein
C Right innominate vein
D Air-filled trachea
E Left innominate vein
F Superior vena cava
G Right atrium
H Atrioventricular region

vessels filled with opacified blood; Fig. 4.2 comes just before Fig. 4.3 in the time sequence of the events.

On radiographs which have been taken with a frontal projection the flow of opacified blood into and then out from the heart produces in the normal a U shape. The arm of this U

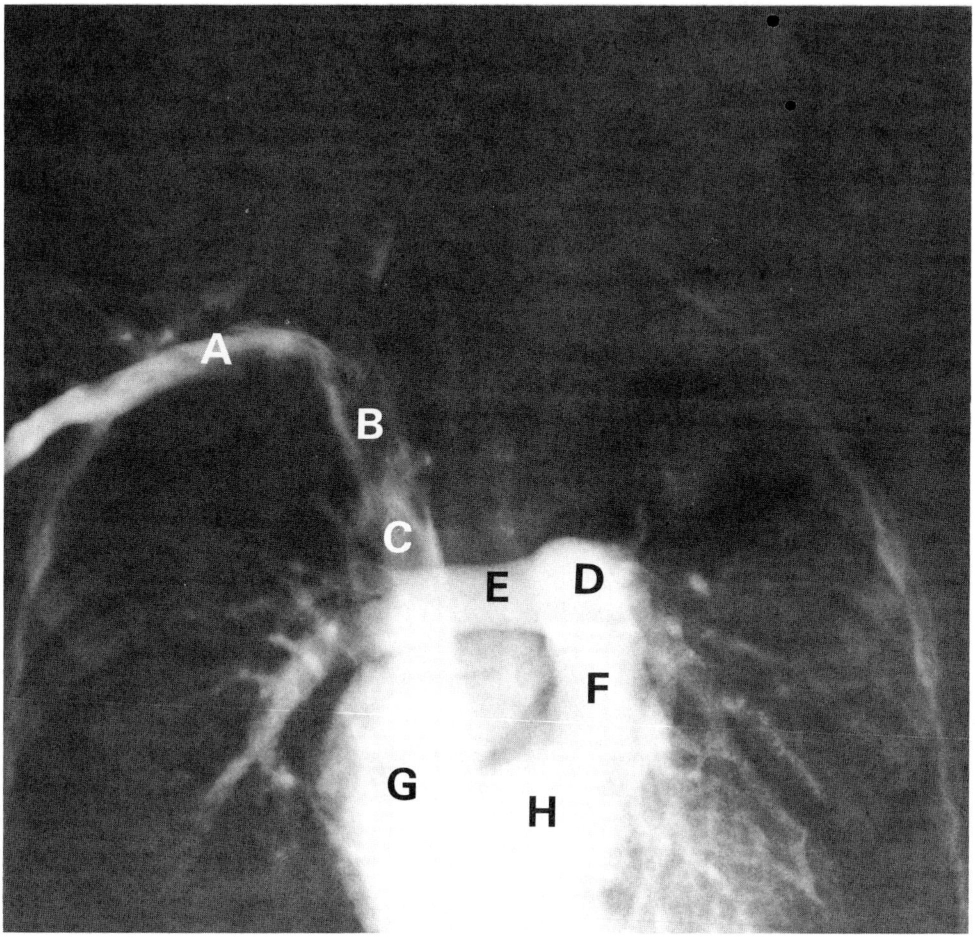

Fig. 4.3. Angiocardiogram of the normal right heart a little later in the series (frontal projection).

A Right subclavian vein
B Right innominate vein
C Superior vena cava
D Left pulmonary artery within the opacity of the pulmonary trunk
E Right pulmonary artery
F Pulmonary trunk
G Right atrium
H Right ventricle

which is to the patient's right is formed by the superior vena cava and then by the right atrium. The bottom curve of the U is the atrioventricular region and the orifice between atrium and ventricle guarded by the tricuspid valve. The half of the U which is towards the patient's left is formed by the right ventricle in its lower part and then by the pulmonary trunk coming off the right ventricle. The pulmonary trunk divides into the right and left pulmonary arteries. The right pulmonary artery is somewhat larger and longer than the left and it runs horizontally to the right behind the ascending aorta; in angiocardiograms it closes the top of the U shape which has been described. The left pulmonary artery is posterior in its situation and runs to the left in front of the descending aorta. Because of its direction it is not well seen on frontal views. A left anterior oblique (or right posterior oblique) position for the patient brings the left pulmonary artery more or less into a line parallel with the film and it can be seen filled in Fig. 4.4.

Fig. 4.2 is an early radiograph in an angiocardiographic series. Opacified blood is seen filling the right subclavian vein which unites with the right internal jugular vein (this has some contrast agent in it here) to form the right innominate vein. The right innominate vein joins with the left innominate vein at the level of the right first costal cartilage to form the superior vena cava; in this radiograph the left innominate vein is not seen filled but a curve on the edge of the column of contrast agent indicates the junction of this vein with its opposite member on the right.

The right atrium is well filled with contrast agent and thus the whole of one side and part of the bottom of the U shape of the normal right heart shows at this time in the sequence. Towards the patient's left side at the bottom of the U, the contrast agent is present in less amount and this part of the curve and the second arm of the U, together with the bar that closes it, do not show so clearly.

Fig. 4.2 shows the trachea outlined by its own natural contrast agent which is air and here it can be followed down to the point of bifurcation. From this point the left main bronchus is discernible going out to the patient's left. Its dark outline is seen superimposed on the white radiopacity of the pulmonary trunk which is in front of it within the thorax.

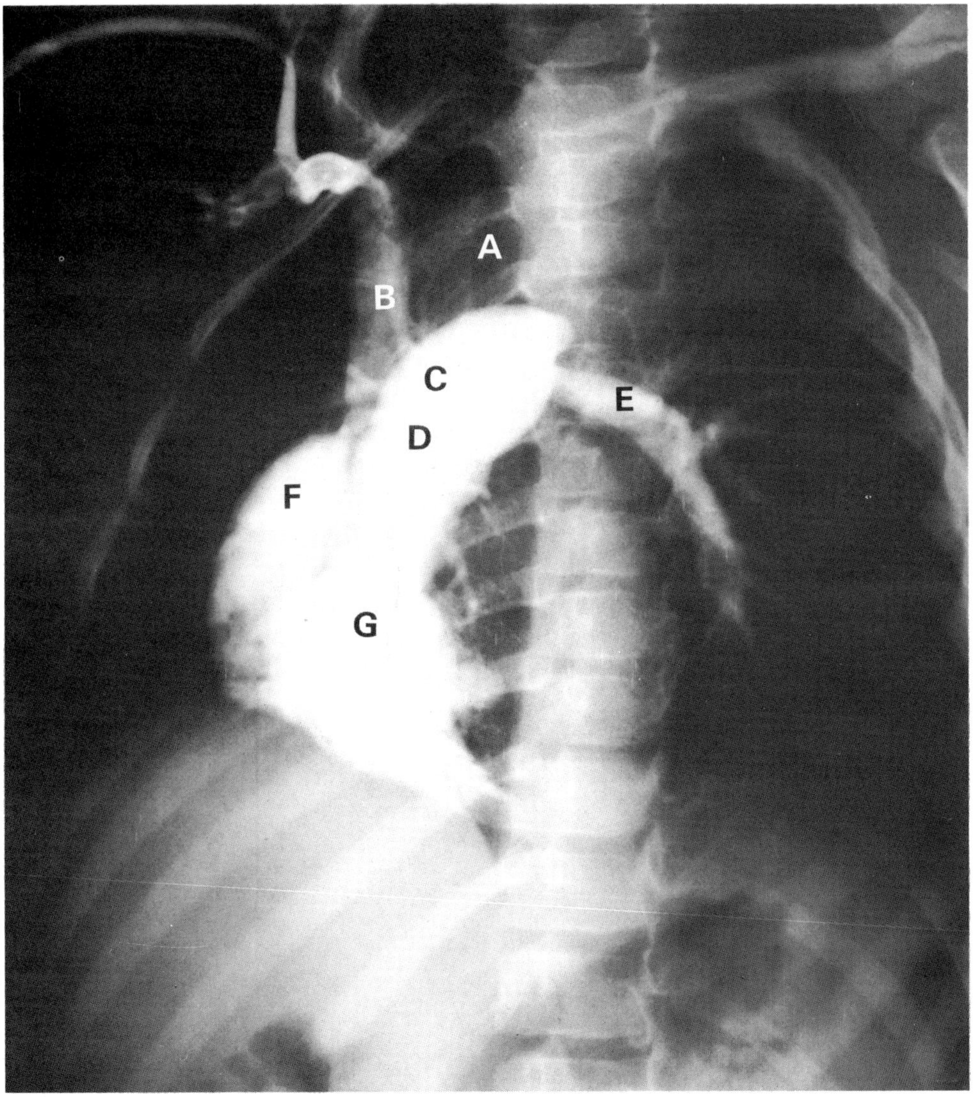

Fig. 4.4. Angiocardiogram showing the normal right heart and vessels in an oblique projection.

A Air-filled trachea
B Superior vena cava
C Right pulmonary artery within the opacity of the pulmonary trunk
D Pulmonary trunk
E Left pulmonary artery
F Right atrium
G Right ventricle

Fig. 4.3 is a radiograph which shows the state of affairs just a little later. The right subclavian vein, the right innominate vein and the superior vena cava now have less contrast agent in them. The opacified blood has moved further on its way and now the right ventricle and the pulmonary trunk are filled. Thus we see the other half of the U completed.

From the top of that arm of the U which is on the patient's left and in Fig. 4.3 shows well filled, the right pulmonary artery is seen running horizontally towards the right lung; it forms the bar across the top of the U which has been mentioned.

Where the outlines of the right pulmonary artery and the superior vena cava are superimposed in the radiograph (in the thorax the artery is behind the vein) the right pulmonary artery is shown dividing into two parts. The upper branch and its ramifications go to the upper lobe of the right lung. The lower and larger branch and its ramifications go to the middle and lower lobes of the right lung.

In this frontal view the left pulmonary artery does not show well but knowledge of anatomy tells us that it is there, going towards the patient's left lung from the pulmonary trunk (at the top of the patient's left side of the U). The left pulmonary artery divides into two branches, one for the upper lobe and one for the lower lobe of the lung. In the radiograph shown in Fig. 4.3 the arteries can be seen ramifying in the tissues of the lung.

Fig. 4.4 is a left anterior oblique (or the equivalent right posterior oblique) projection taken at a stage in the angiocardiographic series which is comparable with that of Fig. 4.3. It was exposed at a time when the superior vena cava is losing the opacified blood and the right heart and the pulmonary arteries are well filled.

This projection places the right heart on the viewer's left hand and the left heart on the viewer's right hand and it brings the left pulmonary artery into a line more or less parallel to the film. In Fig. 4.4 the left heart is not seen because it is not filled with opacified blood; it is present unseen in the space between the right heart and the patient's spine. The position of the patient for the radiograph shown in Fig. 4.4 is only slightly oblique and this accounts for the heart shadow's appearance so close to the spine. There is a good demonstration of the left pulmonary artery running out and down from the pulmonary trunk across the image of the spine and dividing into its main branches in the left lung.

The right pulmonary artery because of its direction is not well seen in this view. It lies within the radiopacity of the pulmonary trunk and thus is undifferentiated, although its branches can be seen ramifying in the lung tissue.

THE LEFT HEART AND ITS VESSELS

The next stage in the angiocardiographic sequence with which we are concerned is the appearances on radiographs when some opacified blood returns from the lungs to the heart. From the pulmonary veins, blood enters the left atrium and thence passes to the left ventricle, from which it is driven out along the aorta to the general systemic circulation.

Fig. 4.5 is a diagrammatic presentation in which the shaded areas indicate the opacified left heart and its vessels as

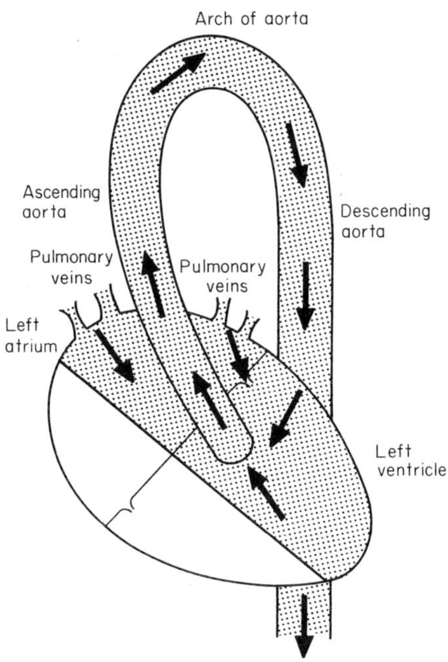

Fig. 4.5. Diagram of the filled left heart and aorta during angiocardiography.

they might be seen from the front. Shown opacified are the following: some pulmonary veins; the left atrium; the left ventricle; the ascending aorta; the arch of the aorta; the descending aorta. The arrows indicate the direction of blood flow.

Searching for a simple description of what it looks like, one finds that the left heart is not as indicative as the right: filled with radiopaque blood, the radiographic shape it produces does not instantly suggest anything to which it may be likened. Perhaps it could be said to look (if you have an active enough imagination) somewhat like a fish diving transversely downwards and towards the patient's left, with the nose of the fish (the left ventricle) resting on the diaphragm and the extension to the tail curving up and towards the patient's left. The tail-end of the body of the fish is the left atrium and the tail itself is the ascending aorta arising from the left ventricle and sweeping upwards.

Comparison of Fig. 4.5 with Fig. 4.1 indicates that in a frontal view the filled left atrium appears in the upper part of the space between the arms of the right-heart U; and that the filled left ventricle appears lower in this space and extends beyond it. Only in abnormal states are the right and the left sides of the heart shown filled together.

Fig. 4.6 is a radiograph exposed in an angiographic series at a time when the blood has returned to the left heart from the lungs. It is a frontal projection, either anteroposterior or posteroanterior. In the hilar regions of both lungs, on each side of the filled left atrium, the pulmonary veins can be seen with some opacified blood within them. The left atrium and the left ventricle are filled, the white shape of the left ventricle merging in the radiograph with the arc of the diaphragm on the patient's left.

At the top, the ascending aorta is seen emerging from the cardiac outline and curving up just to the left of the midline. As it emerges, the direction is towards the patient's right but thereafter the curving course of the ascending aorta carries it towards the patient's left.

The arch of the aorta can be discerned and is marked in Fig. 4.6. Just above the letter B which is used to identify the arch of the aorta, the first branch of the arch can be glimpsed

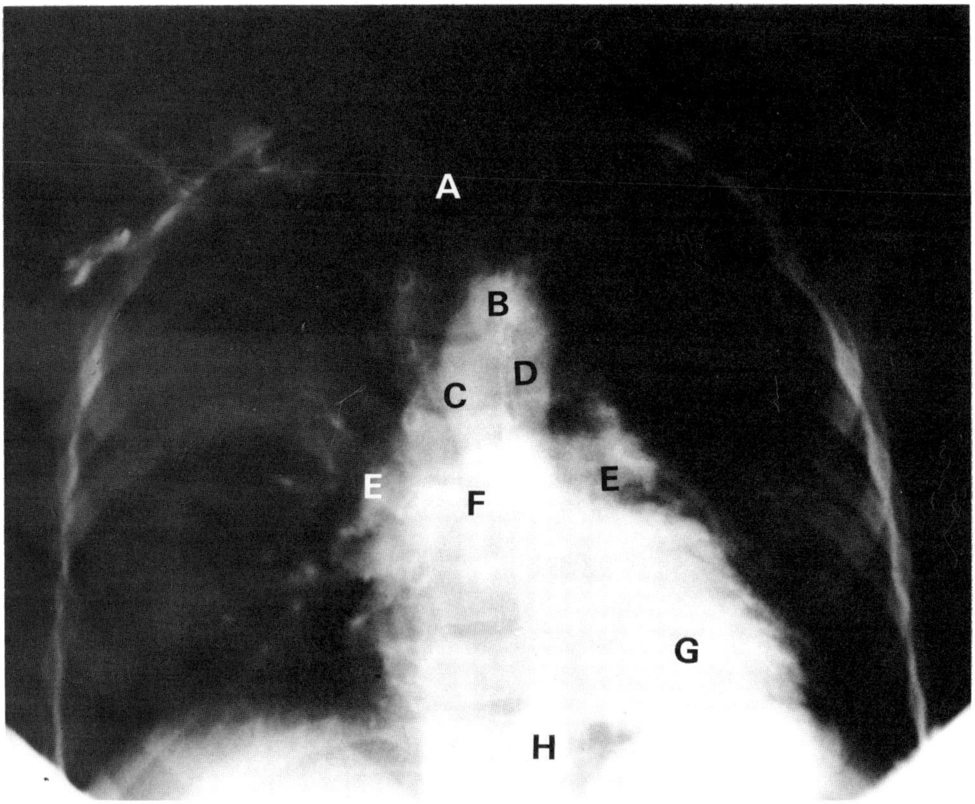

Fig. 4.6. Angiocardiogram of the normal left heart (frontal projection).

A	Air-filled trachea	E	Pulmonary veins
B	Arch of aorta	F	Left atrium
C	Ascending aorta	G	Left ventricle
D	Descending aorta	H	Aorta

curving up towards the patient's right. This is the innominate artery and it ends anatomically behind the right sterno-clavicular joint by dividing into the right common carotid artery and the right subclavian artery. In the radiograph of Fig. 4.6 the innominate artery is not very well filled. It disappears from sight just to the patient's right of the letter A, which has been used over the second thoracic vertebra to identify the trachea.

The arch of the aorta has two further branches arising to the left of the innominate artery. These are the left common carotid artery (which is the second branch of the arch) passing up on the left of the trachea to the base of the neck; and the left subclavian artery (the third branch of the arch) which arises behind the left common carotid artery and goes up to the root of the neck and then laterally to supply the left upper limb. In Fig. 4.6 to the patient's left of the letter B marking the arch of the aorta, there is a glimpse of two vessels which are just filled and partially superimposed. These are the left common carotid and the left subclavian arteries, completing the branches of the arch of the aorta.

From the arch, the descending aorta which is continuous with it can be seen in Fig. 4.6. It goes down through the thorax to the left of the midline and on the left edges of the shadows of the vertebral bodies. The aorta can just be discerned in this radiograph behind the shadow of the left heart filled with contrast agent.

Fig. 4.7 is a radiograph taken with the patient turned slightly oblique from the frontal position to give a left anterior oblique or right posterior oblique projection. As has been noted previously this view puts the left heart towards the spine on the viewer's right and the right heart towards the sternum on the viewer's left. In Fig. 4.7 the left heart is filled. It overshadows, and is not separated from, the spine because the degree of obliquity of the subject is very slight; he is *just* turned from the frontal position.

The left atrium above and the left ventricle below can be seen, together with the ascending aorta passing up from the heart. In this projection of the subject the arch of the aorta is opened up to the viewer, which is in contrast to the frontal view shown in Fig. 4.6. The arch is well demonstrated in Fig. 4.7, curving from before backwards and then downwards, and becoming thereafter the descending aorta as it goes through the thorax.

The three branches of the arch of the aorta are filled and demonstrated. The innominate artery which is the first can be seen in this radiograph to divide into the right common carotid artery ascending into the neck and the right subclavian artery running out across the shadows of the inner end of the right clavicle and the scapula.

Moving to the patient's left and the viewer's right in the radiograph, we see next the second branch of the arch of the

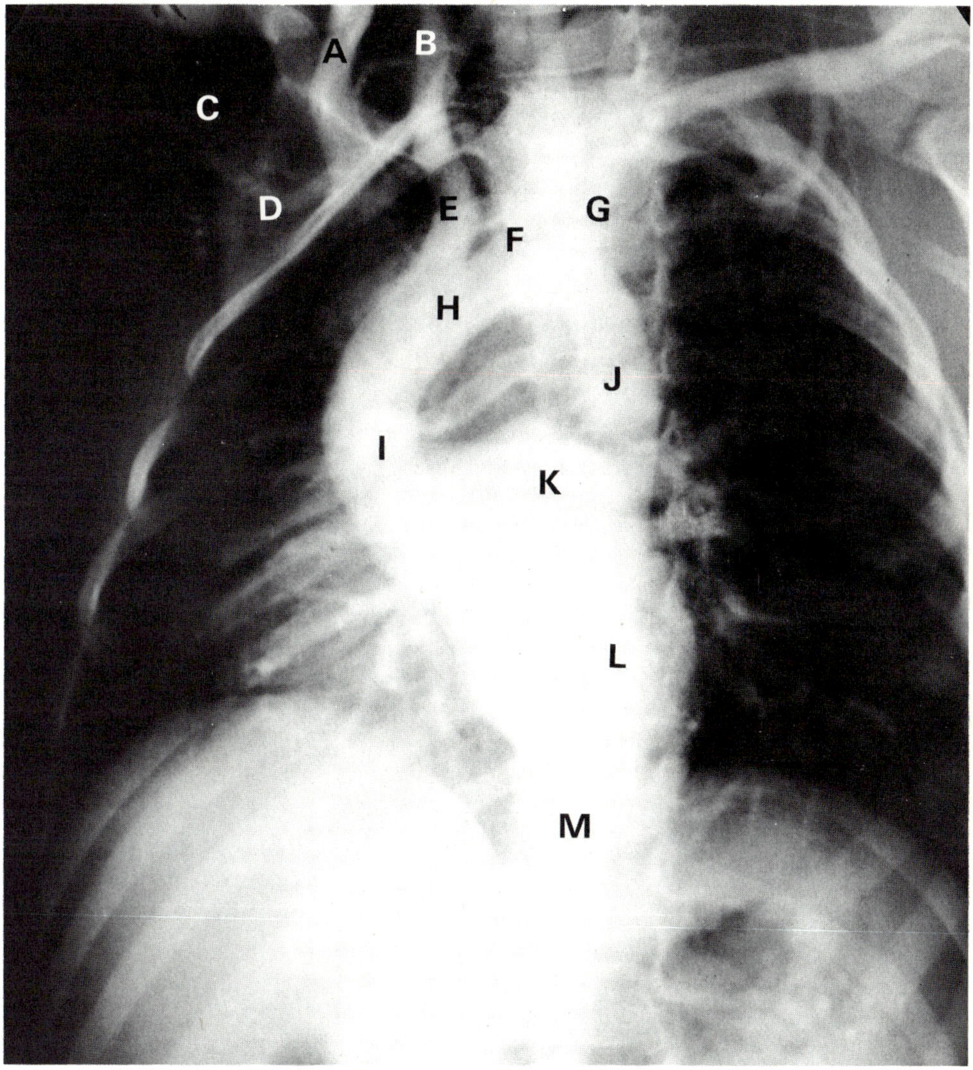

Fig. 4.7. Angiocardiogram of the normal left heart in an oblique projection.

A Right clavicle
B Right common carotid artery
C Right scapula
D Right subclavian artery
E Innominate artery
F Left common carotid artery
G Left subclavian artery
H Arch of aorta
I Ascending aorta
J Descending aorta
K Left atrium
L Left ventricle
M Descending aorta

aorta, the left common carotid artery ascending the neck, and then the third branch of the arch. This is the left subclavian artery running out towards the left clavicle.

Beyond the arch, the descending aorta which is continuous with it is seen superimposed on the shadows of the thoracic vertebrae as it goes down through the thorax. The anatomical course of the aorta takes it down behind the heart and in front of the spine, somewhat to the left of the midline. Because the subject in Fig. 4.7 has been turned from a position which was frontal to one which is of only shallow obliquity, the descending aorta has the shadow of the filled left heart superimposed upon it; further obliquity in the subject separates from each other the radiographic shadows of the spine, the descending aorta and the heart. The most separation of the three structures is obtained when the patient is turned so far from the frontal position as to be lateral to the film; a lateral view of these structures is shown in Fig. 4.8 and is discussed below.

In Fig. 4.7, below the heart the aorta may be just discerned through the superimposed spinal shadows as, having passed through the diaphragm, it continues its course as the abdominal aorta.

The lateral projection in Fig. 4.8 is one of an angiocardiographic series at a stage comparable with that shown in Fig. 4.7. The left heart is filled with opacified blood, as is the thoracic aorta. It can be seen that this position of the subject results in separation of the radiographic shadows of the spine, the aorta and the heart.

The ascending aorta, the arch of the aorta and the descending aorta form a shadow shaped like a shepherd's crook, the tip of the crook being lodged in the left ventricle where the aorta arises. Beneath the curve of the crook, filling the open end of the inverted U which it makes, is the shadow of the left atrium outlined by its content of opacified blood. Just above this are shadows made by the pulmonary veins which are carrying blood and contrast agent back to the left atrium on the return journey from the lungs. Some traces of contrast agent in the vessels of the lungs make their striated pattern visible in the lung fields as background to the cardiac and aortic outlines.

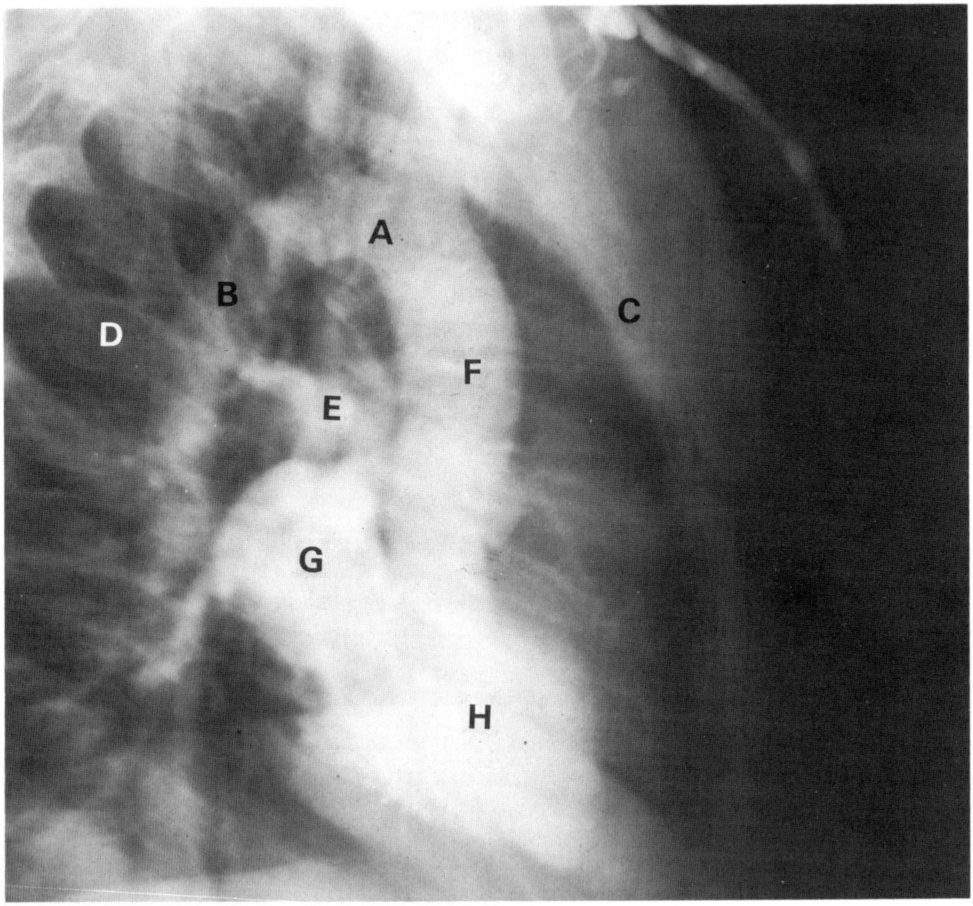

Fig. 4.8. Angiocardiogram of the normal left heart and aorta in a lateral view.

A Arch of aorta
B Descending aorta
C Sternum
D Body of thoracic vertebra
E Pulmonary veins
F Ascending aorta
G Left atrium
H Left ventricle

Bronchographic appearances

Bronchography is the radiographic examination of the bronchial tree with the aid of a positive contrast agent (that is, one producing white shadows) to outline the structures concerned. By this examination abnormal dilatations and narrowings of the bronchi can be revealed. We deal here with

the anatomical appearances shown in normal bronchograms and the projections considered are as follows:
(i) a frontal projection (anteroposterior or posteroanterior);
(ii) oblique projections;
(iii) a lateral projection.

THE FRONTAL RADIOGRAPH

Fig. 4.9 shows a bronchogram undertaken on a child. The projection is either anteroposterior or posteroanterior, giving a frontal view of the thorax. The bronchi in both the right and the left lungs have been filled with contrast agent and are well displayed.

Running down from the top edge of the radiograph is seen a white shadow, superimposed more or less in the midline over the shadows of the lower cervical and upper five thoracic vertebrae. This white shadow is produced by the trachea filled with contrast agent: the small narrowed part above the sixth cervical vertebra is in fact the larynx but all the rest of the white band from the sixth cervical vertebra to the point of division at the fifth thoracic vertebra is the trachea.

It can be seen that what the anatomists tell us of the course of the trachea is at least in this case true. The part in the neck is in the midline but within the thorax the trachea is slightly to the right, being displaced in that direction by the arch of the aorta.

At the level of the fifth thoracic vertebra the trachea divides into the right and the left main bronchi, which each enter the appropriate lung; the right main bronchus enters at the level of the fifth thoracic vertebra while on the left side the main bronchus enters its lung at the lower level of the sixth thoracic vertebra. Again the radiograph demonstrates anatomical facts and it can be seen that the right main bronchus in comparison with the left is shorter and wider and is inclined at an angle nearer to the vertical. The more horizontal left main bronchus is about twice as long as its fellow on the right. The more vertical angle of inclination of the right main bronchus makes an inhaled foreign body which passes down the trachea more likely to continue down the right side and enter the right lung than to turn off towards the left.

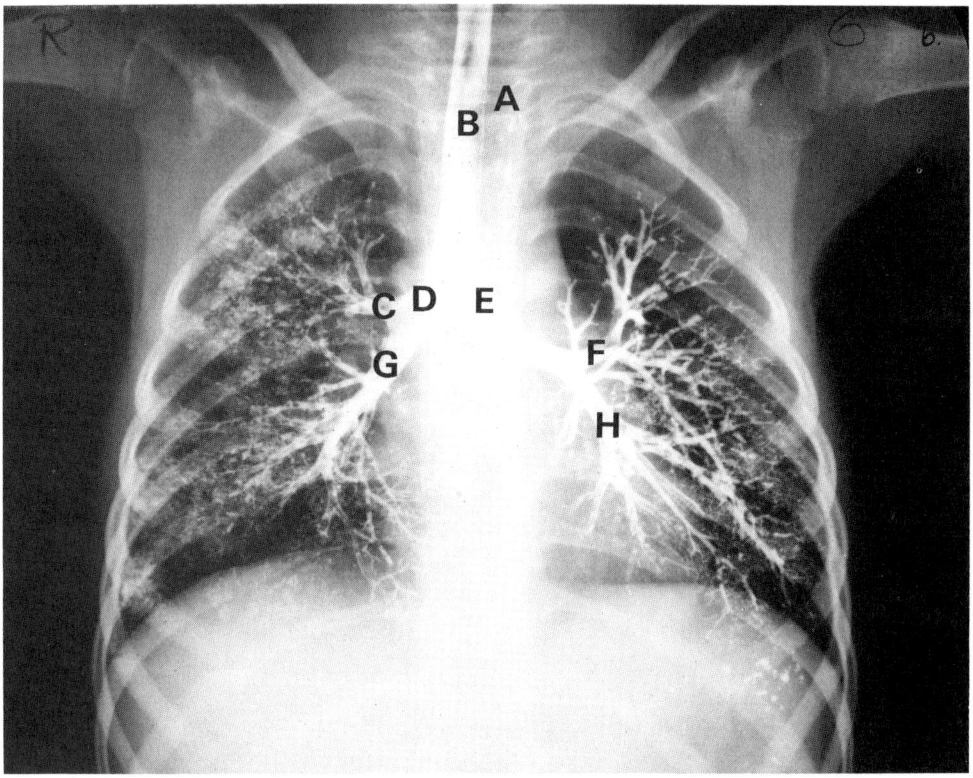

Fig. 4.9. A frontal projection of a bronchogram undertaken on a child.

A Thoracic vertebra I
B Trachea
C Eparterial bronchus
D Right main bronchus
E Left main bronchus
F Bronchus to the upper lobe of the left lung
G Hyparterial bronchus
H Bronchus to lower lobe of the left lung

On the right side at the level of the fifth thoracic vertebra, the right main bronchus shows its first division in the lung. This bronchus is for the upper lobe of the lung and it is called the eparterial bronchus because it arises above the right pulmonary artery. The eparterial bronchus is seen to run laterally for a short distance and then to divide into smaller branches in the upper zone of the right lung field.

Below the right pulmonary artery the continuation of the right main bronchus is known as the hyparterial bronchus. It is seen in the radiograph to run downwards and laterally and soon to divide into a multiplicity of branches. These branches

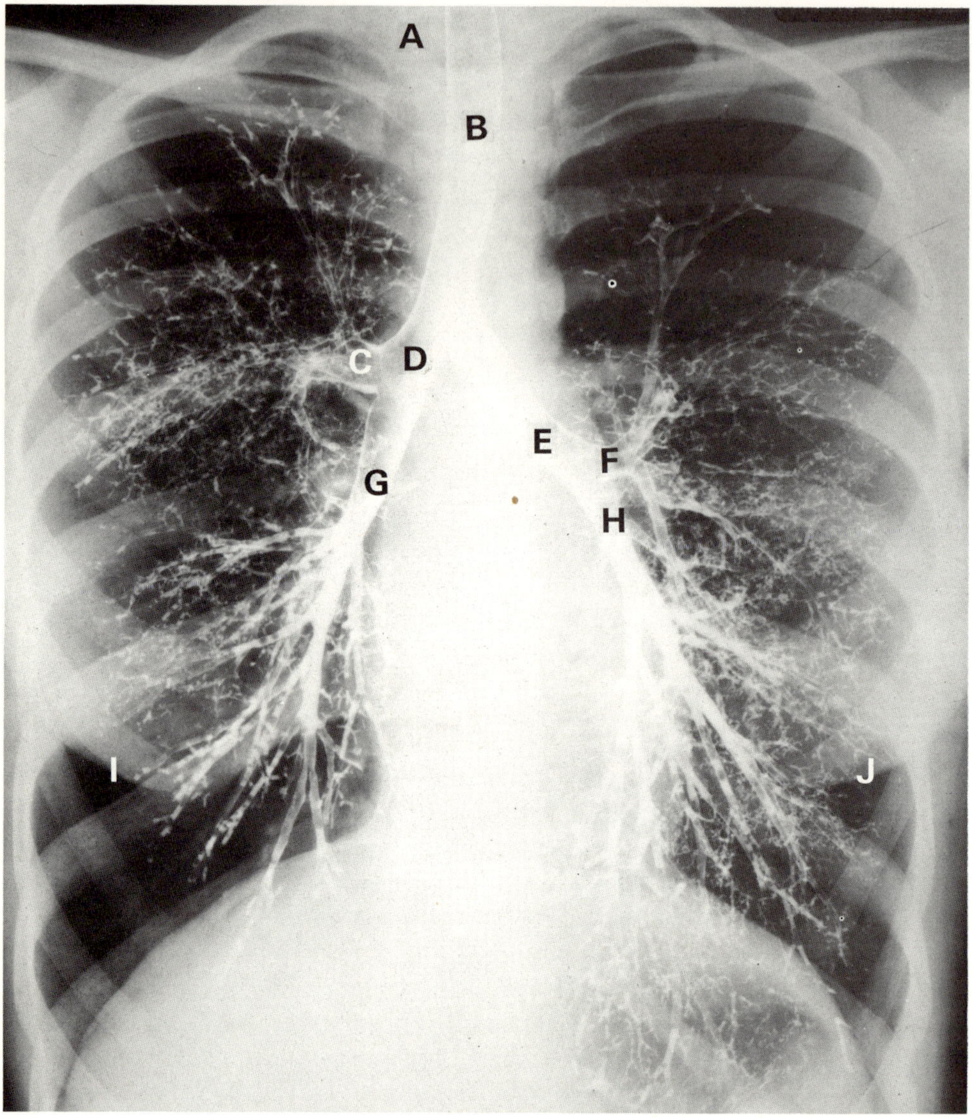

Fig. 4.10. A frontal projection of a bronchogram undertaken on an adult.

A Thoracic vertebra 1
B Trachea
C Eparterial bronchus
D Right main bronchus
E Left main bronchus
F Bronchus to left upper lobe
G Hyparterial bronchus
H Bronchus to left lower lobe
I Right breast shadow
J Left breast shadow

are to various parts of the middle and lower lobes of the right lung.

On the left, the main bronchus runs laterally for a few centimetres and then gives off a large branch which divides into two smaller bronchi. Thereafter these two smaller bronchi give rise to smaller and smaller divisions. This first large branch of the main bronchus and its subsequent divisions are for the upper lobe of the left lung.

The shadow of the left main bronchus continues downwards and laterally on the radiograph and then divides into smaller branches: these ramify into smaller vessels for the lower lobe of the left lung.

Fig. 4.10 is a radiograph comparable with the one shown in Fig. 4.9, the subject in this case being an adult female. The radiographic anatomy of the bronchial tree which is shown is similar in both radiographs.

LEFT ANTERIOR OBLIQUE PROJECTION

Fig. 4.11 is a radiograph taken with the patient in the left anterior oblique (or the equivalent right posterior oblique) position. The trachea and the bronchi of both lungs are filled with contrast agent. This projection results in radiographic appearances as follows:
(i) the patient's spine is to the right hand of the viewer and the patient's sternum is to the left hand of the viewer;
(ii) the patient's left side of her thorax is closed up for the viewer, with the shadows of the vertebral bodies falling across it, while the right side of the thorax is opened up;
(iii) the filled bronchi in the right lung are displayed clear of the spine, while those of the left lung are superimposed over the shadows of the thoracic vertebrae.

When both sides have been filled with contrast agent a lateral projection is of limited value because the two sides are superimposed and in this case an oblique projection must be used instead. The left anterior oblique (or right posterior oblique) is chosen to display the bronchi of the right side.

In Fig. 4.11 the filled trachea is seen as a prominent white band running down from the thoracic inlet at the top of the radiograph. The band passes across the shadow of the inner

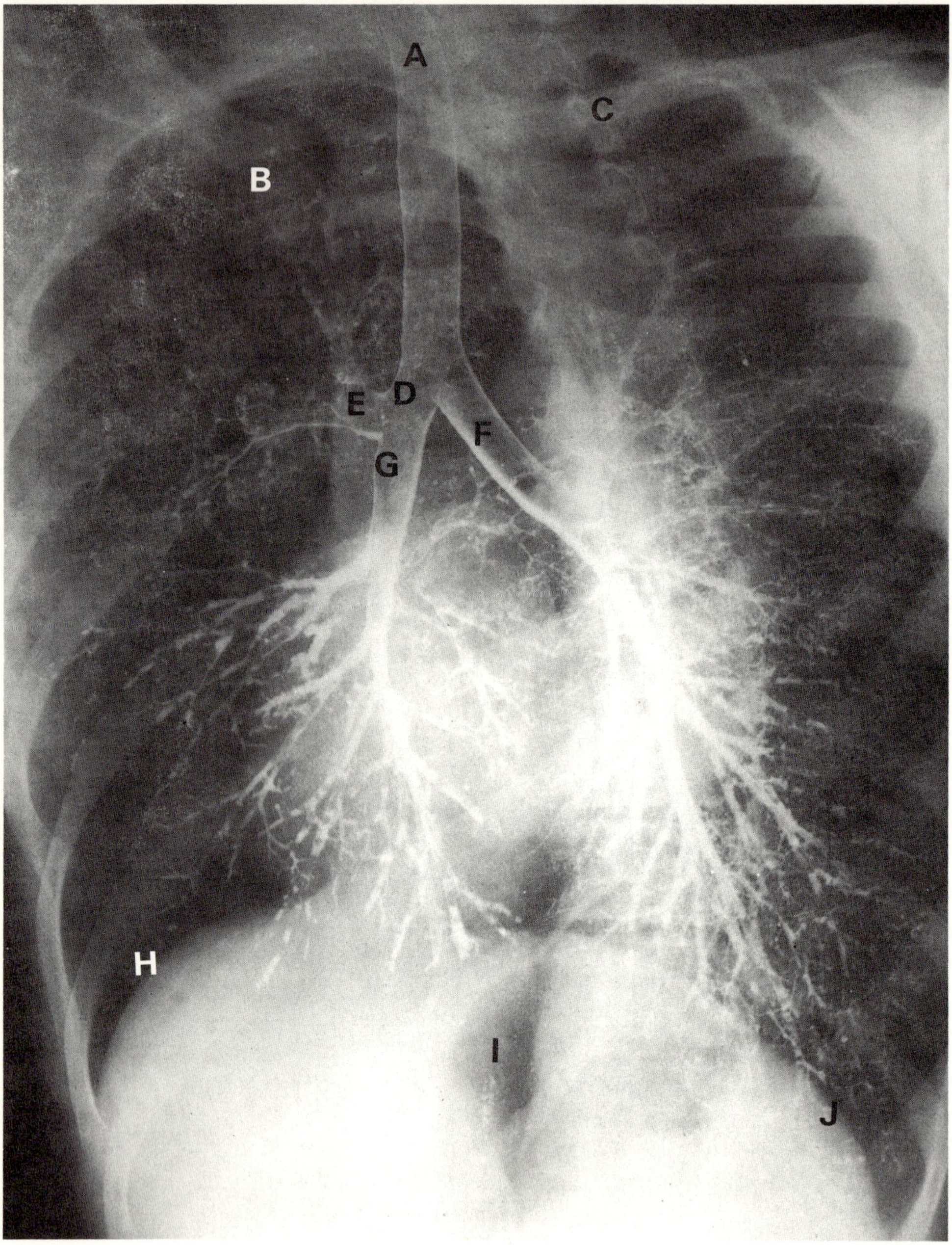

Fig. 4.11. Left anterior oblique projection of a bronchogram undertaken on an adult.

A Trachea
B Right sternoclavicular joint
C Left clavicle
D Right main bronchus
E Eparterial bronchus
F Left main bronchus
G Hyparterial bronchus
H Right arc of diaphragm
I Gas in the fundus of the stomach
J Left arc of diaphragm

end of the patient's left clavicle and goes down through the thorax to the viewer's left of the spine. Further to the viewer's left on the radiograph the inner end of the patient's left clavicle and the sternoclavicular joint can be seen.

Further down the thorax, the white band of the trachea is seen to bifurcate and to form the right and the left main bronchi; this division is placed anatomically at the level of the fifth thoracic vertebra but on the radiograph this vertebra is not separately identifiable. In this projection the right main bronchus is seen as a nearly vertical continuation of the trachea, the shadow running down through the thorax to the viewer's left of the subject's spine. Almost immediately after the bifurcation, the first division within the lung comes off the right main bronchus. This division is the eparterial bronchus branching to supply the upper lobe of the lung. It runs laterally for a short distance and then the shadow splits into many divisions and subdivisions, ramifying in the upper zone of the lung field.

Reverting to the right main bronchus on the radiograph, we can follow its continuation downwards as the hyparterial bronchus. Very soon the shadow of the heart becomes superimposed on it but the bronchial pattern is nevertheless well displayed because the contrast agent used to outline it is more absorptive of X-rays than is the heart muscle itself.

The hyparterial bronchus shows several main branches. These go to supply the middle and lower lobes of the right lung in various sections: the bronchi run anteriorly, posteriorly, out laterally towards the axilla and medially towards the heart. The main branches divide into smaller bronchi within the lung substance.

In Fig. 4.11 at the point of bifurcation of the trachea the left main bronchus is shown well, coming off at an angle to the generally vertical line of the trachea. The white band of this bronchus runs toward the viewer's right on the radiograph and soon reaches the shadows of the vertebral bodies. Partly because of the superimposition of the spine (and of some left breast shadow in this case) and partly because of the directions of some of the divisions, a full display of the bronchial pattern within the left lung is not provided by this projection. It can, however, be seen that there are many divisions and subdivisions within the lung tissue, some to supply the upper lobe and some to supply the lower lobe of the left lung.

In the radiograph the pattern of white lines produced by the contrast agent within the lungs is seen to extend apparently below the diaphragm: both on the right and the left sides of the subject traces show close to the dark area which represents gas in the fundus of the stomach. It is *not* a fact that these bronchial divisions pass through the diaphragm since the lungs are normally entirely contained within the thorax. The radiographic appearance (misleading to the anatomically uninformed) arises because of the limitation mentioned earlier: the projection of the structures by the X-ray beam shows the highest parts of the diaphragm as two arcs with the radiolucent lung fields above and the radiopaque region of the abdomen beneath them. Intrathoracic structures which are in fact above the diaphragm but below its highest parts do not appear above these arcs in certain radiographic projections. This is the situation of these filled bronchi which can be seen straggling below the diaphragmatic curves in Fig. 4.11.

RIGHT ANTERIOR OBLIQUE PROJECTION

Fig. 4.12 is a radiograph taken with the patient in the right anterior oblique (or the equivalent left posterior oblique) position. The trachea and the bronchi in both lungs are filled with contrast agent. This projection results in radiographic appearances which are as follows:

(i) the patient's spine is to the viewer's left hand and the patient's sternum is to the viewer's right;

(ii) the patient's right side of her thorax is closed up for the viewer with the shadow of the vertebral bodies falling across it, while the left side of the thorax is opened up;

(iii) the filled bronchi in the left lung are displayed clear of the spine while those of the right lung are superimposed over the shadows of the thoracic vertebrae. When both sides have been filled with contrast agent, the oblique projections of choice to display the bronchi of the left side are the right anterior and its equivalent left posterior oblique.

In Fig. 4.12 the filled trachea shows as a light band, first seen at the top of the radiograph in the thoracic inlet. It goes

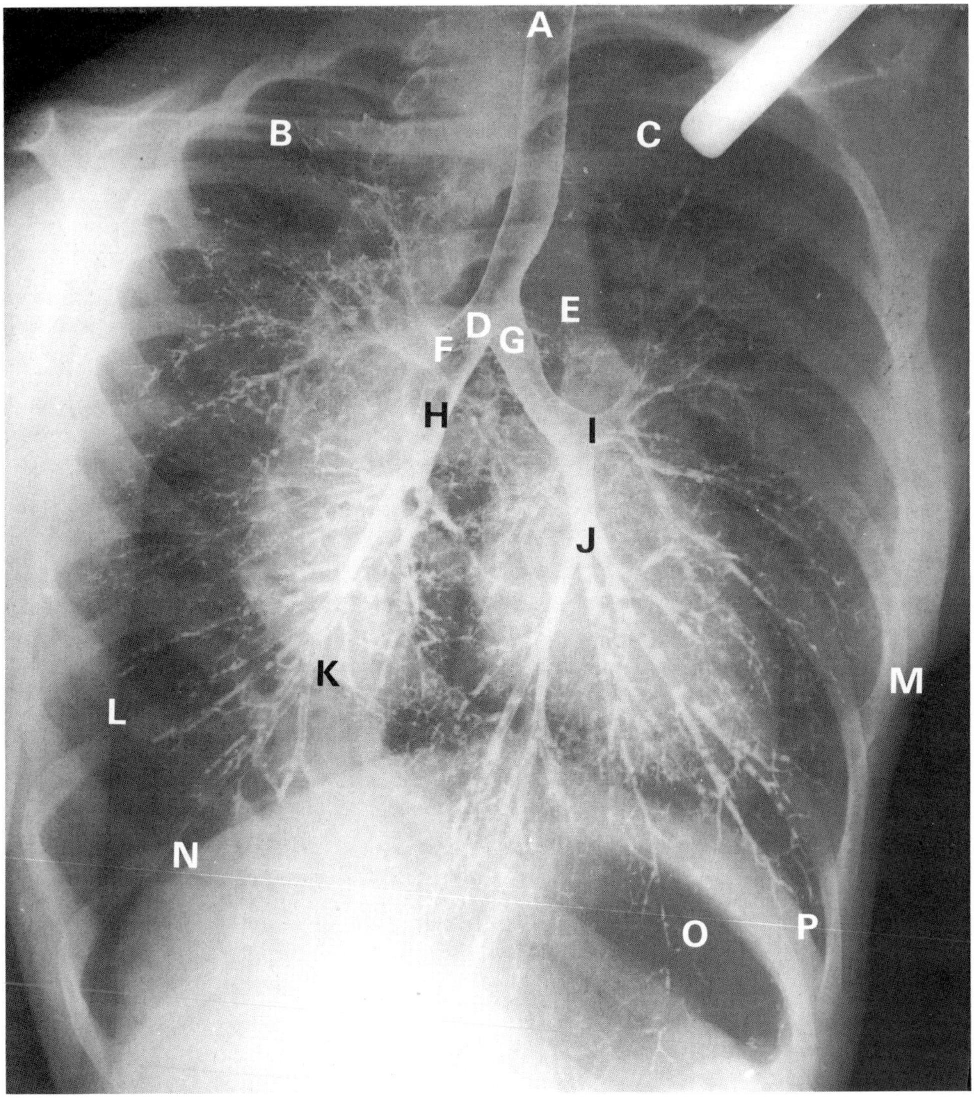

Fig. 4.12. Right anterior oblique projection of a bronchogram undertaken on an adult.

A Trachea
B Right clavicle
C Left sternoclavicular joint
D Right main bronchus
E Ascending aorta
F Eparterial bronchus
G Left main bronchus
H Hyparterial bronchus
I Division to supply upper lobe of left lung
J Division to supply lower lobe of left lung
K Right breast shadow
L Shadow of the soft tissues of the right arm
M Left breast shadow
N Right arc of diaphragm
O Gas in the fundus of the stomach
P Left arc of diaphragm

down into the thorax, passing close to the inner end of the subject's right clavicle. The subject's spine appears to the viewer's left of the trachea and to the viewer's right of the trachea the subject's left sternoclavicular joint can be discerned.

Somewhat lower down, just above the bifurcation of the trachea, a greyish soft-tissue shadow shows superimposed on the trachea and extending to the viewer's right of it: this shadow is formed by the ascending aorta. The line of its edge can be followed down and seen to merge with the anterior outline of the heart shadow.

From the bifurcation of the trachea, the left main bronchus goes out towards the viewer's right on the radiograph across the shadow of the aorta which has been noted. Anatomically it is closely related to the aorta, passing below the arch on its way to the left lung. In Fig. 4.12 most of the divisions and subdivisions of the bronchi in the left lung are seen with the cardiac shadow superimposed upon them. Nevertheless they are well displayed because the contrast agent used is more absorptive of X-rays than is the heart muscle itself.

The first division of the left main bronchus extends laterally in the radiograph, running towards the patient's left axilla for a very short distance before branching into what appear to be three smaller divisions. These smaller bronchi ramify within the lung tissue to supply the upper lobe of the left lung.

The left main bronchus, having put out its first main division, can be followed down through the thorax for a short distance; it shows as a nearly vertical white band superimposed on the heart shadow. Shortly it ends by dividing into three main branches. These are to supply anterior, axillary and posterior regions of the base of the left lung. In the radiograph their ramifications can be seen towards the basal region of the lung field.

From the point of bifurcation of the trachea, the right main bronchus can be followed in Fig. 4.12 as a continuation downwards of the white band of the trachea. On the radiograph it runs towards the viewer's left: it is clear of the heart shadow and goes towards the shadow of the spine. The eparterial bronchus supplying the upper lobe of the lung can be seen as a branch coming off the right main bronchus. The downwards continuation of the main bronchus as the hyparterial bronchus is visualised, together with the ramifying vessels within the middle and lower lobes of the right lung. The hyparterial bronchus and its main divisions become in this projection superimposed upon the spine and in this case also upon the shadow of the patient's right breast.

We noted before (p. 94) the falsely apparent descent of some bronchi to the region below the diaphragm. This feature is seen here in Fig. 4.12 as well as in Fig. 4.11.

RIGHT LATERAL PROJECTION

Bronchograms are usually undertaken bi-laterally, one side being filled first with contrast agent to be followed by the filling of the other. A common technique used to display the middle lobe of the right lung most advantageously is to fill the right side first and while that is the only side filled to take a right lateral radiograph in addition to the frontal and oblique views. The side to side superimposition of the two lung fields in the lateral view does not matter because the bronchi of the left lung are not filled with contrast agent and hence are not displayed on the radiograph. Once both sides are filled the lateral view is of little or no value and oblique projections replace it.

Fig. 4.13 is a lateral projection of a bronchogram carried out on a child. The radiograph shows only the right side filled. Some prominent bony landmarks noted before are seen, the spine being on the viewer's left and the sternum to the viewer's right. The ribs form fairly prominent shadows, superimposed from side to side and slanting across the lung fields from a higher level posteriorly to a lower level anteriorly. Below, the diaphragm closes the thoracic outlet and shows as a shallow arc outlining a lower boundary for the thorax. Its span extends from the back of the anterior chest wall (in the radiograph from just above the shadow of the anterior ends of the sixth ribs) to the thoracic vertebrae posteriorly. In the radiograph the arc skirts across the top of the body of the tenth thoracic vertebra and loses itself at a slightly lower level posteriorly in the shadows of the pedicle and the laminae.

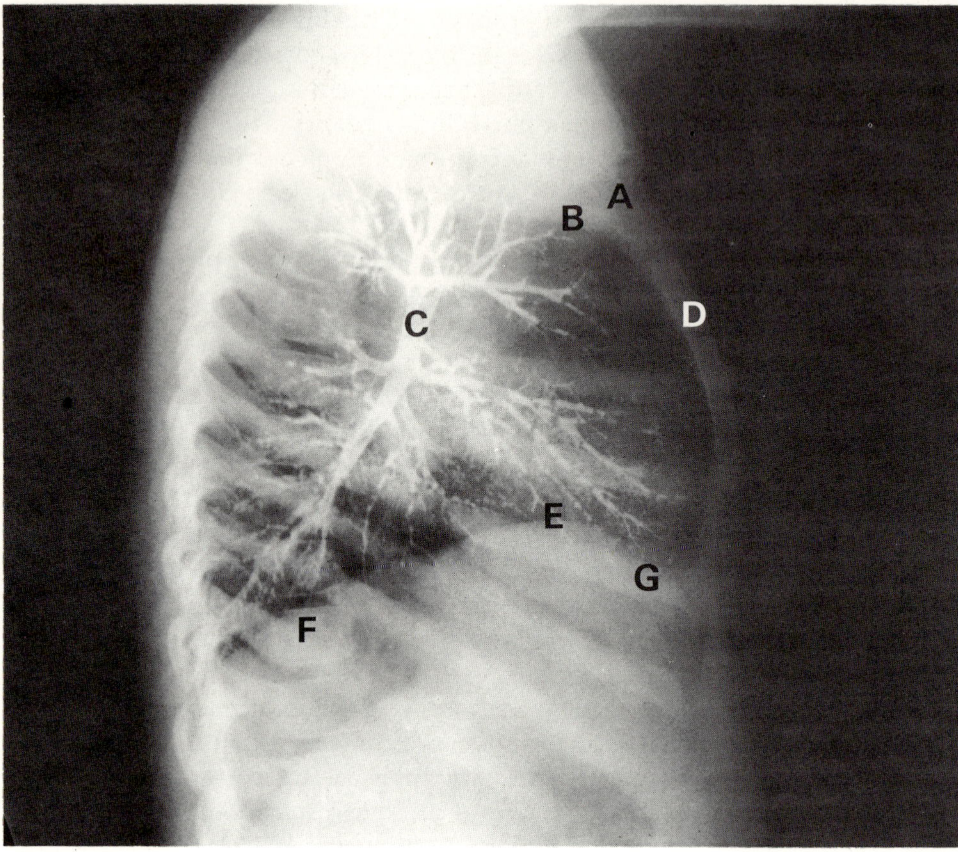

Fig. 4.13. A lateral projection showing the right side filled in a bronchogram undertaken on a child.

A	Manubrium sterni	E	Diaphragm
B	Right and left ribs 2	F	Thoracic vertebra 10
C	Hyparterial bronchus	G	Right and left ribs 6
D	Body of sternum		

The filled bronchial tree is seen from a lateral aspect superimposed over bony shadows and the air-containing lungs. The hyparterial bronchus shows as a white band to the viewer's right of the vertebral bodies. Above are the divisions and subdivisions which derive from the first branch of the main bronchus and supply the upper lobe of the right lung. Shown at the levels of the lower border of the fifth thoracic vertebra and the upper border of the sixth are the divisions of the hyparterial bronchus which supply the middle lobe of the right lung. Below are the divisions which go to the lower lobe of the right lung.

All these ramifications can be seen extending through the lung tissue both anteriorly and posteriorly. Some run in another direction, laterally or medially, but the line of view in a lateral projection is not such as to display these clearly in their full extent.

THE OESOPHAGUS OUTLINED WITH BARIUM SULPHATE

The normal thoracic oesophagus with no contrast agent in it is unseen on radiographs of the region. Its tissues are not sufficiently absorptive of X-rays to cast a discernible shadow and it is not a structure which contains air (as the trachea does) to outline its lumen as a dark radioparent band. Unless food, drink or any other substances which may be swallowed are passing down it, the oesophagus in fact contains nothing: its front and back walls are in contact with each other and the space within it is potential rather than actual.

If the material filling it is radiopaque, the oesophagus appears as a white shadow and it can be seen clearly in the thorax on radiographs taken of this region. Barium sulphate is a radiographic contrast agent with a high degree of radiopacity and the oesophagus is easily visualised throughout when it is so filled.

The course of the oesophagus down the thorax is through the superior and posterior mediastinum just in front of the spine. Its general direction is vertical but it does not follow a completely straight line. At its point of entry from the neck into the thorax the oesophagus is just to the left of the midline. It follows a slightly curving course which brings it to the midline at the level of the fifth thoracic vertebra. Two vertebrae lower down, the oesophagus begins to curve towards the left again. This causes it to cross the aorta just above the diaphragm. At this point the oesophagus is directed from the midline towards the left while the aorta (descending through the thorax just on the left of the spine) approaches the midline as it goes and when it pierces the diaphragm it is in front of the spine. So the oesophagus is going from the midline towards the left and the aorta is going from the left towards the midline:

they are bound to cross and they do this just before they both separately pass through the diaphragm.

In a frontal projection, the upper part of the thoracic oesophagus when filled with barium sulphate appears as a white shadow superimposed on the greyer shadows of the vertebral bodies and of the vessels occupying the mediastinum. Lower down, the filled oesophagus is superimposed on the cardiac and spinal shadows. At about the level of the tenth thoracic vertebra the oesophagus pierces the diaphragm to enter the abdomen and ends at the cardiac opening of the stomach.

Along its length the oesophagus is constricted and indented in certain places by the closeness of other structures. In its thoracic part there is a constriction where the oesophagus is crossed by the arch of the aorta; there is another about 5 cm lower down where it is crossed by the left main bronchus. For the last part of its length within the thorax the oesophagus is immediately behind the heart and the presence of the left atrium in front indents the anterior oesophageal wall in a long shallow curve.

These indentations which have been mentioned can be seen on radiographs of the thorax when the oesophagus is filled with barium sulphate. A study of the curves and indentations of the filled oesophagus may be helpful in elucidating abnormalities not only of the oesophagus itself but of the structures which produce the indentations. For example, enlargement of the left atrium deepens the curve which it puts on the anterior oesophageal wall. Enlargement or displacement of the aorta can alter the indentations which it makes on the oesophageal outline.

Fig. 4.14 is a frontal projection of the thorax showing the oesophagus filled with barium sulphate and appearing on the radiograph as a white shadow. Its general course down through the thorax is demonstrated, from the thoracic inlet at the top almost to the point where it ends at the cardia of the stomach below the left arc of the diaphragm. The shadow of the oesophagus is superimposed on those of the vertebral bodies, the mediastinal structures and the heart. At the level of the aortic knuckle the indentation which the arch makes in the oesophagus shows prominently. It narrows the band of the

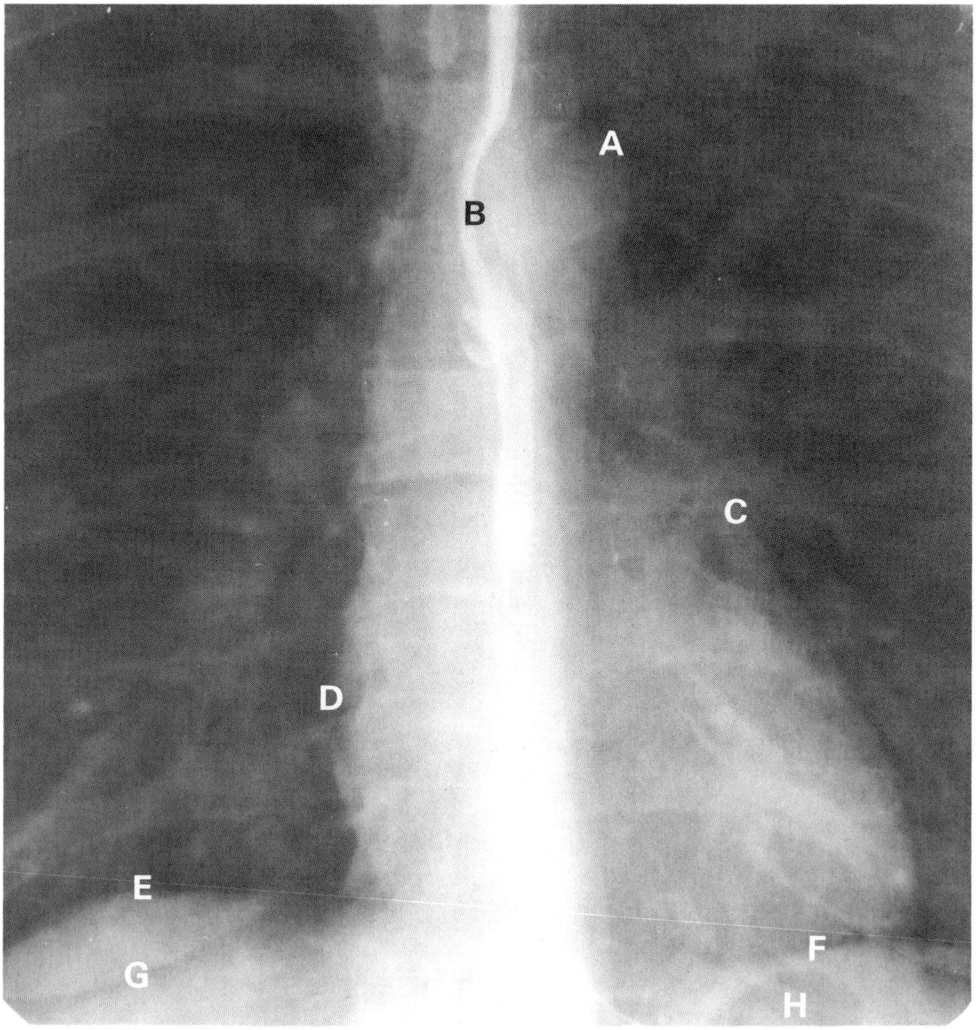

Fig. 4.14. A frontal projection showing the oesophagus outlined with barium sulphate.

A Aortic knuckle
B Indentation produced by the arch of the aorta
C Left margin of the cardiac shadow
D Right margin of the cardiac shadow
E Right arc of diaphragm
F Left arc of diaphragm
G Right breast shadow
H Gas in the fundus of the stomach

oesophageal shadow and puts in it a pronounced curve which is convex to the subject's right. In this particular case there is an abnormality present in the oesophagus. Just below the indentation produced by the arch of the aorta a diverticulum is demonstrated.

Fig. 4.15 is a radiograph of another patient taken as a right anterior oblique projection. Bony landmarks noted earlier are seen: the spine to the viewer's left and the sternum to the viewer's right. The prominent shadow of the oesophagus filled with barium sulphate is seen at the thoracic inlet crossing the shadow of the inner end of the subject's right clavicle. The general course of this white band of the oesophagus is down through the thorax, between the shadows of the thoracic vertebrae on the viewer's left and the shadows of the heart and the great vessels on the viewer's right.

Constrictions which were mentioned earlier show themselves as arcs indented at the edge of the band which is towards the viewer's right. The first starts at the level of the lower border of the fifth rib; this is the indentation produced by the arch of the aorta. The next lower arc is shallower. It begins in the space between sixth and seventh ribs on the radiograph, ends at the lower border of the seventh rib and is caused by the left main bronchus. The third indenting arc is the longest and shallowest. It begins on the radiograph in the space between the eighth and ninth ribs and continues along the remaining extent of the thoracic oesophagus. It is caused by the close application of the oesophagus to the pericardium and the left atrium of the heart.

As it goes down the thorax the shadow of the oesophagus veers further to the viewer's right away from the spine (that is, it is directed anteriorly in the subject's thorax). At its most anterior (in the radiograph in front of the lower edge of the eleventh thoracic vertebra) the oesophagus is seen to cross the right arc of the diaphragm; this is a radiographic superimposition of shadows misleading to the uninformed and it is *not* the point where the diaphragm is pierced. Anatomically the oesophageal opening in the diaphragm at the level of the tenth thoracic vertebra is to the left of the midline, as can be seen in the frontal projection of Fig. 4.14. On the right anterior oblique radiograph shown in Fig. 4.15 the left arc of the dia-

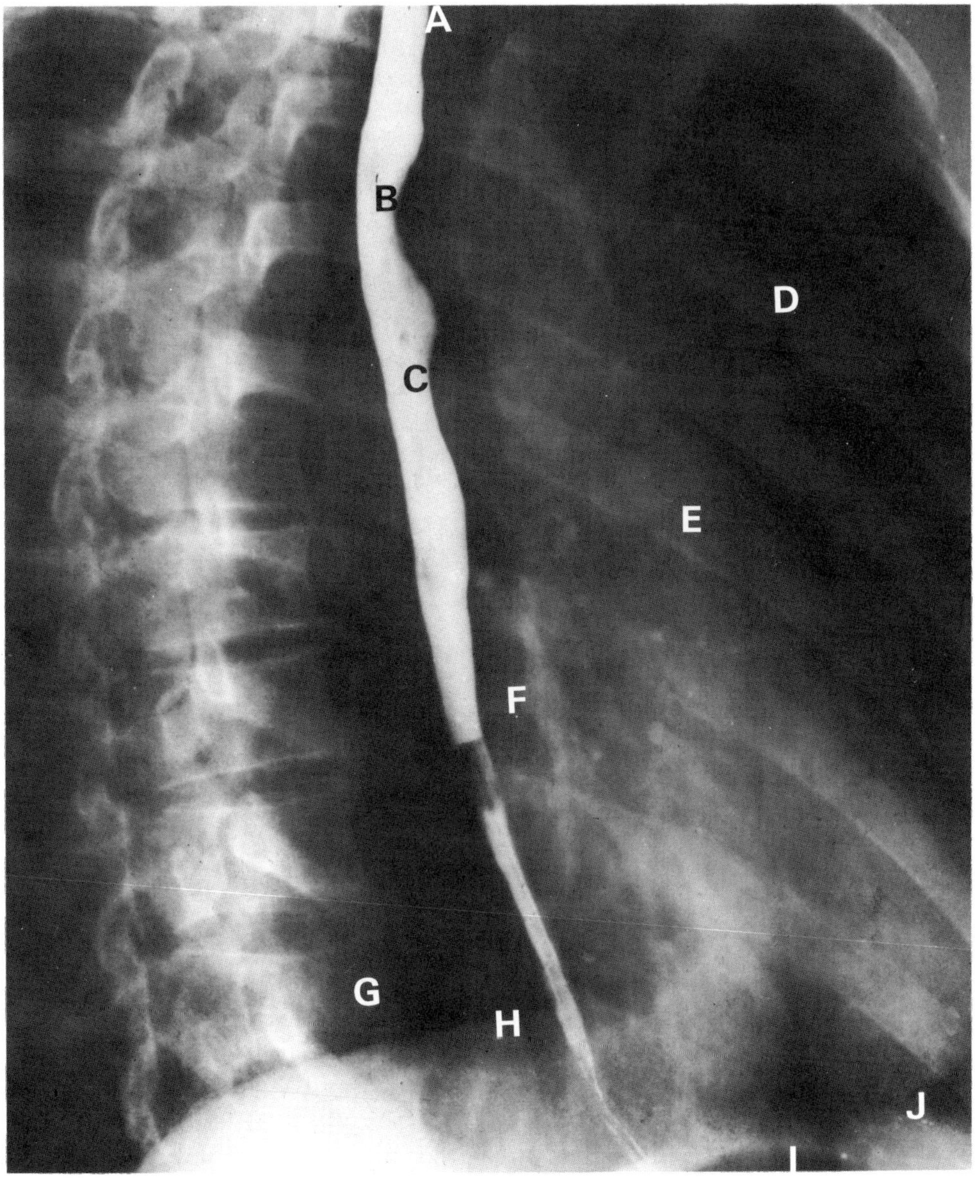

Fig. 4.15. Right anterior oblique projection showing the oesophagus outlined with barium sulphate.

A Inner end of the right clavicle
B Indentation produced by the arch of the aorta
C Indentation produced by the left main bronchus
D Left rib 5
E Left rib 7
F Left atrium
G Thoracic vertebra 11
H Right arc of diaphragm
I Gas in the fundus of the stomach
J Left arc of diaphragm

phragm and gas in the fundus of the stomach are discernible at the lower edge of the illustration. The oesophagus piercing the diaphragm in the left arc can just be seen.

Lymphangiographic appearances

In recent years techniques have been developed for demonstrating radiographically parts of the lymphatic system of the body. Lymphatic structures can be filled with a radiographic contrast agent which makes them visible on radiographs; the procedure is called lymphangiography. Chapter 12 of this book gives some explanation of this and of the lymph system and the structures which comprise it. In the present chapter we concern ourselves with lymphangiographic appearances within the thorax.

The principal lymphatic structure to be shown within the thorax is the thoracic duct. This is the main lymph vessel of the body conveying the chyle and lymph into the blood. It is the common trunk of nearly all the lymph vessels; the exceptions are those of the right side of the head, neck and thoracic wall, the right upper limb, the right lung, the right side of the heart and part of the liver.

The thoracic duct in fact begins just below the diaphragm as a continuation of the cisterna chyli (see Chapter 12, p. 264) near the lower border of the twelfth thoracic vertebra. It enters the thorax through the aortic opening in the diaphragm and then goes up in the posterior mediastinum on the right side of the aorta and behind the oesophagus.

At the level of the fifth thoracic vertebra, the thoracic duct runs towards the left, enters the superior mediastinum and reaches the thoracic inlet on the left of the oesophagus. At this level the duct is behind the left common carotid artery and the left internal jugular vein. It arches laterally and then ends by opening into the venous system at the left subclavian vein, close to the point where the left subclavian vein and the left internal jugular vein unite behind the clavicle to form the left innominate vein.

Just before this point of termination it is usual for the thoracic duct to be joined by two lymphatic trunks opening into it: these are (i) the left subclavian trunk draining lymph from the left arm; and (ii) the left jugular trunk draining lymph from the left side of the head and neck. Sometimes these two trunks may open, not into the thoracic duct, but independently into the venous system.

Fig. 4.16 is a frontal radiograph of the thorax showing the thoracic duct filled with contrast agent. It appears as a very narrow white band on the radiograph, just to be glimpsed at

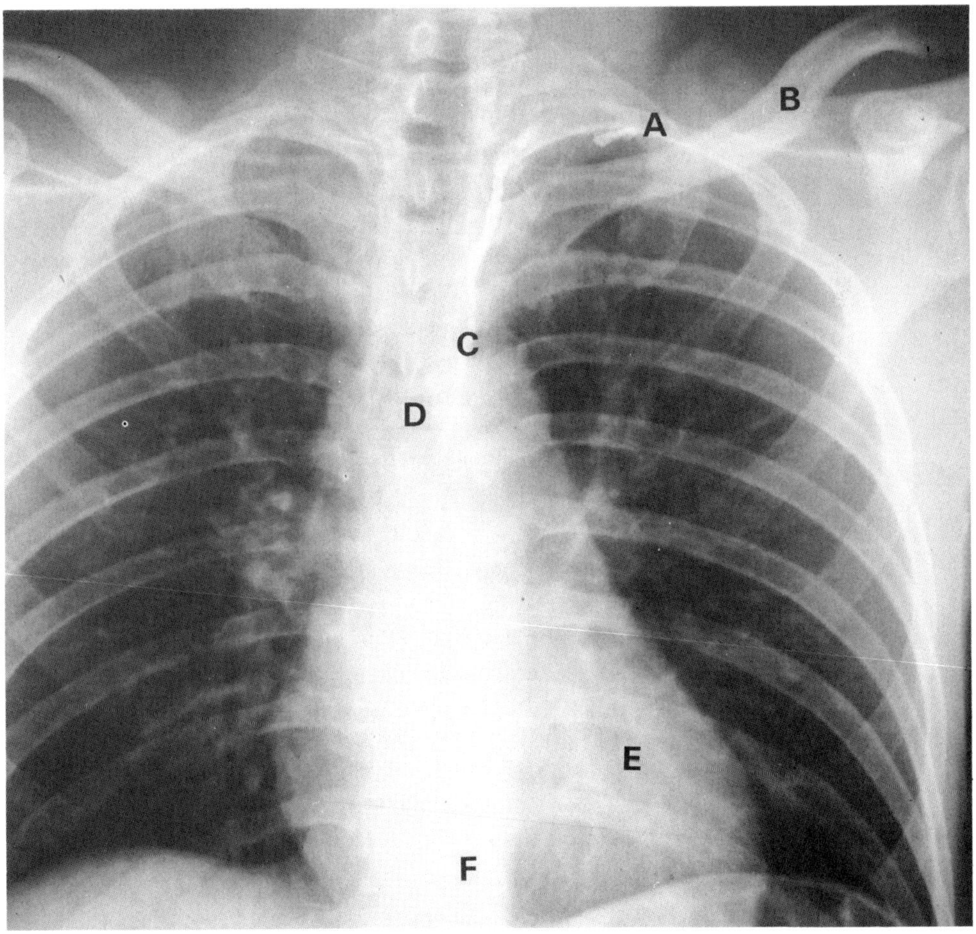

Fig. 4.16. A lymphangiogram showing the thoracic duct in a frontal projection.

A Left rib 2
B Left clavicle
C Thoracic duct
D Thoracic vertebra 5
E Cardiac shadow
F Thoracic vertebra 10

the level of the tenth thoracic vertebra with the mass of the cardiac shadow superimposed. At this level the thoracic duct appears to be almost at the midline (perhaps very slightly to the right of it). The narrow white shadow can be traced upwards in the thorax: as it goes the duct is seen to become more distinctly radiopaque relative to its surroundings.

At the level of the fifth thoracic vertebra the outline of the duct is to the left of the spine and it remains on the left as it ascends to the thoracic inlet.

At the level of the inner end of the left clavicle on the radiograph, the shadow of the thoracic duct becomes fragmented. Nevertheless its arch in a lateral direction can be distinguished and the outline of the duct ends over the shadow of the left second rib.

In this radiograph some contrast agent is dispersed into the lungs, making their radiographic pattern more prominent than usual. The opaque agent has reached the lungs because the thoracic duct opens into the venous system at the left subclavian vein. The pathways for the contrast agent thereafter are: the left innominate vein; the superior vena cava; the right atrium of the heart; the right ventricle of the heart; and then out along the main pulmonary arteries to the lungs.

Fig. 4.17 is another frontal view of a lymphangiogram showing a normal variation in appearance. The thoracic duct can be followed up the thorax from the level of the ninth thoracic vertebra at the foot of the radiograph. Again the white shadow becomes more distinct as it goes upwards and its change of direction towards the left at the level of the fifth thoracic vertebra is seen. From the third thoracic vertebra upwards the thoracic duct is shown most clearly. In this case, the laterally directed arch of the duct takes place at a higher level than the previous one and it is seen over the transverse process of the seventh cervical vertebra. This is the level which a classical anatomical description assigns to it.

Fig. 4.18 is a lateral projection of a lymphangiogram. The thin white band which represents the thoracic duct outlined by contrast agent can be seen ascending in the posterior mediastinum. It is just in front of the spine and behind the heart. The general curvature of the white line is concave anteriorly. As it enters the superior mediastinum at the level

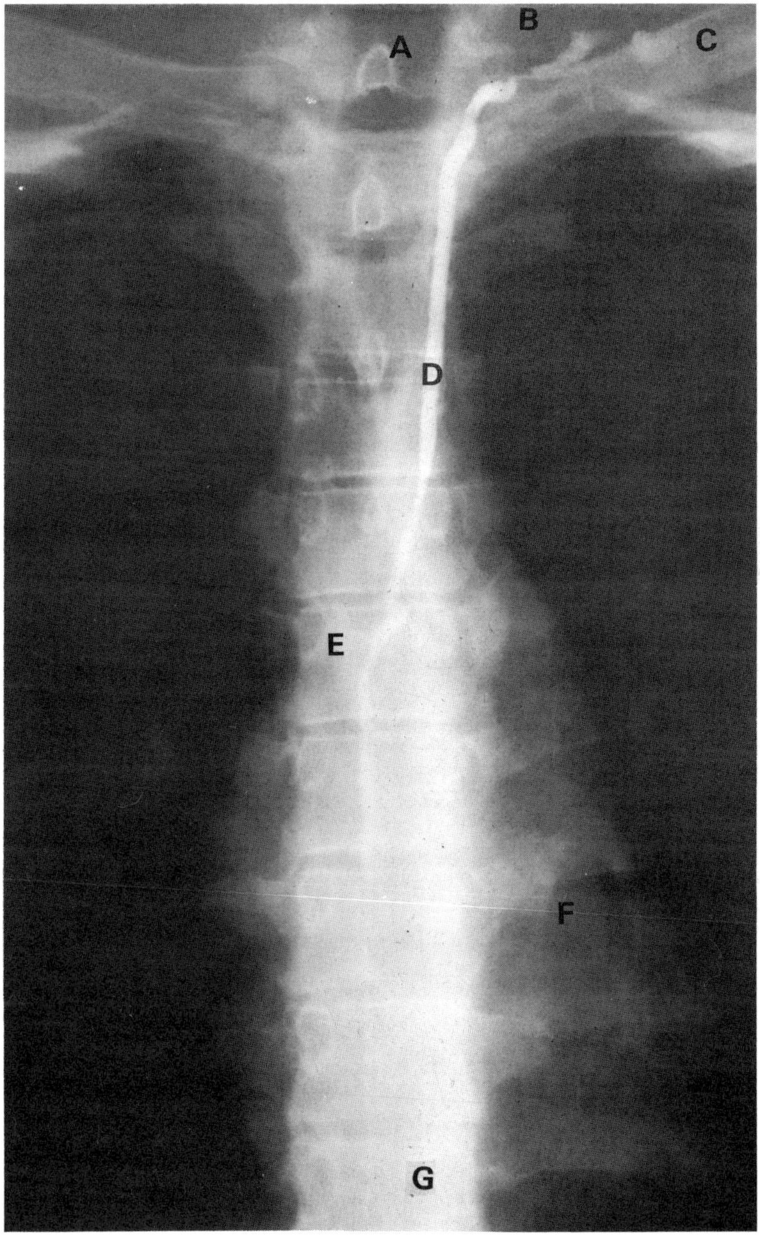

Fig. 4.17. A lymphangiogram showing the thoracic duct in a frontal projection.

A Cervical vertebra 7
B Transverse process of cervical vertebra 7
C Left clavicle
D Thoracic duct
E Thoracic vertebra 5
F Cardiac shadow
G Thoracic vertebra 9

of the top of the heart shadow, there is a reverse curve in the outline of the thoracic duct: it is convex anteriorly. Here the duct is very close to the arch of the aorta which crosses it in passing from the front towards the back of the thorax.

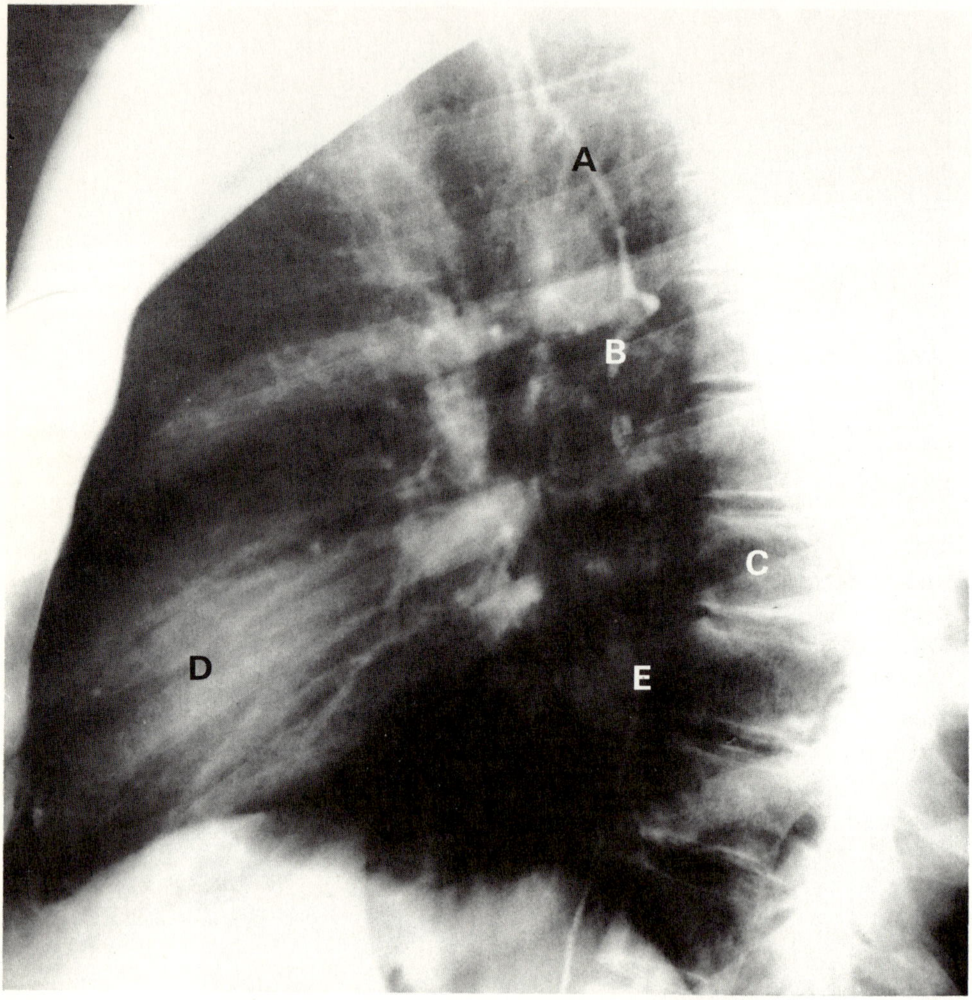

Fig. 4.18. A lymphangiogram showing the thoracic duct in a lateral projection.

A Thoracic duct in superior mediastinum
B Thoracic duct close to the arch of the aorta
C Thoracic vertebra
D Cardiac shadow
E Thoracic duct in posterior mediastinum

Chapter 5
The Plain Radiograph of the Abdomen

The basic radiograph of the abdomen is the anteroposterior (AP) view taken while the patient is lying on his back. The area which the radiograph should include is demarcated by the diaphragm on the superior boundary and the pubic symphysis below. In practice on some radiographs of the abdomen the diaphragm is not fully seen, especially if the film has been exposed on expiration, during which the diaphragm rises. This is often the case of control radiographs before intravenous urography: the subdiaphragmatic region is usually adequately demonstrated for the examination concerned but the film 'stops short' of the diaphragm itself.

Abdominal organs are visible radiographically because the X-ray beam is absorbed differentially by several tissues present: thus varying intensities of radiation reach the film and various film-blackenings result. The appearances concerned on a plain radiograph are of (a) bone, (b) fat, (c) gas, (d) the soft tissues of the abdominal viscera and other structures.

Distinct from the plain radiograph is the one depicting a particular abdominal organ or system after the introduction of a radiological contrast agent. These contrast examinations will be considered in subsequent chapters. Just now we will refer in more detail to the appearances which have been listed above but first it may be helpful to define what is meant by the abdomen.

The abdomen is the region of the trunk between the thorax and the pelvis, its upper and lower parts being continuous at the plane of the pelvic inlet. Essentially the abdomen is a cavity containing the abdominal viscera and other organs, separated by the diaphragm from the thorax and enclosed by the abdominal wall. Whilst possessing some skeletal elements (the lumbar vertebrae and pelvic bones), the abdominal wall is constituted mainly by the anterolateral and posterior groups of abdominal muscles. Thus, its tone may vary considerably between individuals, it is readily distended by the organs it encloses and it moves with respiration. The abdomen is considered as possessing a number of regions which are listed and depicted in Fig. 5.1. The regions of the abdomen are demarcated by four planes which are defined as follows:

(i) the transpyloric plane, a line drawn horizontally across the abdomen; it runs half-way between the suprasternal notch

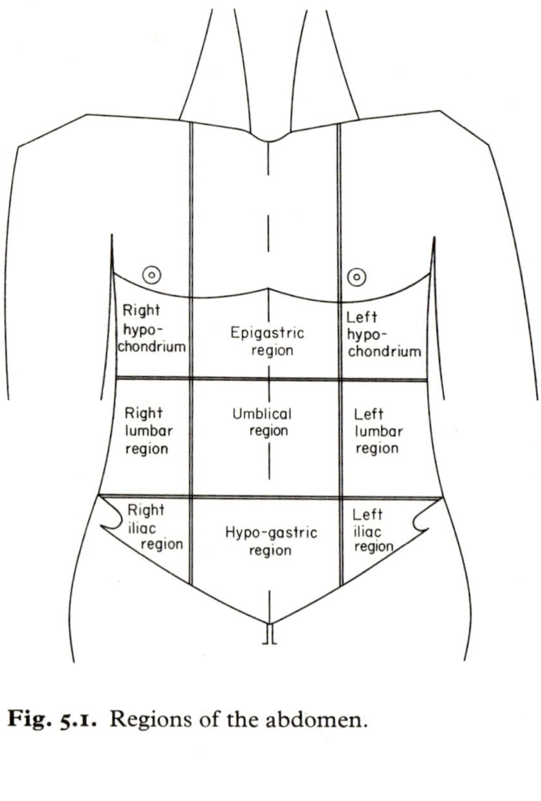

Fig. 5.1. Regions of the abdomen.

and the pubic symphysis (the median plane of the body) and passes through the first lumbar vertebra;
(ii) the transtubercular plane, a line drawn horizontally across the upper surface of the iliac crests at the level of the highest point of each which is visible from the front and corresponding to the upper border of the fifth lumbar vertebra;
(iii) and (iv) the right and left lateral vertical planes; these are lines drawn parallel to the median plane, half-way between that plane and the anterior superior iliac spine on each side.

The skeletal appearances

The authentic anatomist would not include regions of the skeleton in an account of the abdomen. However, in a description of radiographic anatomy we are bound to do so because of the composite nature of the X-ray image. A plain radiograph of the abdomen is a record of superimposed anatomical structures: it depicts parts of the spine and pelvis no less—and actually rather more obviously—than the abdominal organs which are the real subjects of the examination. Student radiographers, whose experience of looking at radiographs is necessarily short, find the skeleton more easily recognisable than are soft-tissue structures such as the kidneys and liver.

The parts of the skeleton usually recorded on the AP view of the abdomen are:
(i) the last two—sometimes three—pairs of ribs;
(ii) the last two—sometimes three— thoracic vertebrae;
(iii) all five lumbar vertebrae;
(iv) the sacrum;
(v) the hip bones.
These appearances are seen on Fig. 5.2.

Features of the lumbar vertebrae which are prominent on the radiograph are:
(a) the bodies;
(b) the transverse processes;
(c) the spinous processes;
(d) the pedicles;
(e) the articular processes, superior and inferior.

Although one or two may be clearly seen, the inter-

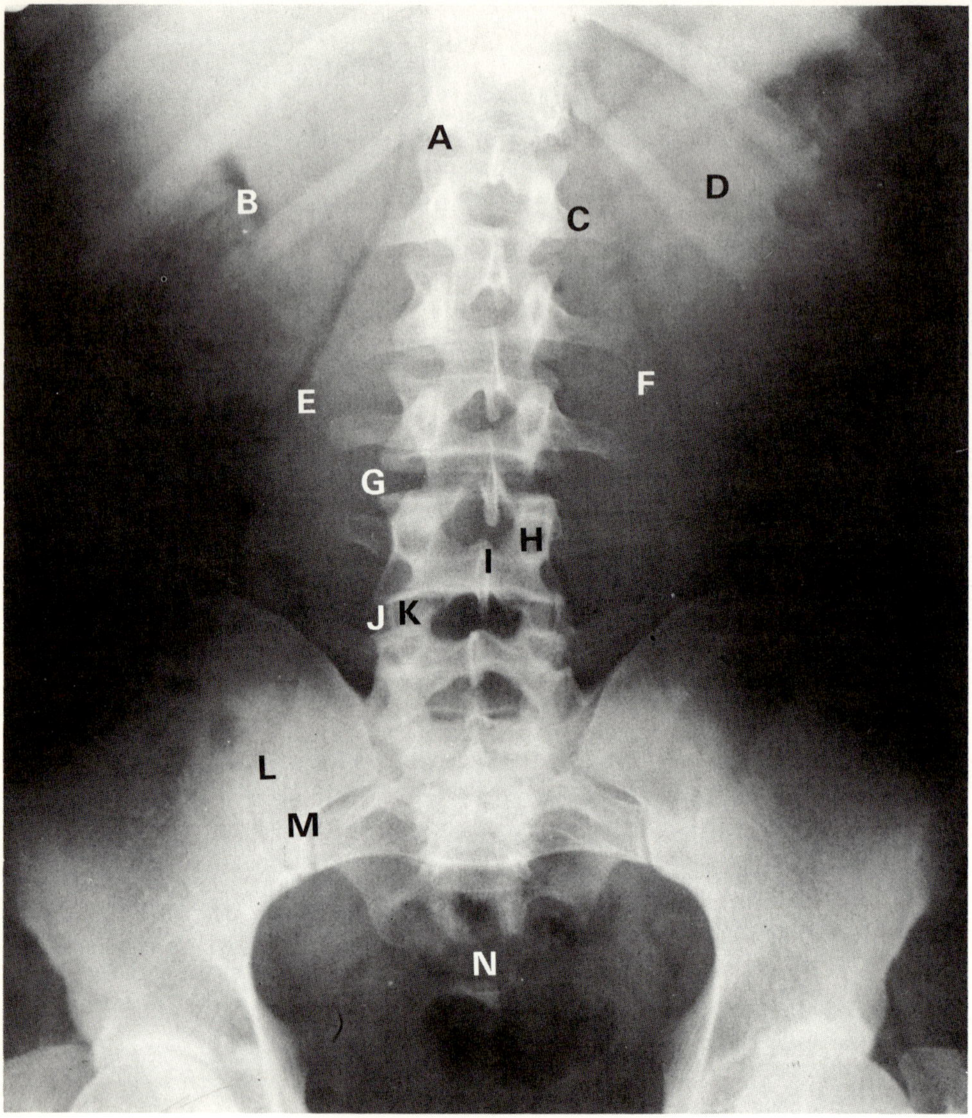

Fig. 5.2. An anteroposterior radiograph of the abdomen.

- A Overlapping images of the superior surface of the body of lumbar vertebra 1 on the inferior surface of thoracic vertebra 12
- B Right kidney
- C Left transverse process of lumbar vertebra 1
- D Left kidney
- E Right psoas muscle
- F Left psoas muscle
- G Disc between lumbar vertebra 3 and 4
- H Left pedicle of lumbar vertebra 4
- I Spinous process of lumbar vertebra 4
- J Superior articular process of lumbar vertebra 5
- K Inferior articular process of lumbar vertebra 4
- L Anterior edge of right sacroiliac joint
- M Posterior edge of right sacroiliac joint
- N Foreshortened image of sacrum

vertebral disc spaces generally cannot be appreciated. The X-ray beam is not at right angles to the majority of them. As a result the upper and lower surfaces of each vertebral body form elliptical images and the bodies appear to overlap.

The sacrum—because it is not either parallel to the film or central to the beam—is foreshortened on the radiograph. The amount of this foreshortening may be pronounced (as it is in Fig. 5.2) or may be quite slight (as it is in Fig. 5.5). To a large extent these differences in projection are sexual. In the male the long axis of the sacrum is almost vertical when he is erect and will be virtually parallel to the film when he is recumbent. In the female the lumbosacral angle is usually more acute and the sacrum consequently more tilted in relation to the film.

The sacroiliac joints are necessarily foreshortened in appearance on the AP radiograph for the same reasons. Not infrequently, each sacroiliac joint presents as a pair of linear translucencies, the curves being concave medially and one

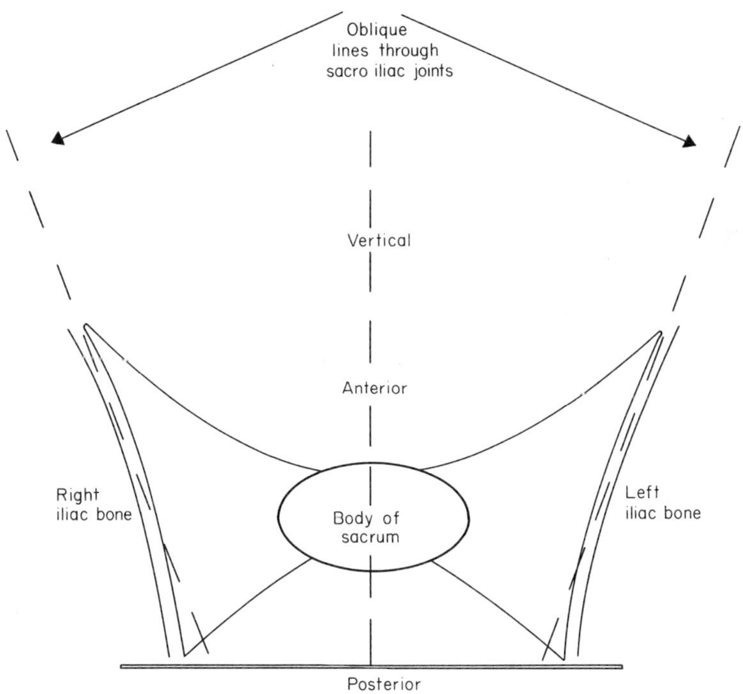

Fig. 5.3. The sacroiliac joints.

more distinct than the other. This effect is particularly marked on Fig. 5.2 because of the foreshortened projection.

The sacroiliac joint is a plane joint, formed between the auricular surface on the lateral aspect of the sacrum and the corresponding area on the internal surface of the hip-bone. Anteroposteriorly the auricular surfaces are inclined inwards (see Fig. 5.3). Thus, on the AP radiograph, the lateral, wider translucency marks the anterior edge of the articulation (and not—as may appear to the new reader of X-ray appearances—a fracture line of some kind); the medial, sharper translucency represents the posterior part of the articulation.

An interesting feature of the hip-bone for the student of radiographic anatomy is the appearance of the ossific centres when the subject is an adolescent or young adult. The hip-bone ossifies from eight centres: three primary (for the ilium, ischium and pubis) and five secondary centres. Ossification occurs in the secondary centres at puberty and is not complete until the age of perhaps twenty or twenty-five years; thus, it is usual to see on the abdominal radiographs of young people the crescentic epiphyses for the crests of the ilia. This feature is demonstrated in Fig. 5.4 at a stage when ossification is almost complete.

The appearances due to fat and muscle

Fat is more radiolucent than are other soft tissues and usually provides sufficient radiographic contrast for the visualisation of certain abdominal organs on a plain radiograph. This is true of the kidneys, for example: they are surrounded by a quantity of fat which results in an area of deeper blackening on the underlying film and highlights the composite tonal density due to (a) the kidney substance, (b) its over-lying incomplete muscle layer, (c) its fibrous capsule, which are not differentiated from each other radiographically. Renal appearances are more fully described on pages 188 and 204.

There are certain fatty planes which form sign-posts on abdominal radiographs of good quality. In each flank—that is in the area between the ribs and the ilium—several translucent bands are to be detected. These vary in width and visibility and—as they are due to fat—are naturally more prominent in an obese mature subject than in a child or old person. These flank stripes are demonstrated in Figs. 5.5, 5.8 and 9.2a, page 214. From the medial to the lateral aspect they are to be identified as follows:

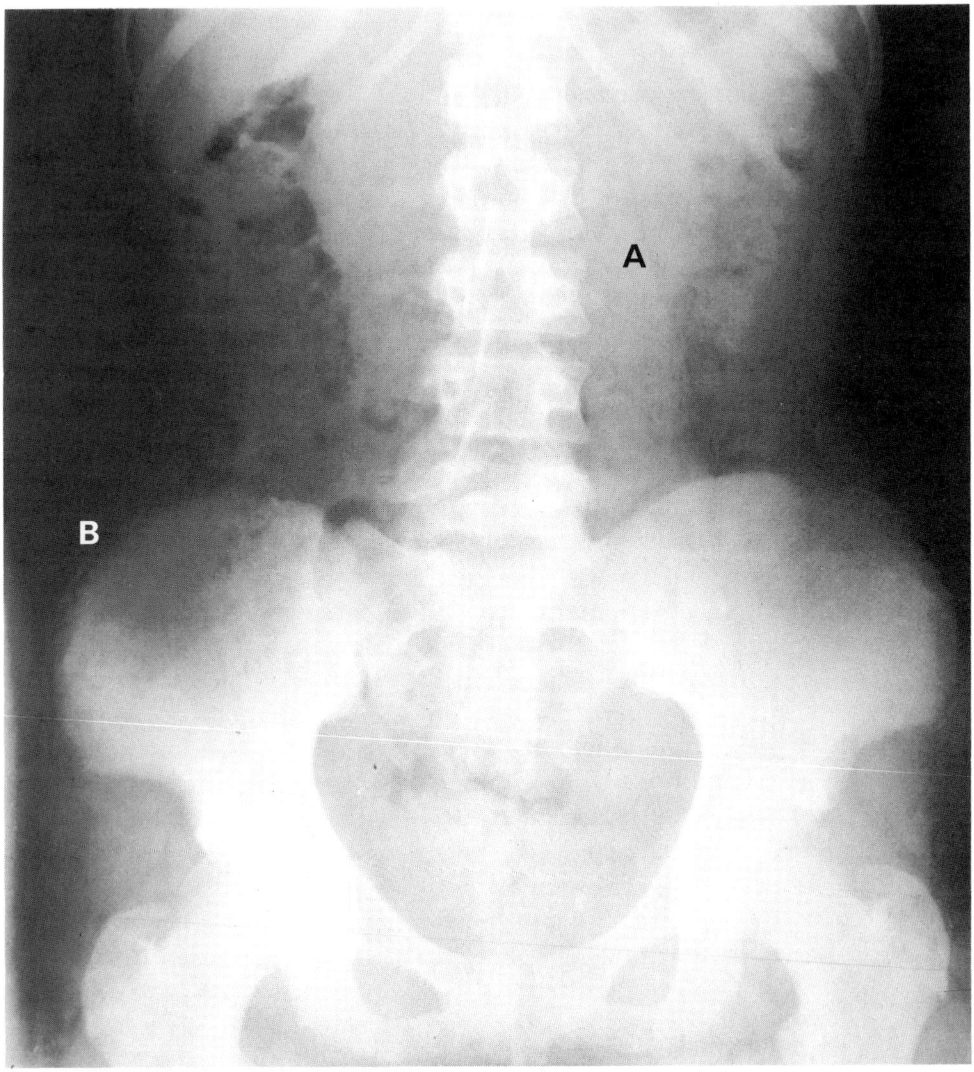

Fig. 5.4. An anteroposterior radiograph of the abdomen of an adolescent subject.

A Left psoas muscle

B Epiphysis for the crest of the right iliac bone

(i) is the extraperitoneal fat layer. It varies in breadth on the radiograph from as little as 1 mm up to several centimetres depending on such factors as:

(a) the build of the individual;

(b) the phase of respiration during which the exposure was made;

(c) posture (for example, because of muscular contraction, a film exposed whilst the patient occupies the lateral decubitus shows the extraperitoneal fat band in the uppermost flank to be shorter, broader and more convex medially, compared with its appearance on a supine radiograph).

(ii) is a layer of fat between the transverse and oblique abdominal muscles. It is about 1 mm or less in breadth on the radiograph and often appears shorter than the extraperitoneal layer.

(iii) is another thin fatty band situated between the external and internal oblique abdominal muscles. It approximates in length to the extraperitoneal layer.

Fig. 5.5 is the radiograph of a very obese subject. The horizontal translucency giving the impression of a 'belt' is caused by folds of subcutaneous fat at the waistline. This effect is seen again on Fig. 5.7b.

In the radiograph of a lean patient, the thin bands of fat between the muscles may be scarcely apparent or virtually non-existent. Diagnostically the important flank stripe is therefore the peritoneal fat line and its presence should be invariably sought by the observer of any abdominal radiograph. For instance, a loss of symmetry between the flank stripes on comparing one side with the other, or a diffuseness of contour, may suggest the presence of a mass or of free fluid in an acute abdominal condition.

As the colon normally lies immediately medial to the peritoneal fat line, the colic haustrations are seen sometimes to give the fat an indented medial border. This can be seen in Fig. 5.5.

One of the posterior muscles of the abdominal wall is easily recognisable on the AP radiograph (see Fig. 5.2).

This is the psoas major which has several origins on the transverse processes and bodies of all the lumbar vertebrae and on the lower margin of the body of the twelfth thoracic vertebra. The muscle proceeds downwards across the brim of the true pelvis, ending in a tendon which is inserted in the

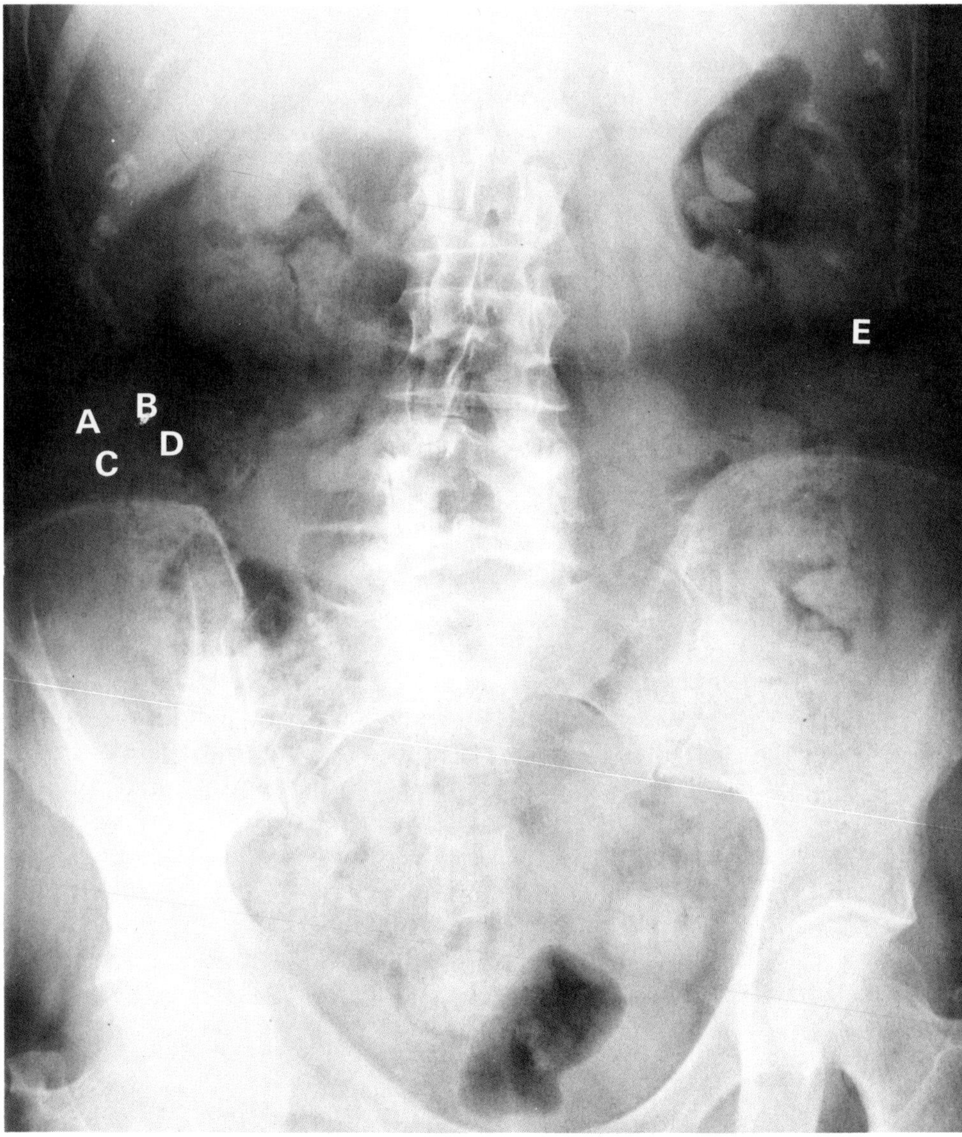

Fig. 5.5. An anteroposterior view of the abdomen.

A, B, C 'Flank stripes' (fat planes)
D Ascending colon
E Fat at the waistline

lesser trochanter of the femur. On the AP radiograph the lateral edge of the psoas major forms a long, radiolucent line on each side, beginning near the neck of the twelfth rib and running obliquely outwards and downwards until it is lost from view somewhere in the iliac fossa. The right and left psoas major normally make together a prominent triangular formation on the AP radiograph.

This feature has diagnostic significance, since loss of the psoas shadow on one or other side may be indicative of the presence of disorder: for example, abscess formation involving a vertebral body may cause pus to track beneath muscle fasciae and obliterate the psoas outline; other instances may occur in appendicitis, perforated duodenal ulcer, or haemorrhage from a kidney if there has been a history of injury. Sometimes obliteration of the psoas is accompanied by a lumbar scoliosis, the curvature being the result of muscular spasm and concave towards the side in question.

The appearances due to gastric and intestinal gas

Bone, soft tissues in general and fat exhibit—in that order—increasing radiolucency to X-ray beams generated at the kilovoltages usually employed in diagnostic medical radiography.

In a gas, however, no absorption of the beam occurs and we have a medium which is radioparent. Whenever it is present among structures exposed to an X-ray beam it creates areas of deeper blackening on the underlying film and provides radiographic contrast; in some radiological procedures it is artificially introduced to body cavities for this purpose. In the alimentary tract variable quantities of gas are found as a normal physiological feature and we may notice its presence at any or all of numerous sites on the plain AP radiograph of the abdomen.

GAS IN THE STOMACH

Most people swallow air at one time or another, some to a greater degree than others. Certain circumstances increase the probability of gas being present in the stomach: a crying child, for example; or accelerated respiration for any reason;

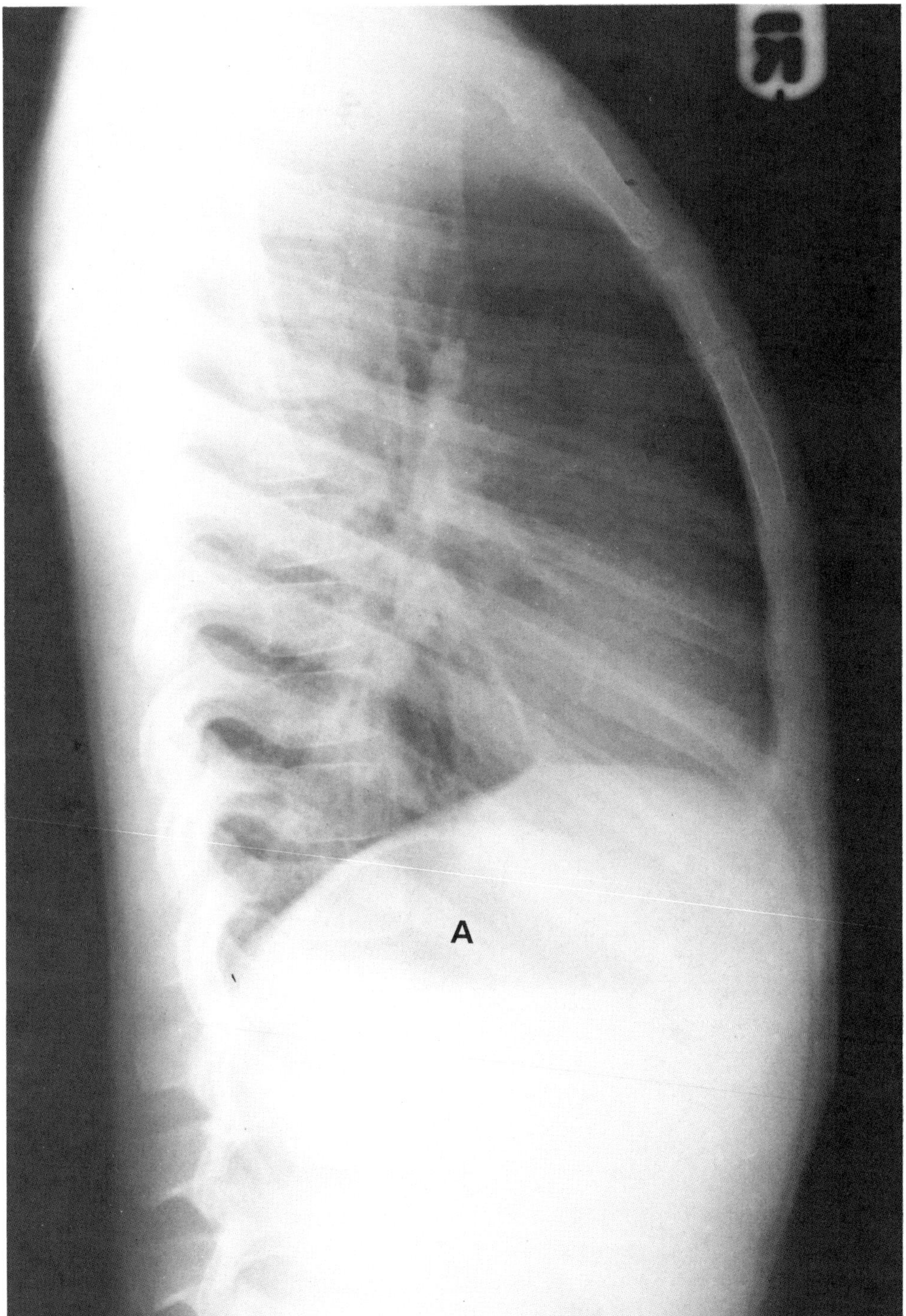

Fig. 5.6. A lateral radiograph of the chest.
A Gas in the gastric fundus outlining the lower surface of the left dome of the diaphragm

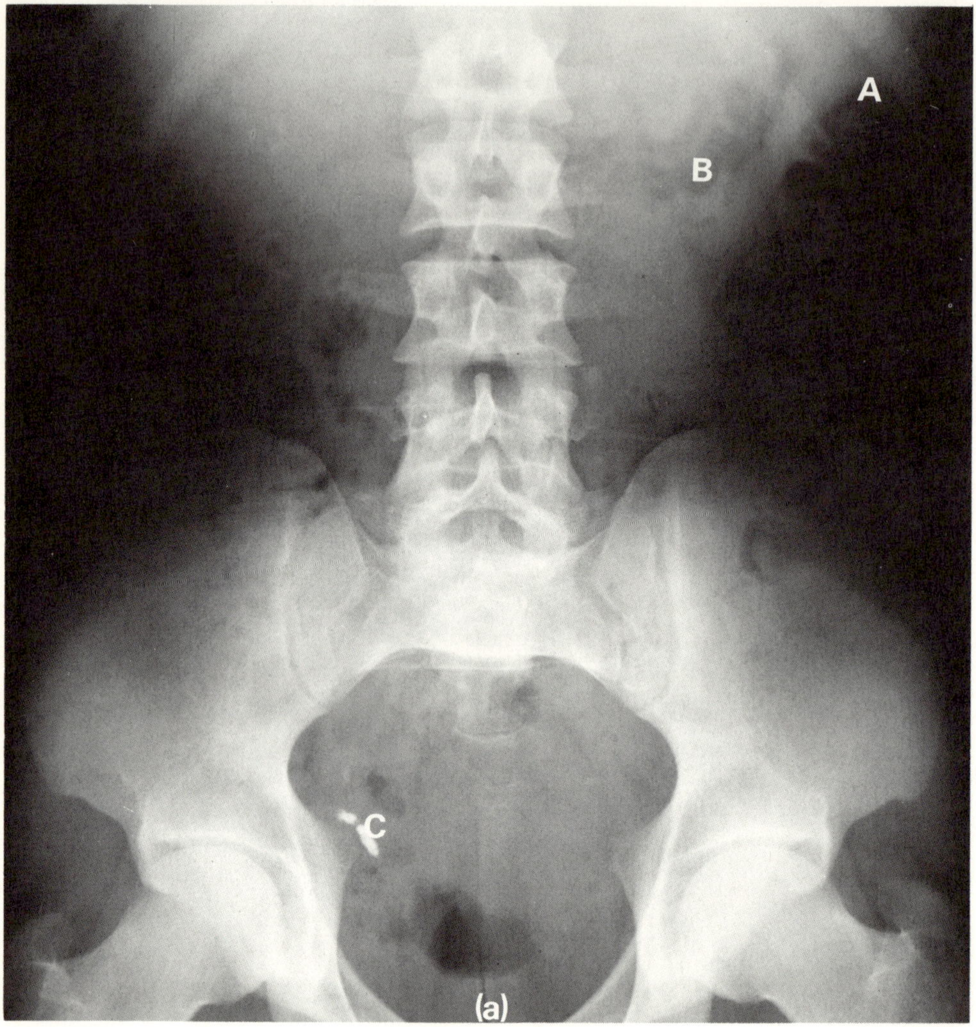

Fig. 5.7.a. An anteroposterior radiograph of the abdomen.

A Splenic flexure delineated (as are other parts of the colon) by gas present in the bowel

B Air in the body of the stomach. Gastric rugae are shown.

C An opaque residue, possibly barium sulphate, in the vermiform appendix

or the taking of an aerated ('fizzy') drink; or even feelings of nervousness which tend to exacerbate a habit of air-swallowing.

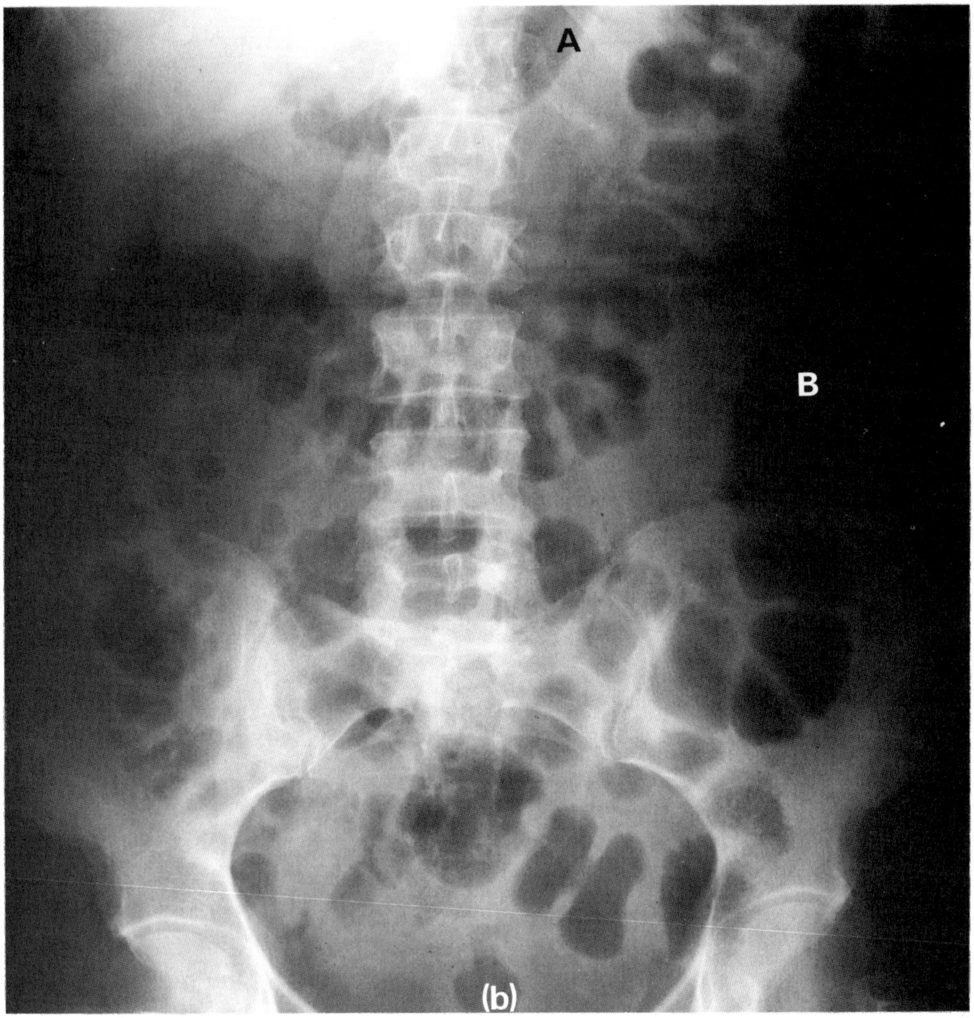

Fig. 5. 7b. A supine anteroposterior radiograph of the abdomen, in which much of the large gut is demonstrated by contained gas.

A Air outlining the body of the stomach

B Descending part of the colon

A bubble of gas in the fundus of the stomach just under the diaphragm is an extremely common finding on radiographs of the chest (see Chapter 1, p. 16) and of the abdomen, if the film was exposed while the patient was erect. Such a bubble is seen from the posteroanterior aspect on Fig. 1.13 and from the lateral aspect on Fig. 5.6.

Air naturally rises and, in both the radiographs mentioned, the fundus was the highest part of the stomach at the moment of exposure. In the case of the abdominal AP radiograph of a supine subject, gastric air—when present—gives a rather different picture. It is spread over the anterosuperior surface of the body of the stomach, sometimes delineating folds of the gastric mucosa (rugae) and even the pylorus and duodenal cap if a large quantity has been swallowed. Fig. 5.7a shows gastric rugae defined on the greater curvature of the stomach by the presence of gas; in Fig. 5.7b there is air in the body and pyloric parts of the stomach.

INTESTINAL GAS

Gas from the stomach may enter the intestines (it is very likely to do so in a recumbent patient), or it may be present there for some other reasons, such as the digestion of gas-producing foods. Gaseous radiographic translucencies are normally to be seen scattered anywhere in the small and large bowels. A rectal 'bubble' is a relatively frequent finding (see, for example, Fig. 5.5) and sometimes most of the course of the colon may be identified by means of its content of gas. Colic haustrations are seen thus demonstrated on Fig. 5.7b.

In the diagnosis of acute abdominal conditions, gas patterns in the abdomen—or their displacement or absence—may be extremely significant. For example, large quantities of gas tend to accumulate in and distend the bowel proximal to an obstruction, while there may be only a few gas shadows—or none—demonstrable in the distal segments of the tract. Similarly, the displacement of gut by an intra-abdominal mass may be inferred when intestinal gas shadows are seen to be abnormal in situation in the abdominal cavity.

UNCONTAINED GAS

Free gas in the abdominal cavity (that is gas which is not contained within the gut), unless it has been introduced deliberately as a diagnostic procedure or coincidentally during abdominal surgery, is evidence of an acute abnormality. Radiographs exposed when the trunk is erect assist the demonstration of uncontained air beneath the dome of the diaphragm (see Chapter 1, p. 15–16).

The appearances of the abdominal organs

In all patients we may expect to see certain abdominal organs on an AP radiograph which is of acceptable diagnostic quality; other organs are demonstrated only in a proportion of subjects and their visualisation cannot be guaranteed.

The organs to be considered are:
(i) the liver;
(ii) the kidneys and bladder;
(iii) the spleen;
(iv) the pancreas.

THE LIVER

The liver, the largest gland in the body, is apparent as a homogeneous density in the right upper abdominal quadrant. Its superior margin is indicated on the plain radiograph by the right diaphragm and the base of the right lung. In fact, the organ is bigger than its radiographic outline suggests: it extends across the upper epigastrium and—not infrequently—into the left hypochondrium as far as the left lateral line. An account of the surface markings of the liver may be found in many textbooks of anatomy.

On the AP radiograph the lower border of the liver is usually well demonstrated in the right flank, near the right costal margin, contrast being provided by adjacent fat. This feature is seen in Figs. 5.8, page 124, and 9.2a, page 214.

THE KIDNEYS AND BLADDER

Perirenal and retroperitoneal fat provide contrast for the visualisation of the kidneys on a plain radiograph (see Figs. 5.2 and 5.9). These two organs lie on the posterior abdominal wall behind the peritoneum, one to either side of the vertebral column. The left kidney—relative to the right—is usually a little larger, narrower, more oblique and nearer to the median plane. The right kidney is normally lower than the left,

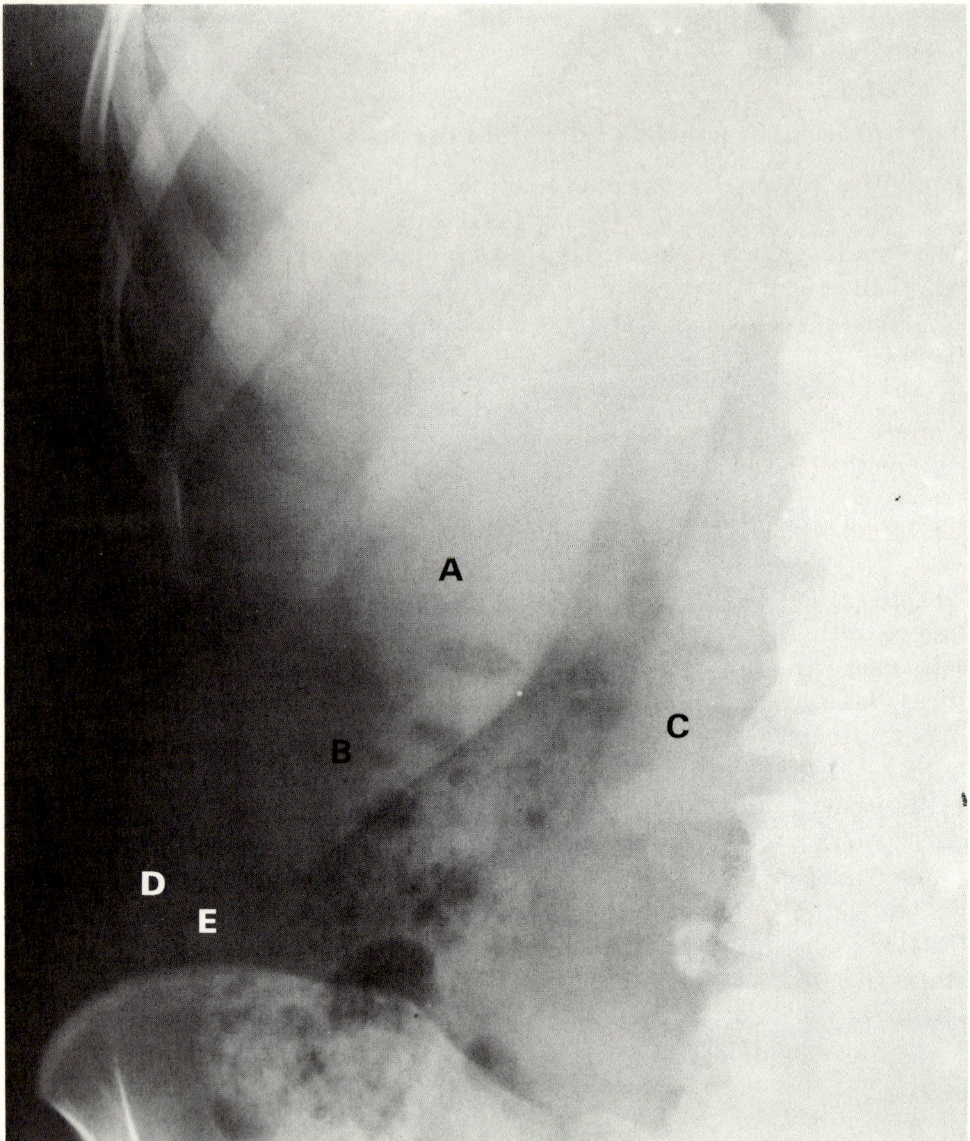

Fig. 5.8. A posteroanterior projection of the gall bladder region.

A Right kidney
B Right lobe of the liver
C Right psoas muscle
D Fat planes between the transverse and oblique abdominal muscles
E The peritoneal fat line

probably because of its relationship to the liver. The long axis of each kidney is directed downwards and laterally; its transverse axis laterally and backwards.

As demonstrated on a plain radiograph, the outer border of the kidney is normally regular and convex and the upper pole more pointed than the lower (see Fig. 9.2a and Figs. 5.2 and 5.9). Approaching the hilum, the renal outline tends to be lost. The renal hila are often described as lying on the transpyloric plane 5 cm from the median line; but radiographers should remember that the kidneys move freely with respiration and that a film exposed on inspiration will show them to lie 1–4 cm lower in the abdomen than they appear on expiration.

The size, shape and position of each kidney may usually be determined from a plain radiograph (see also p. 188) but the organ's structural and functional elements are not apparent because of insufficient radiation contrasts in the subject. Renal calculi which contain calcium are readily detectable (see p. 130). However, only a proportion of urinary calculi have such radiopacity. For these reasons plain radiographs of the urinary tract are not very informative and are seldom taken in isolation. A procedure using an appropriate radiological contrast agent is much more likely to be the chosen investigation of the urinary tract (see Chapter 8).

The ureters, the tubes conveying urine from the kidneys to the bladder, normally are not seen on the plain radiograph, again because of insufficient contrast between them and adjacent tissues. An observer of the film may easily project the course of each ureter along a line beginning approximately on the transpyloric plane (level of the first lumbar vertebra) 5 cm from the median plane; this line is continued downwards over the lumbar transverse processes, medial to their tips on each side, and crosses the pelvic brim just medial to the relevant sacroiliac joint. Running downwards and backwards on the posterolateral pelvic wall, the ureter turns at the level of the ischial spine, passing medially and forwards to the lateral angle of the trigone on the base of the urinary bladder. It is useful for the student to compare such an imaginary line with the appearances of the ureters during intravenous urography (see Chapter 8). Fig. 5.12 is a plain

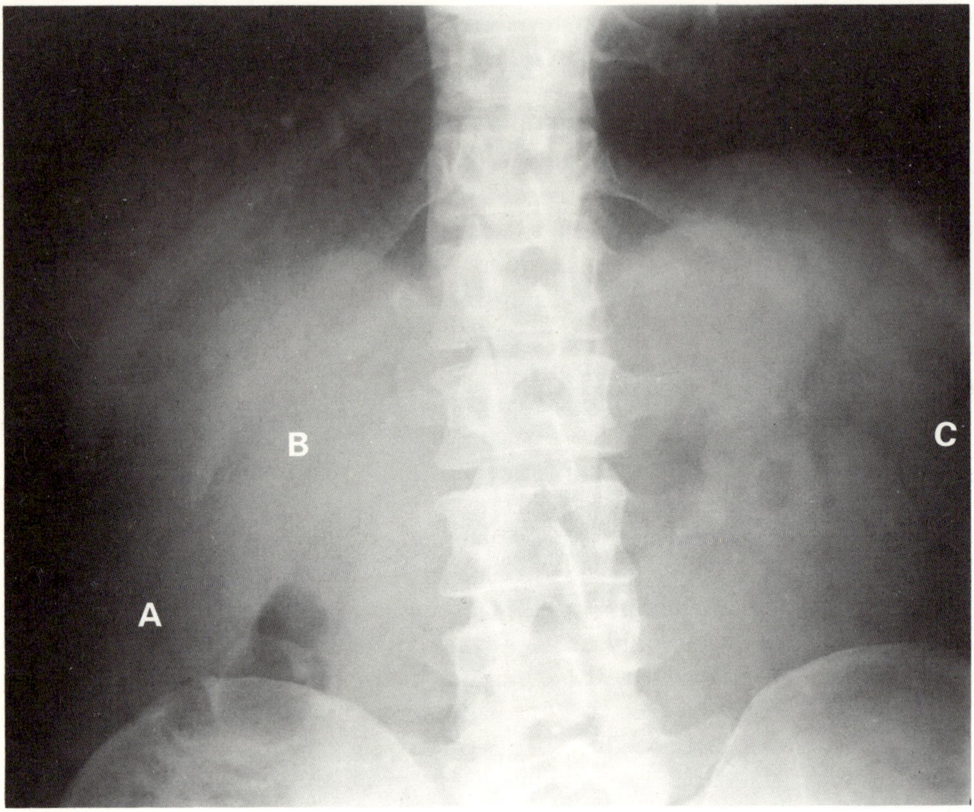

Fig. 5.9a. An anteroposterior radiograph of the upper abdomen.
A The peritoneal fat line
B The right kidney
C The spleen

radiograph which reveals a radiopaque stone at the lower end of the left ureter (see also p. 192).

If it is empty of urine the bladder is not normally visualised on a plain radiograph. When it is full, its faint rounded outline may be detected in the pelvis, particularly if this area of the film is free of gas shadows (see Fig. 5.10). The radiographic appearance of the bladder is further discussed in Chapter 8.

THE SPLEEN

Visualisation of the spleen on a plain radiograph of the abdomen cannot be guaranteed and in fact is relatively unusual.

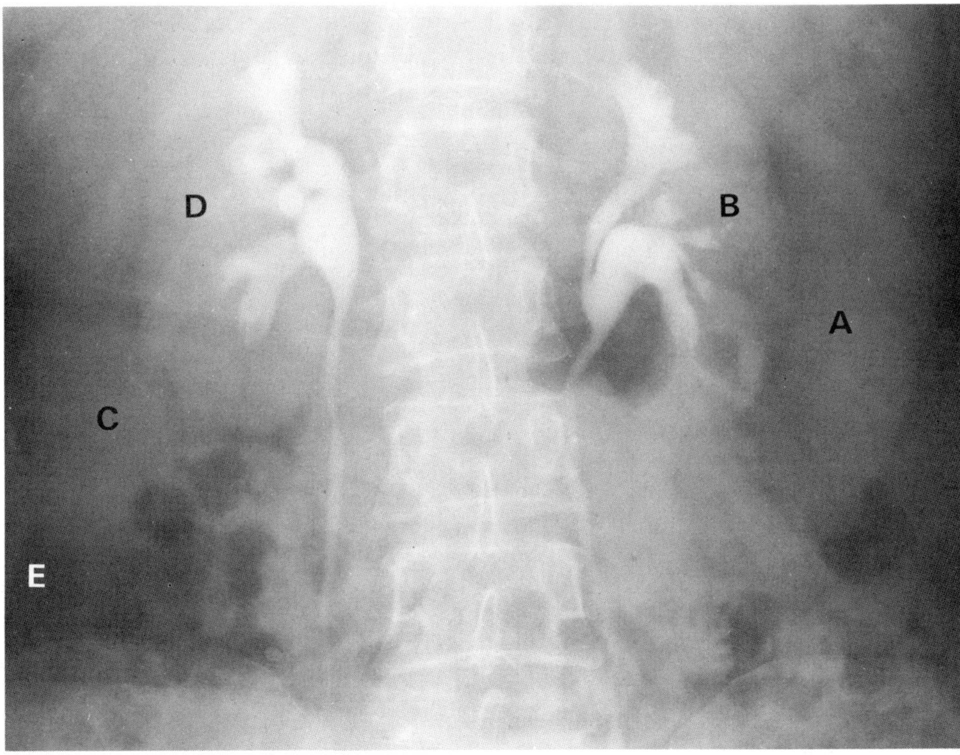

Fig. 5.9b. A radiograph taken during intravenous urography which coincidentally has well demonstrated the spleen and liver.

A Spleen
B Left kidney
C Liver
D Right kidney
E The peritoneal fat line

The largest of the ductless glands, the spleen mainly occupies the left hypochondrium, its upper end extending into the epigastrium. It is situated between the diaphragm and the fundus of the stomach, where the coincidental presence of air may assist delineation of its upper pole (this has happened in the case illustrated on Fig. 5.9a; fat surrounding the colon may perform a similar office for the splenic lower pole (see Fig. 5.9b).

The spleen is a pulpy vascular organ, of rounded oblong shape; its visceral aspect is flattened and characterised by four impressions (gastric, renal, pancreatic and colic); superiorly the spleen is convex and smooth. On the inferior surface, near to the lower edge of the gastric impression, is a long fissure, the hilum of the spleen, carrying the splenic vessels and nerves.

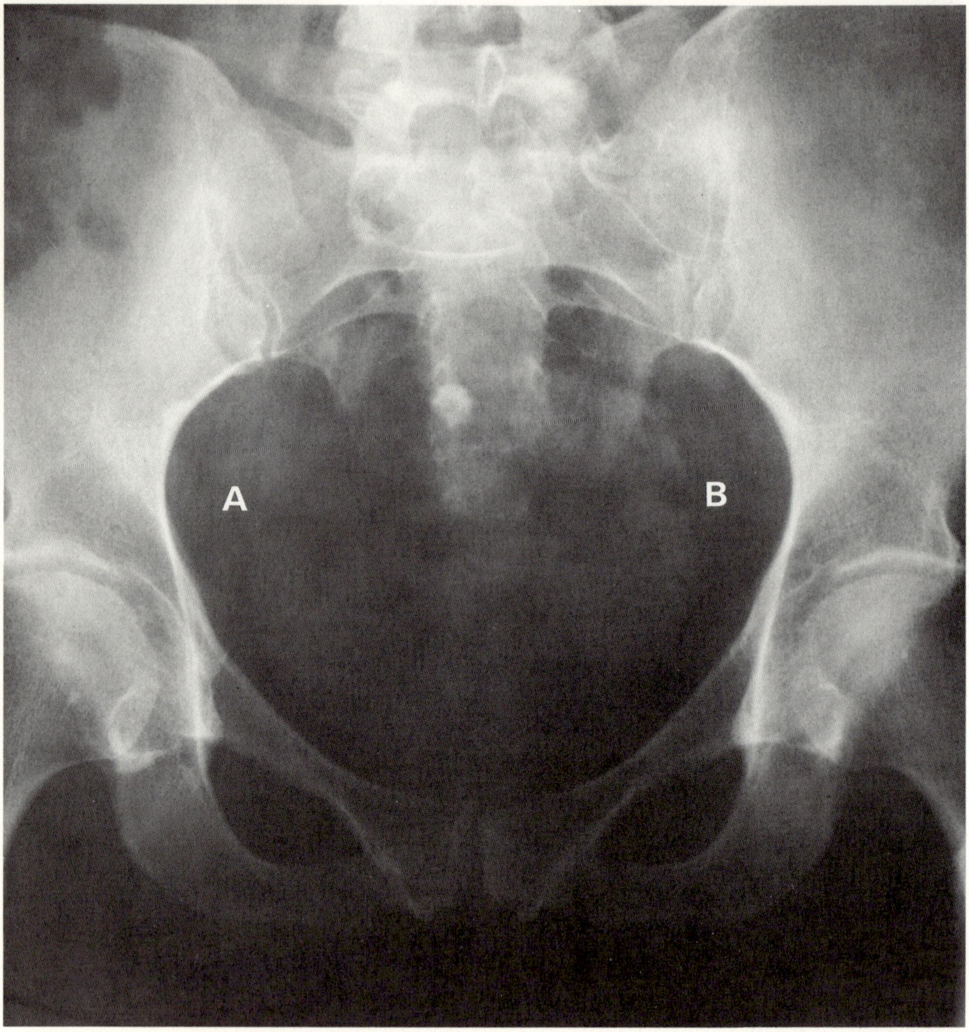

Fig. 5.10. A plain radiograph of the pelvis which shows the bladder.
A The right wall of the bladder B The left wall of the bladder

THE PANCREAS

Plain radiographs do not show the normal pancreas, although radiopaque stones in the pancreatic ducts are an occasional finding (Fig. 5.13a and b). The pancreas is a flattened,

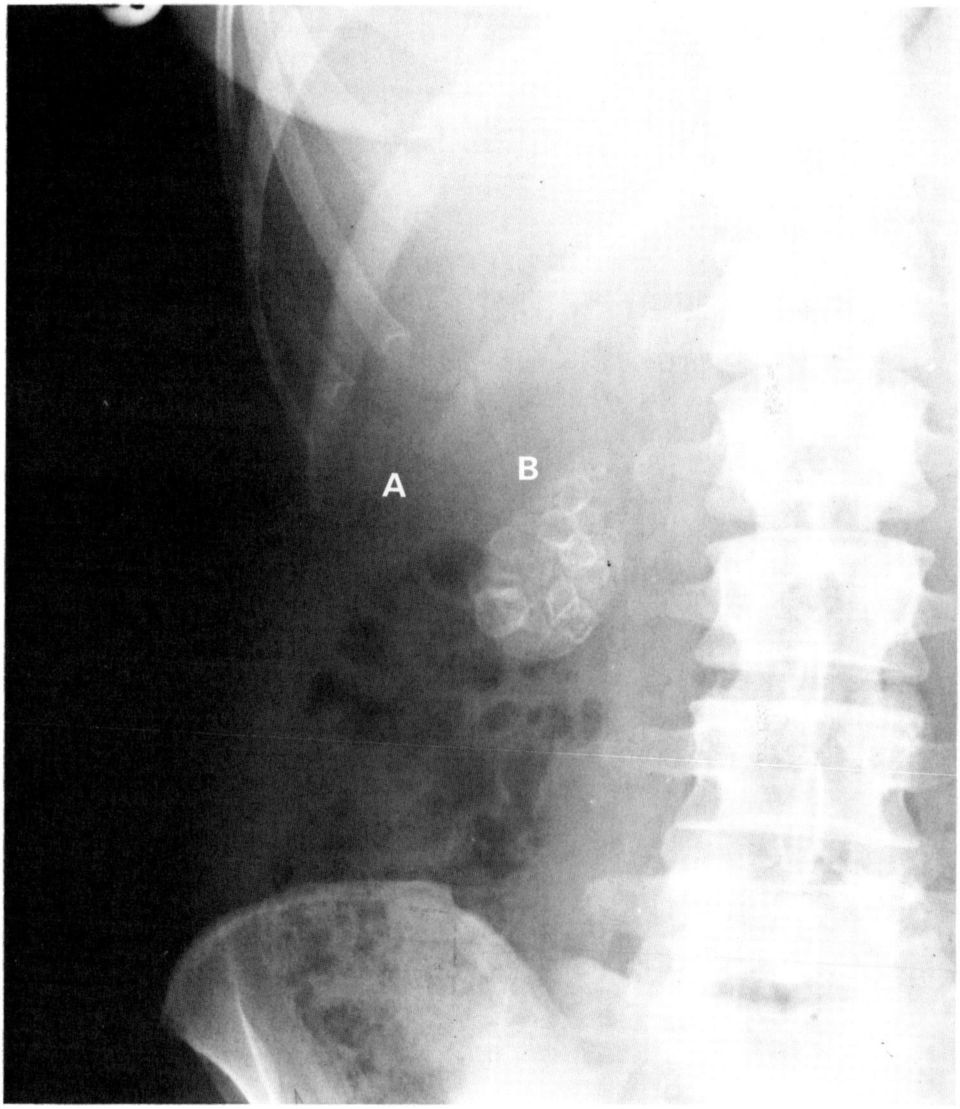

Fig. 5.11. A plain radiograph of the gall bladder region.

A Right lobe of the liver

B The gall bladder, demonstrated by the presence of stones which contain calcium elongated gland, situated on the posterior abdominal wall at the back of the epigastrium and the left hypochondrium.

The head of the pancreas is tucked beneath the curve of the duodenum, sometimes a small part being actually embedded in the duodenal wall. Because of such an intimate relationship, an abnormality of the pancreas—which often offers no sign on a plain radiograph—may be capable of diagnosis by means of barium studies of the gastrointestinal tract (the duodenum displaying deformity or invasion).

The appearances due to calcified structures

Calcium is an element of high atomic number. Consequently its presence anywhere in the body results in radiographic opacities which are detectable, although they may be difficult to perceive if the calcium content is small. Fig. 5.11 shows stones in the gall bladder which are obvious but vary in the amount of calcium in their composition: many are only slightly radiopaque but about half-a-dozen of them consist severally of a relatively dense outer calcific ring (in some, partially complete), which renders their radiographic visualisation plain.

Like gallstones, calculi in the urinary tract may or may not contain calcium and on this will depend their demonstration on plain radiographs. In Fig. 5.12 the small calcific oval shadow medial to the left ischial spine is a stone at the lower end of the left ureter.

Fig. 5.13b is a left posterior-oblique projection showing the left side of the abdomen. Opacities visible within a triangle formed between the eleventh left rib and lumbar vertebral bodies 1 and 2 are due to the presence of calcification within the pancreas.

In elderly people, calcification of certain structures is a generally insignificant and almost expected finding, since it represents degenerative changes likely to occur with increasing bodily age. Thus, on Fig. 9.2a we notice calcification of part of the right costal cartilages, visible in the area of the tenth and eleventh right ribs. Fig. 5.14 shows a number of small, rounded opacities in the lower pelvis. These are phleboliths; that is, calcified thrombi or clots in the pelvic veins.

Calcification is sometimes seen within the walls of sclerotic (hardening) arteries. The abdominal aorta is a likely candidate for the exhibition of such changes, which are best demonstrated in a lateral projection (Fig. 5.15a). The aorta descends in front of lumbar vertebral bodies 1–4, deviating a little to the left of the median plane at the artery's division into the right and left common iliac arteries. Thus, from the anteroposterior

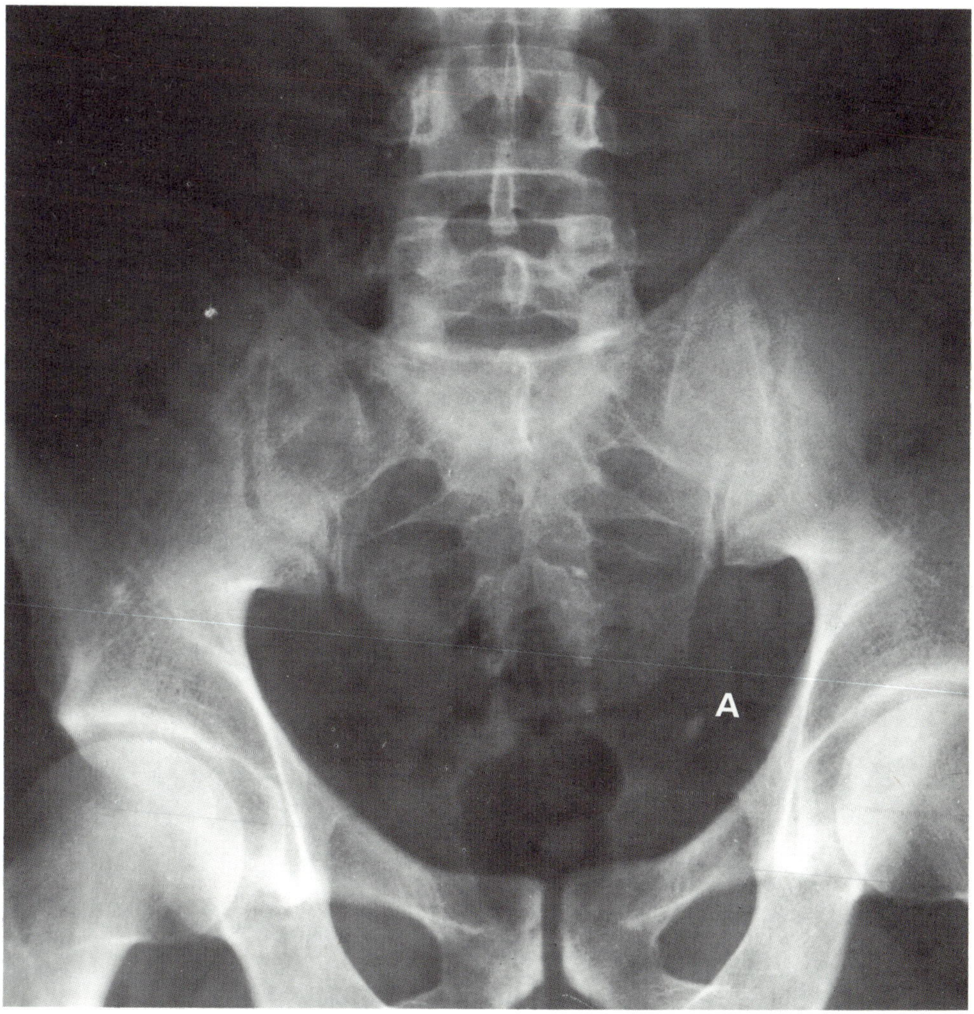

Fig. 5.12. A plain radiograph of the pelvic area.
A A calcific calculus at the lower end of the left ureter

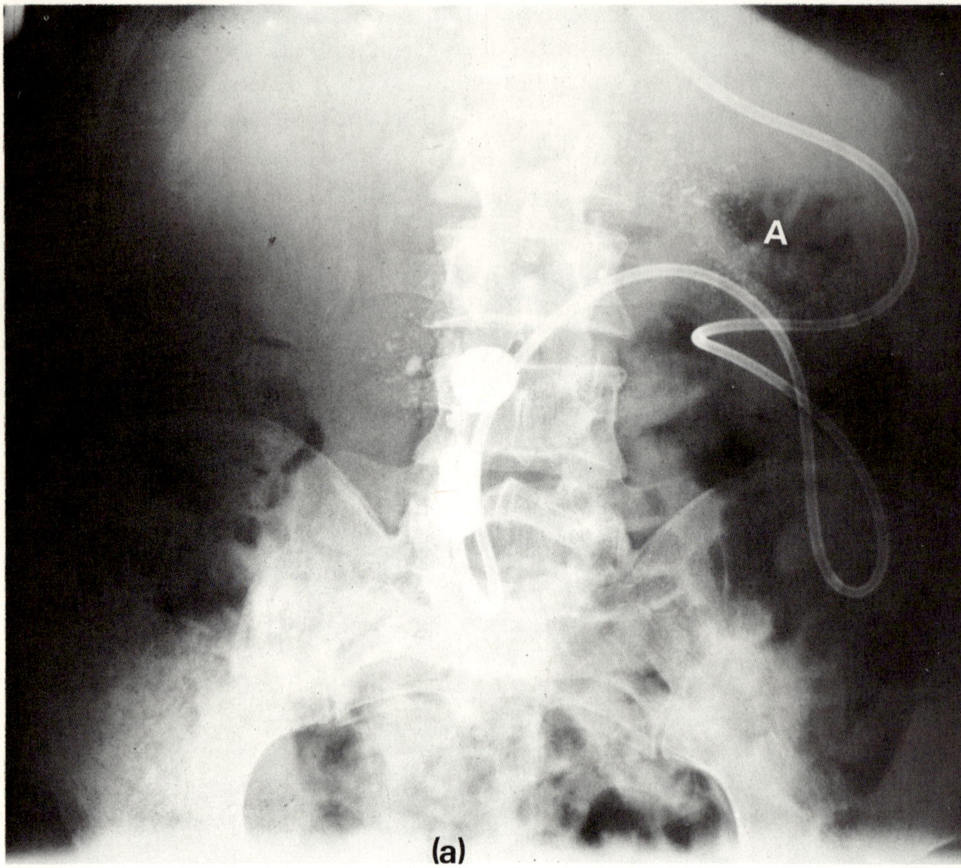

Fig. 5.13a. An anteroposterior radiograph of the upper abdomen. A radiopaque tube is present in the alimentary tract for the purpose of medical investigation.
A Calcification within the pancreas

aspect, the vessel is largely obscured by the vertebral column. Fig. 5.15b shows such calcification in the walls of pelvic arteries which was an incidental finding during radiography.

Other appearances in the abdomen

Opaque swallowed foreign bodies provide various appearances on the plain radiograph of the abdomen which are abnormal, though usually mild enough in consequence. Indeed, for some reason, they often add a certain 'entertainment value' to the

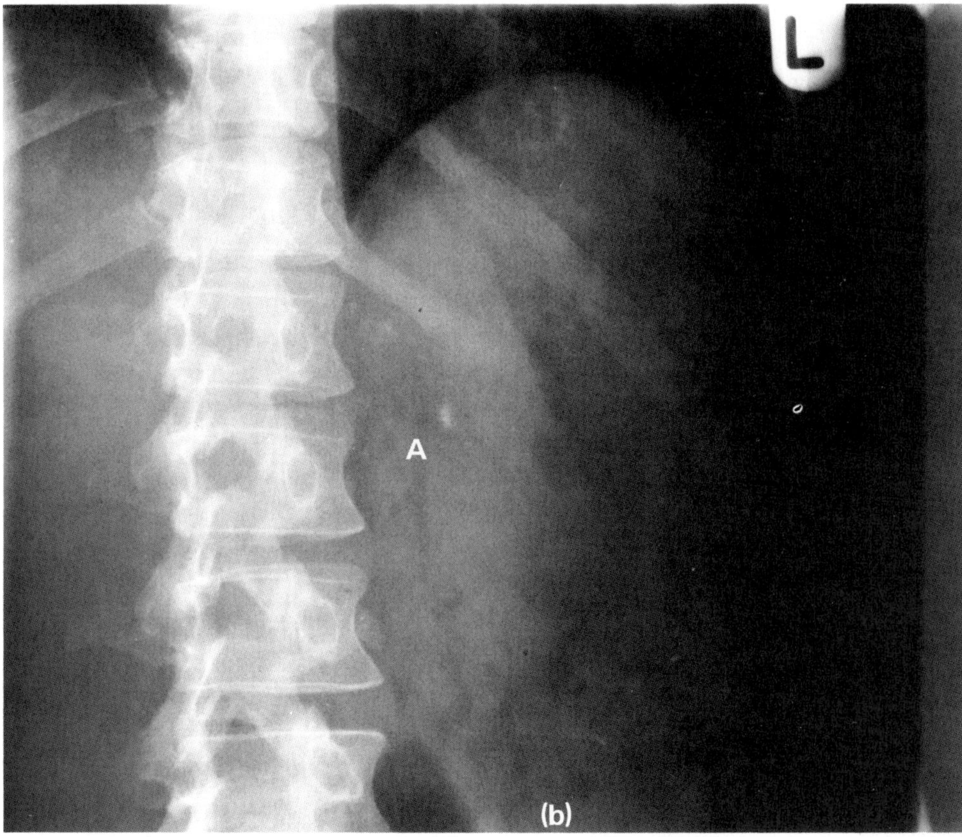

Fig. 5.13b. A left posterior oblique projection of the left upper abdomen.
A Calcification within the pancreas

radiograph: Fig. 5.16, for example, may demonstrate the little-documented, though widely recognised, condition known as 'butterflies in the stomach'.

However, it is normal—and this book is concerned with the normal—from time to time to notice on the abdominal film structures which an anatomist would not recognise as accepted features of the abdominal cavity. Nor are they such. We include them here as they may otherwise provide the student reader of radiographs with an occasional puzzle.

On Fig. 5.17 the sausage-shaped radiolucency lying medial to the right ischial spine is a tampon (for example Tampax) in the vagina. It is demonstrated because—rather unusually—air has entered the vagina during its insertion and is sur-

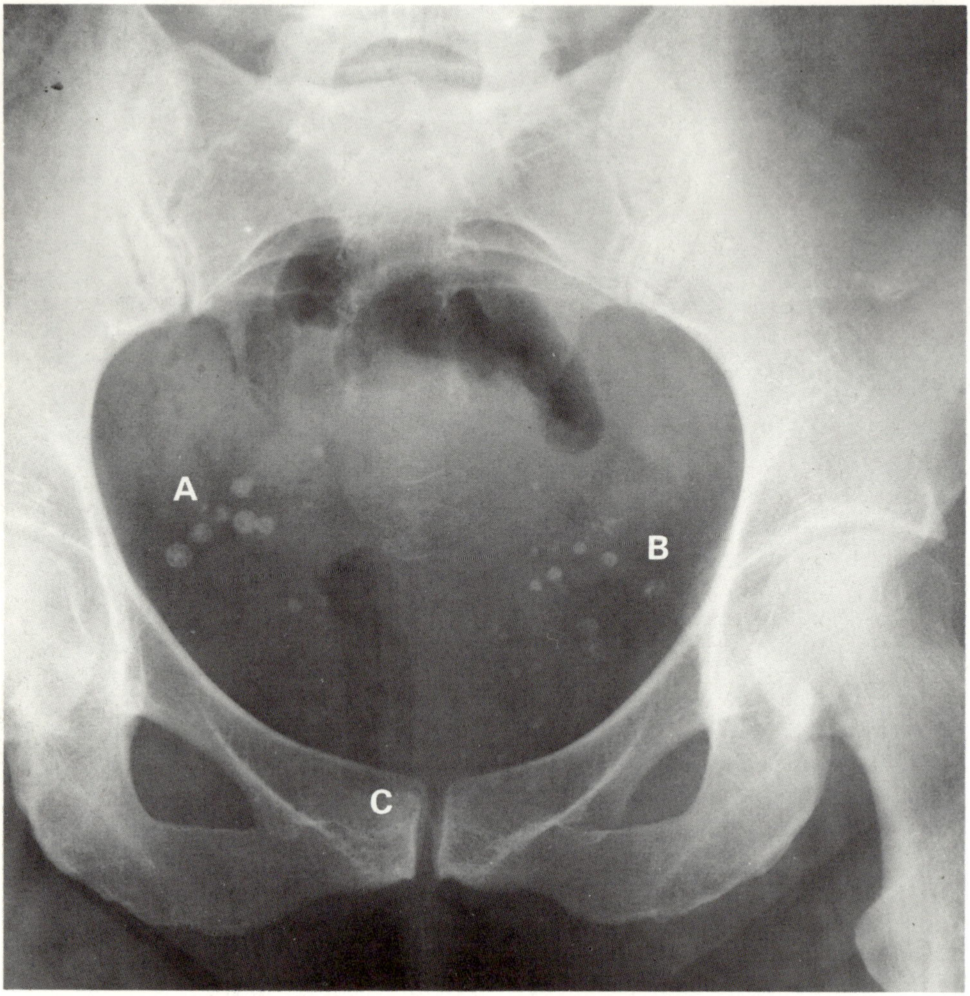

Fig. 5.14. An anteroposterior radiograph of the pelvis.
A, B Pelvic phleboliths
C Vaginal tampon outlined by surrounding air

rounding it. Generally such a tampon provides no radiographic evidence of its presence and there is no need for a menstruating patient to remove it because of an X-ray examination. A similar appearance is to be noticed in Fig. 5.14.

A large annular density is a prominent feature of the pelvic cavity shown on Fig. 5.18. This is a pessary, an instrument which at one time was often placed in the vagina for the

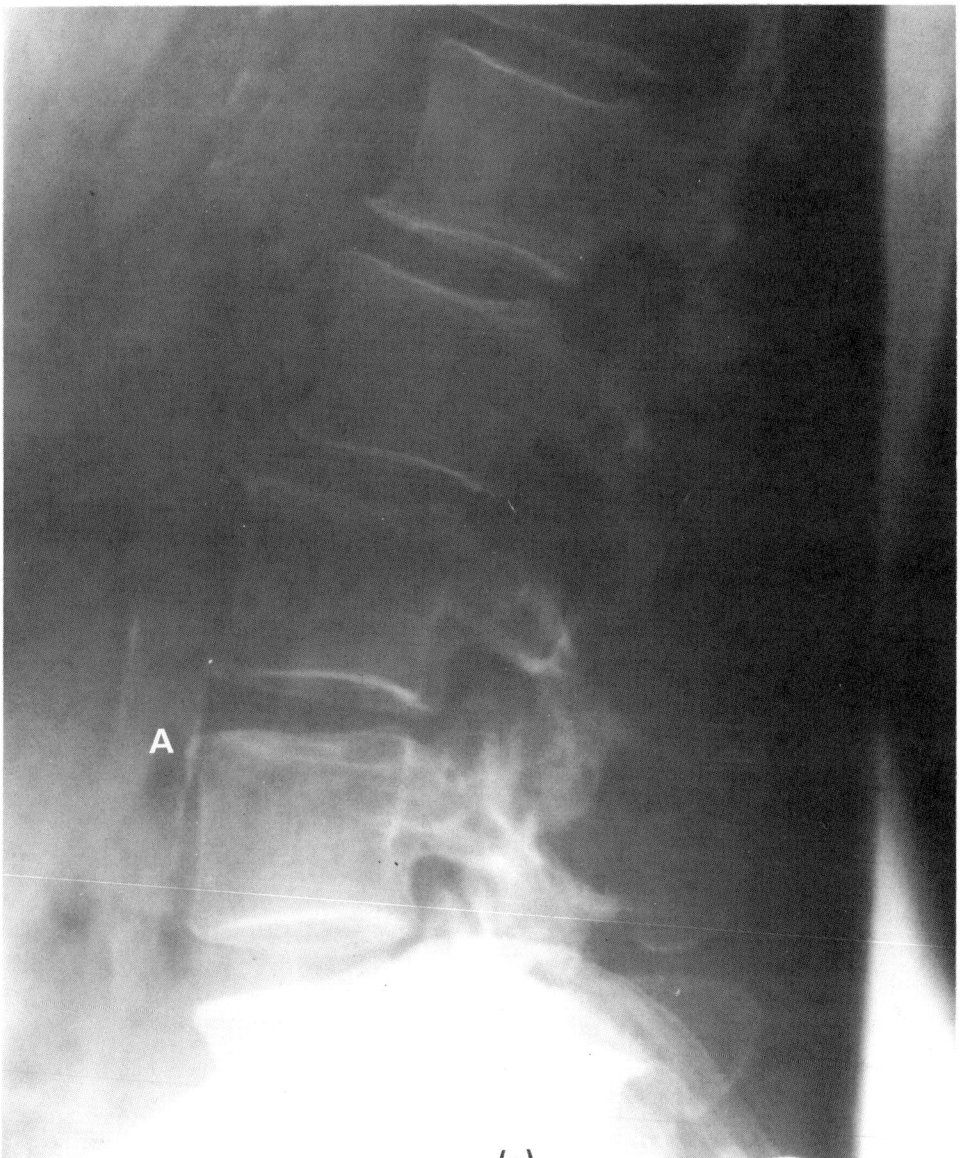

Fig. 5.15a. A lateral radiograph of the lumbar vertebrae.

A The abdominal aorta, demonstrated because its walls contain deposits of calcium (a degenerative change)

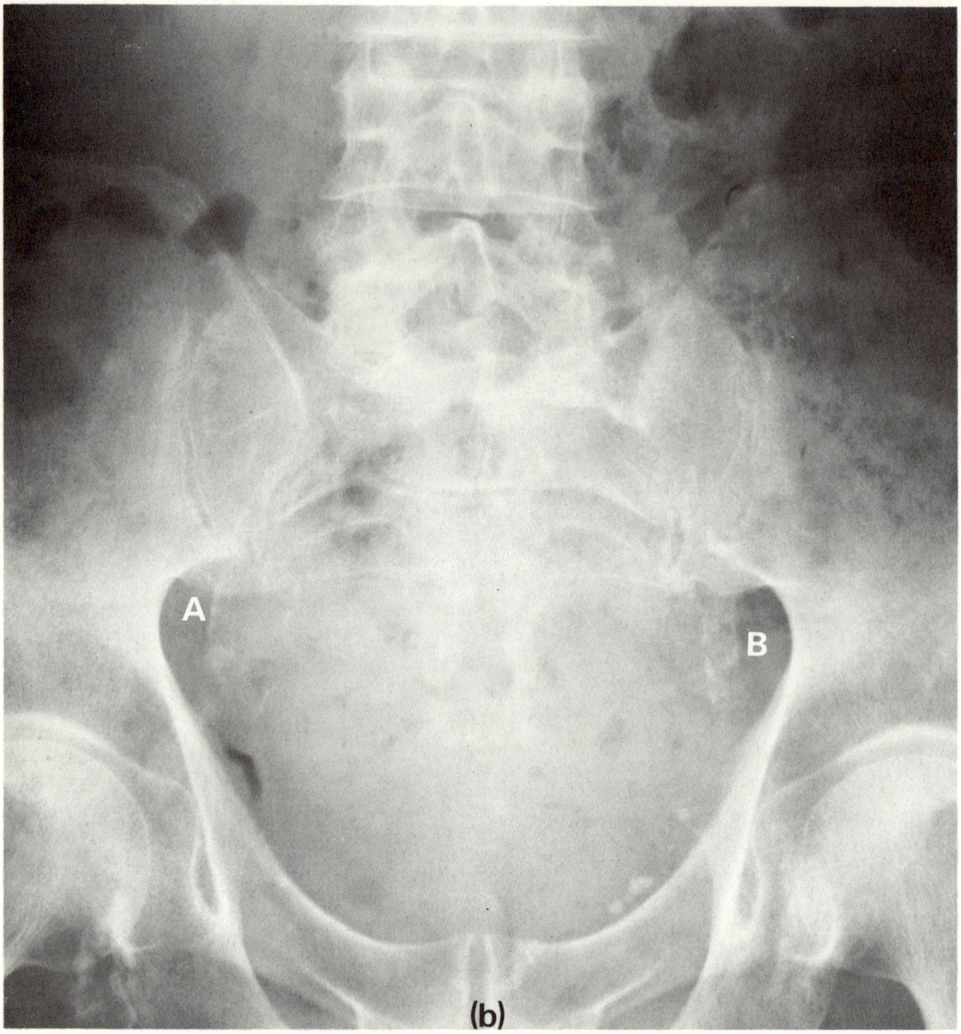

Fig. 5.15b. An anteroposterior radiograph of the pelvis.
A, B Calcium deposits in the walls of pelvic blood vessels

purpose of supporting a prolapsed uterus or rectum. It is now largely in medical disfavour (one of the reasons against it, for example, is that it may establish an infection) and consequently it makes only a rare appearance on contemporary radiographs. When it does so, the patient is virtually certain to be an elderly woman.

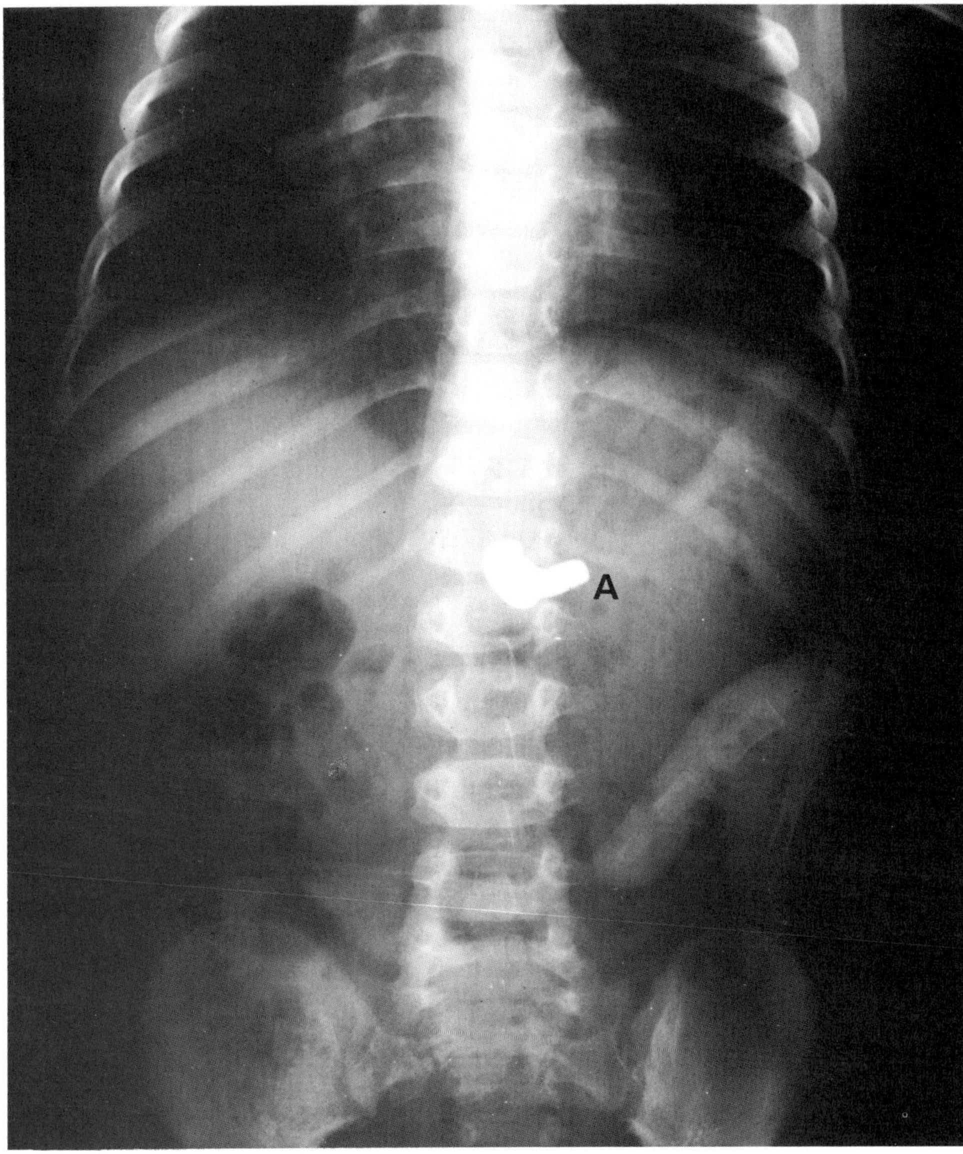

Fig. 5.16. An anteroposterior radiograph of the alimentary tract of a child.
A The image of a butterfly nut which has been swallowed
The image of the patient's left thumb is seen on the left side of the abdomen because his hand was not drawn clear of his trunk before exposure of the radiograph.

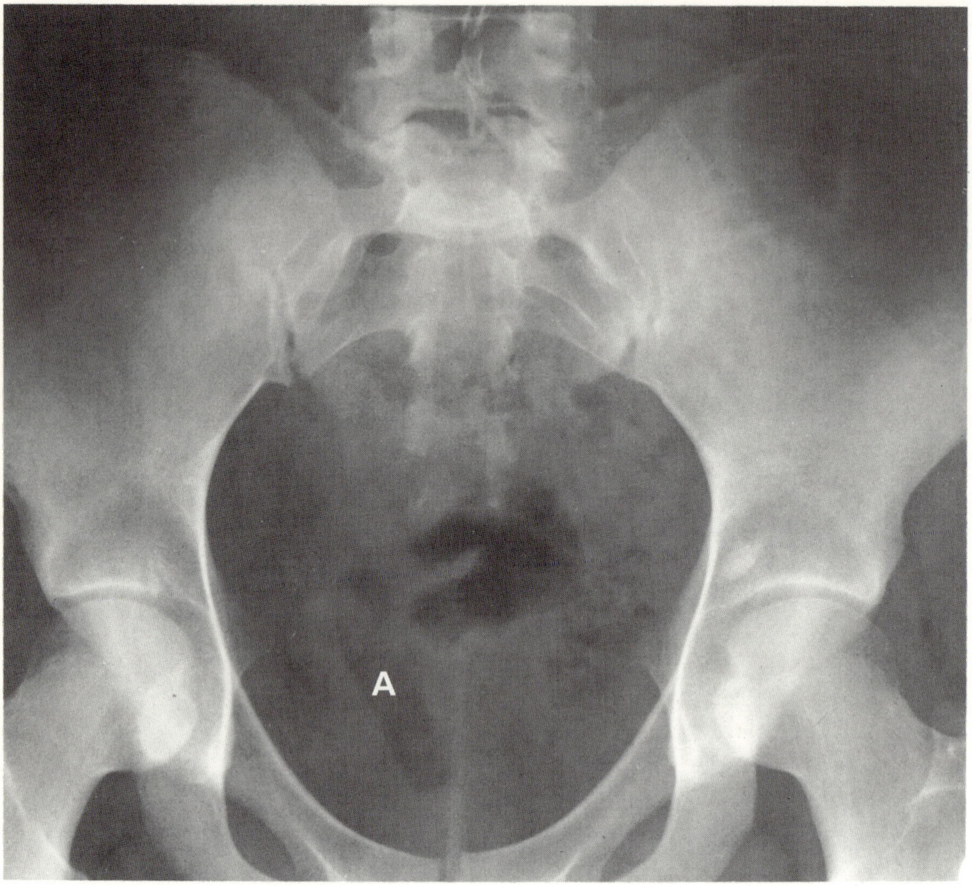

Fig. 5.17. An anteroposterior radiograph of the female pelvis.
A A vaginal tampon, outlined because there is air surrounding it

On Fig. 9.2 two large semi-circular opacities are noticeable in the upper part of each radiograph. These shadows are due to overlap on the abdomen of the female breasts and are likely to be seen on the radiographs of a big-breasted woman who was either prone (Fig. 9.2a) or erect (Fig. 9.2b) during the exposure.

On Fig. 5.19 the dense circular opacity superimposed on the pubic symphysis does not represent a variety of large stone in the bladder. It is due to the chance, end-on projection of the penis of a young male.

Intra-uterine contraceptive devices (IUCD), which are

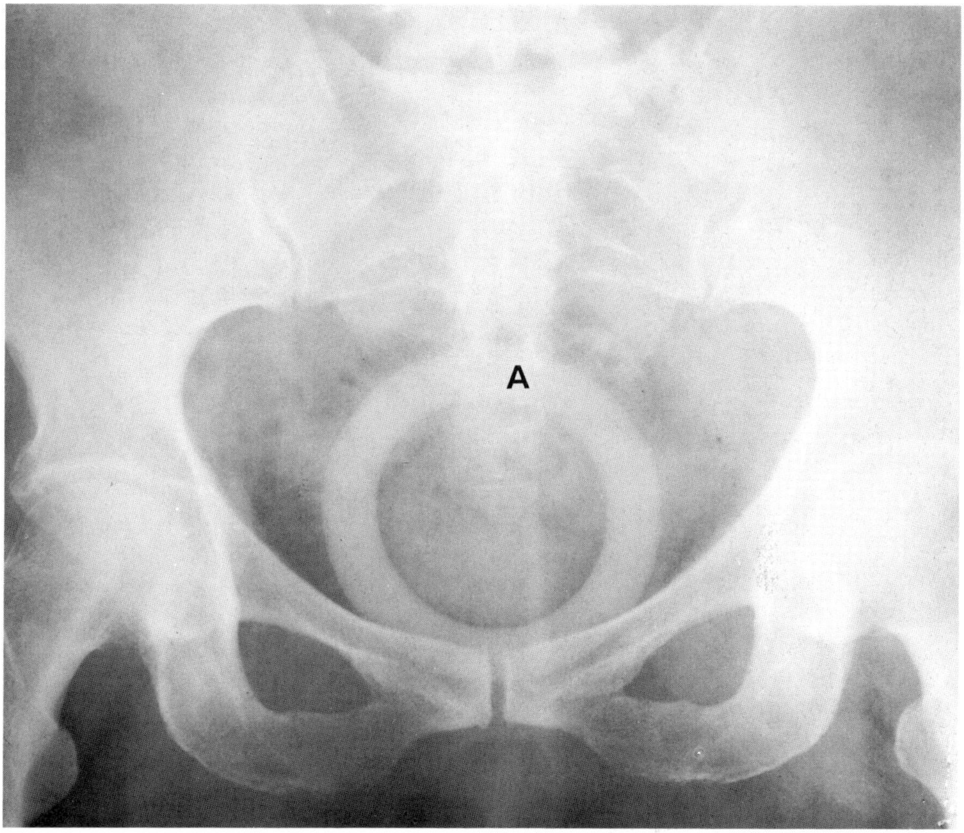

Fig. 5.18. An anteroposterior radiograph of the female pelvis.
A A pessary in the vagina

formed from loops of thin metal, possess expectedly some degree of radiopacity. This characteristic means that a radiograph of the abdomen is an obvious method of locating the device when its 'tail' is not to be seen on vaginal inspection. Sometimes, at X-ray examination of a pregnant woman, an IUCD is to be found occupying the uterus together with a full-term fetus; it is not unknown for there to be even two IUCD's alongside the youngster! In other patients the presence of an IUCD may be noticed as an incidental appearance during radiography of the abdomen, lumbosacral vertebrae or hip bones. Fig. 5.20 shows one variety of such a device from both anteroposterior and lateral aspects.

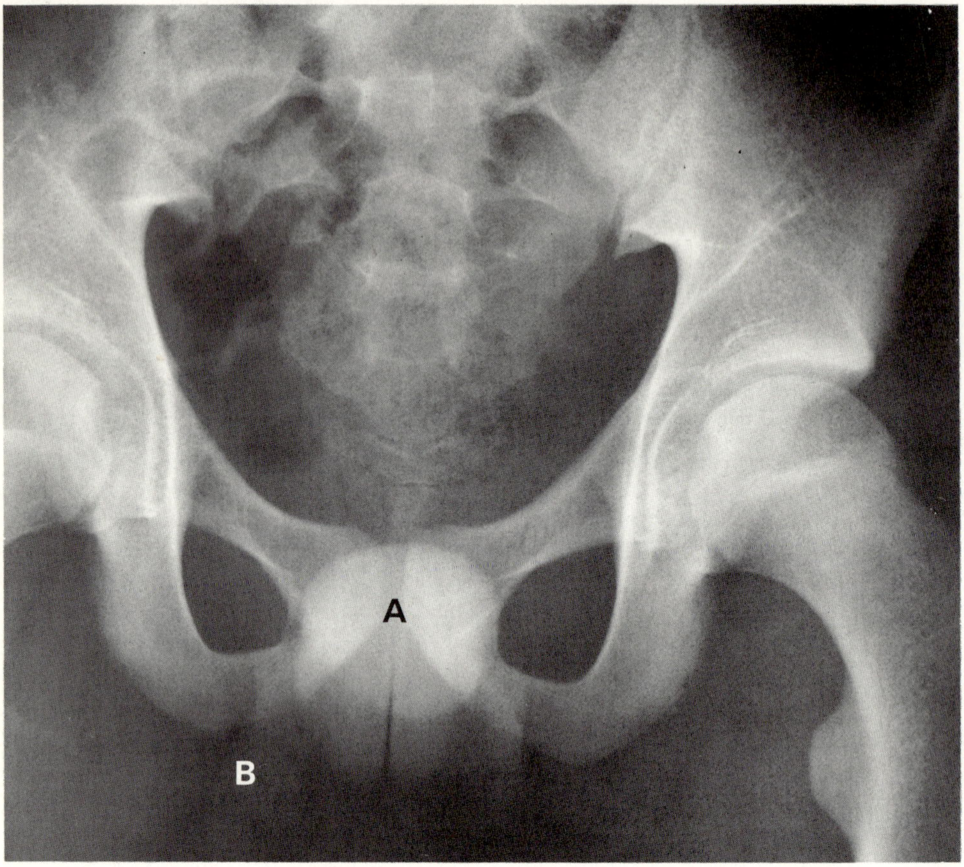

Fig. 5.19. An anteroposterior radiograph of the male pelvis.
A The penis projected 'end-on' by the X-ray beam
B The scrotum

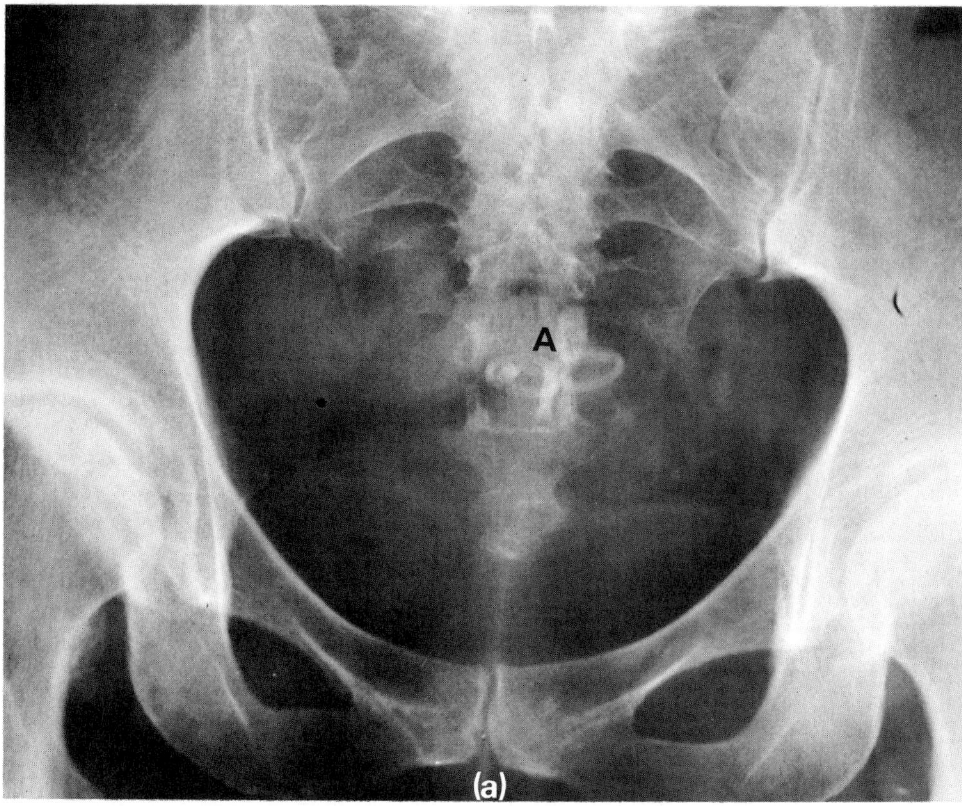

Fig. 5.20a. An anteroposterior radiograph of the female pelvis.
A An intra-uterine contraceptive device

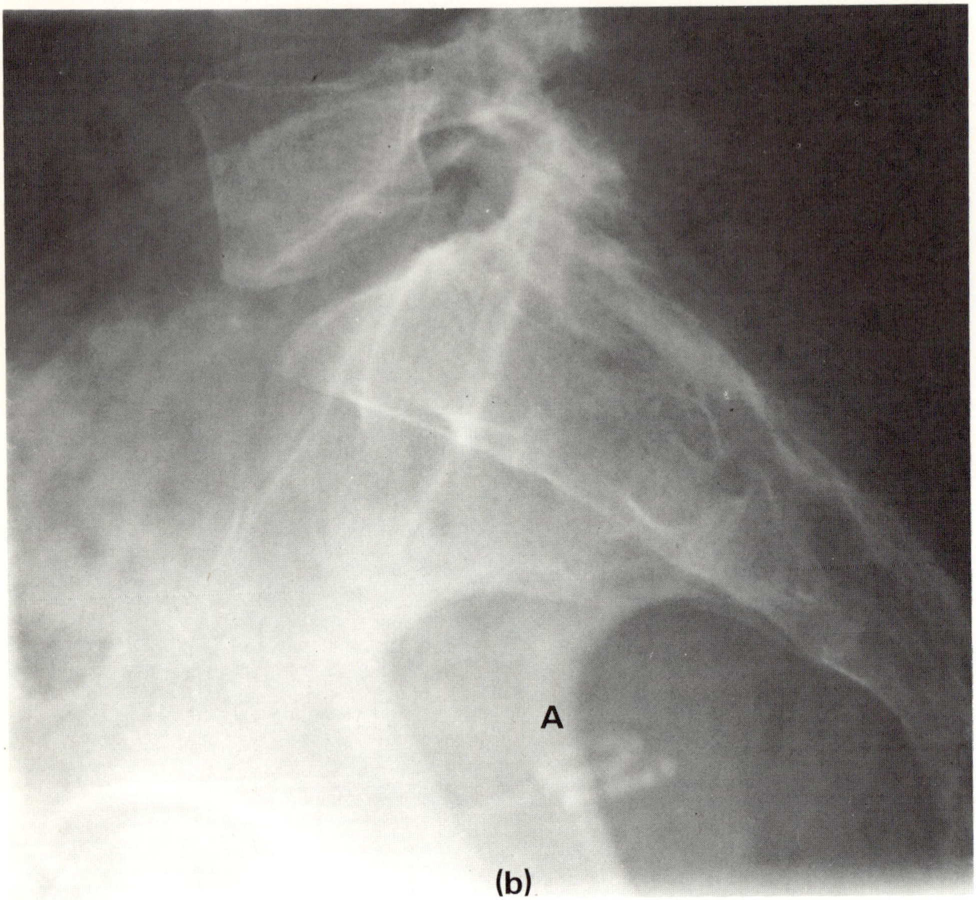

Fig. 5.20b. A lateral radiograph of the lumbosacral region of a woman.
A An intra-uterine contraceptive device

Chapter 6
Contrast Examinations: The Stomach and Small Bowel

The stomach

X-ray examination of the stomach is usually made by means of a barium meal; this term is doubly a misnomer, since the contrast agent given is not barium but barium sulphate and certainly provides no food to the patient. It is, however, taken by mouth in the form of a drink, the procedure being observed radiologically on a fluoroscopic screen.

Without the introduction of a contrast agent, the alimentary tube as a whole is not distinguishable on a radiograph of the abdominal cavity. When air is swallowed—as it naturally is in many circumstances—gastric mucosal patterns may often be recognised (see Chapter 5, p. 118) but this is a matter of chance and results in no more than a fragmentary demonstration of the organ.

The stomach is a length of the digestive tube between the oesophagus and the small bowel and is its most dilated part: the volume of the stomach varies within the limits of health probably more than is true of any other viscus. As a rule the stomach occupies some part of the following abdominal regions: the epigastrium; the umbilical region; the left hypochondrium. However, the position and shape of the stomach are greatly affected by changes in the organ itself and in surrounding viscera: it is hardly possible to describe one position and one form as totally characteristic.

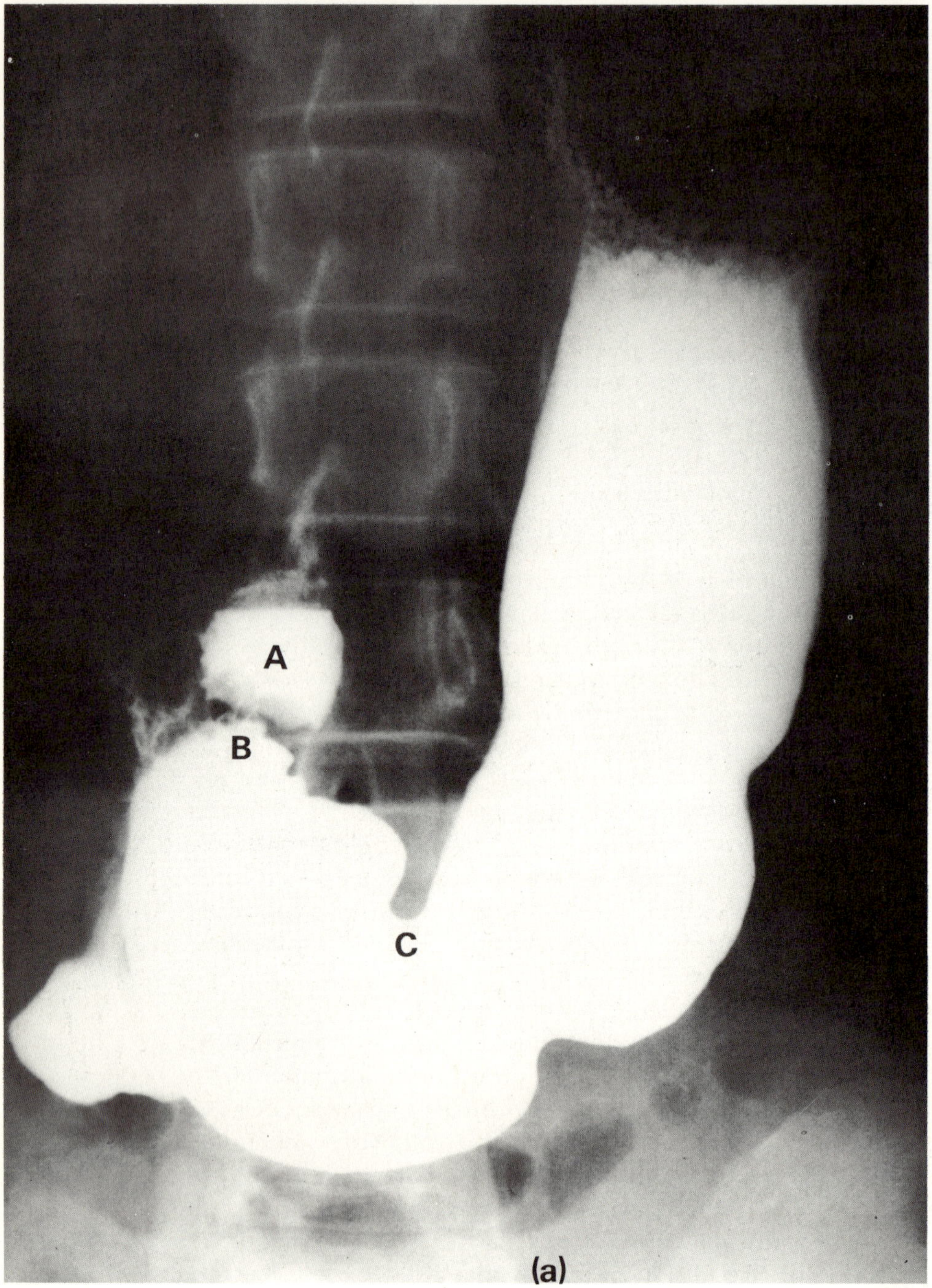

Fig. 6.1a. An erect anteroposterior immediate radiograph of the stomach after a barium meal.

A 1st part of duodenum
B Pylorus
C Incisura

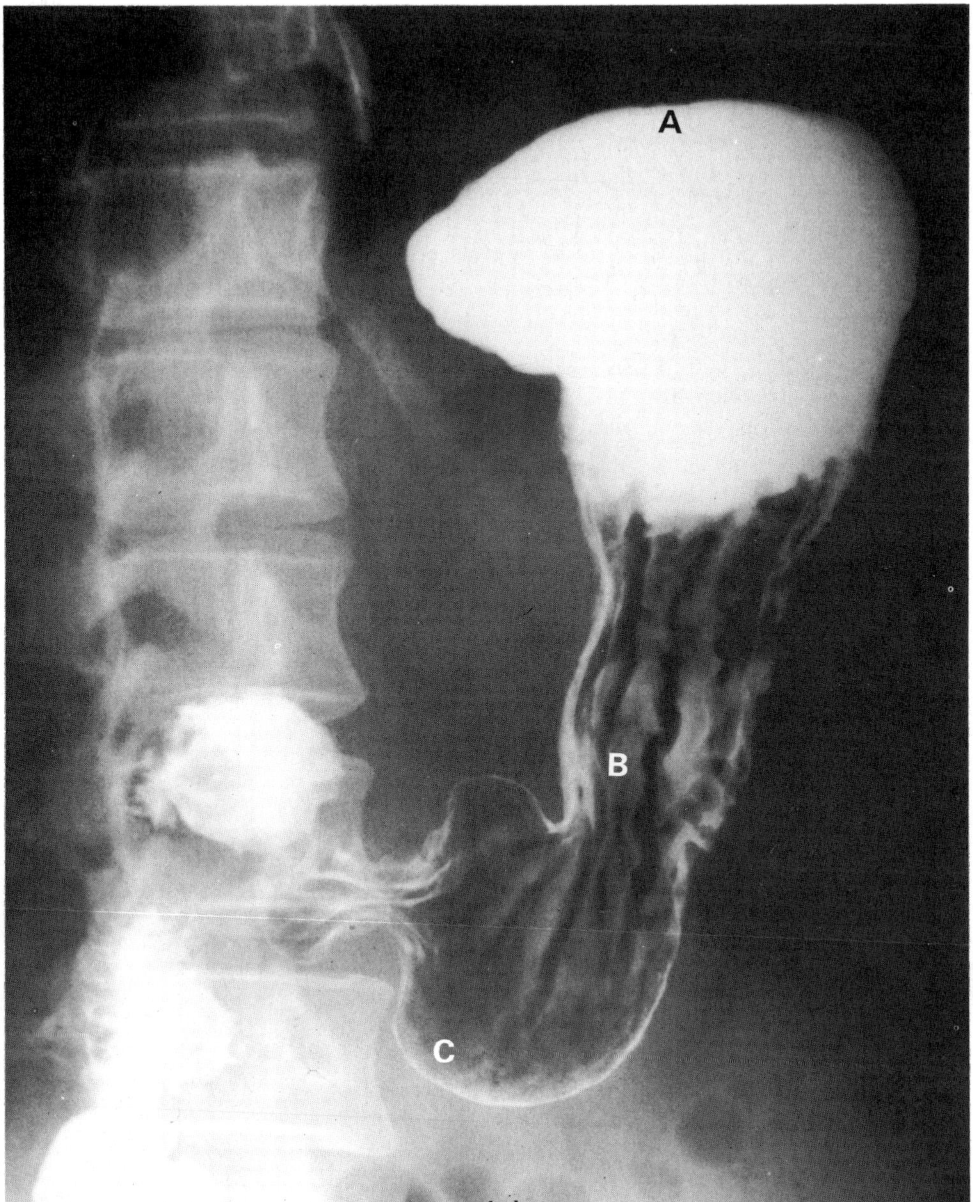

Fig. 6.1b. A supine oblique immediate radiograph of the stomach after a barium meal.

A Gastric fundus
B Rugae in the body of the stomach
C Pyloric part of the stomach

Fig. 6.1a is a posteroanterior radiograph of the barium-filled stomach, exposed when the patient was standing erect. The stomach is seen here to be more or less J-shaped. Its upper limit is at the level of thoracic vertebra 12 and its lowest part overlies lumbar vertebra 5. Other normal gastric forms have been described: there is the steer-horn stomach which takes a transverse position across the abdomen; another example is the elongated stomach, dependent to the pelvic part of the abdominal cavity and sometimes described as having a fish-hook shape.

In Fig. 6.1b the same patient as in 6.1a was X-rayed whilst lying supine and rotated to the left. The stomach appears to be narrower because it contains much less barium. Although its upper end is mainly fixed by the relationship of this part to the oesophagus and the left dome of the diaphragm, the body of the stomach in this instance is some two or three inches higher than in Fig. 6.1a.

We may at this point usefully compare and contrast the features of Fig. 6.2a, b and c which illustrate what may happen to the apparent form of the stomach when a patient changes from the erect position to supine and then to prone recumbency.

Erect. Posteroanterior projection, Fig. 6.2a. Configuration and contours of the stomach are generally well seen.

Upper surface of the contrast agent makes a fluid level, with the normal air bubble in the gastric fundus (see p. 121) lying above it.

The stomach appears relatively long.

Supine. Posteroanterior projection, Fig. 6.2b. The stomach appears relatively shorter and has divided to either side of the vertebral column because of the pull of gravity. This effect makes it easy to distinguish such a radiograph from another taken when the patient was prone.

Barium now fills the fundus of the stomach beneath the diaphragm. The gastric air bubble disappears from the fundus and moves towards the distal part of the stomach.

Prone. Anteroposterior projection, Fig. 6.2c. When the patient lies face downwards a self-compression of the abdominal tissues is obtained.

Barium flows towards the pylorus (see p. 153), filling and

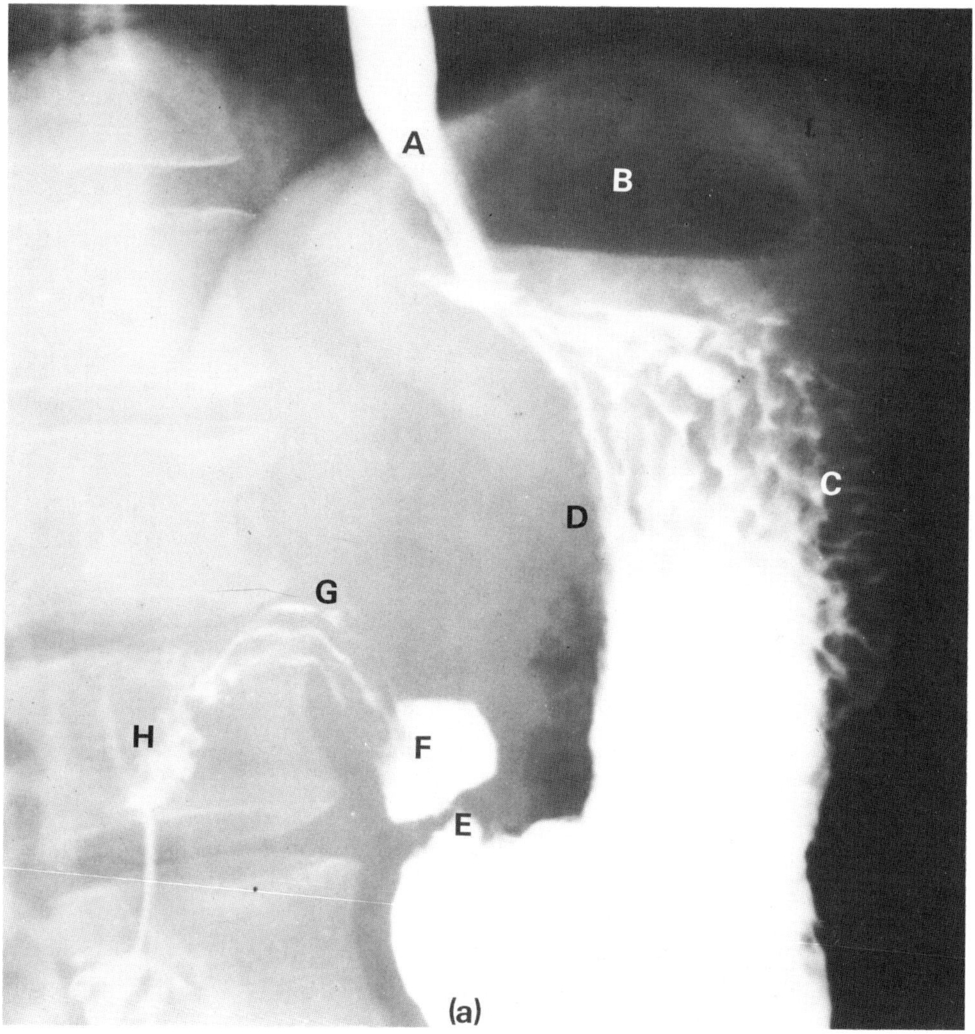

Fig. 6.2a. An erect oblique radiograph taken during the administration of a barium meal.

A Oesophagus
B Gastric fundus containing swallowed air
C Rugae on the greater curvature of the stomach
D Lesser gastric curvature
E Pyloric canal
F 1st part of duodenum
G Superior duodenal flexure
H 2nd part of the duodenum

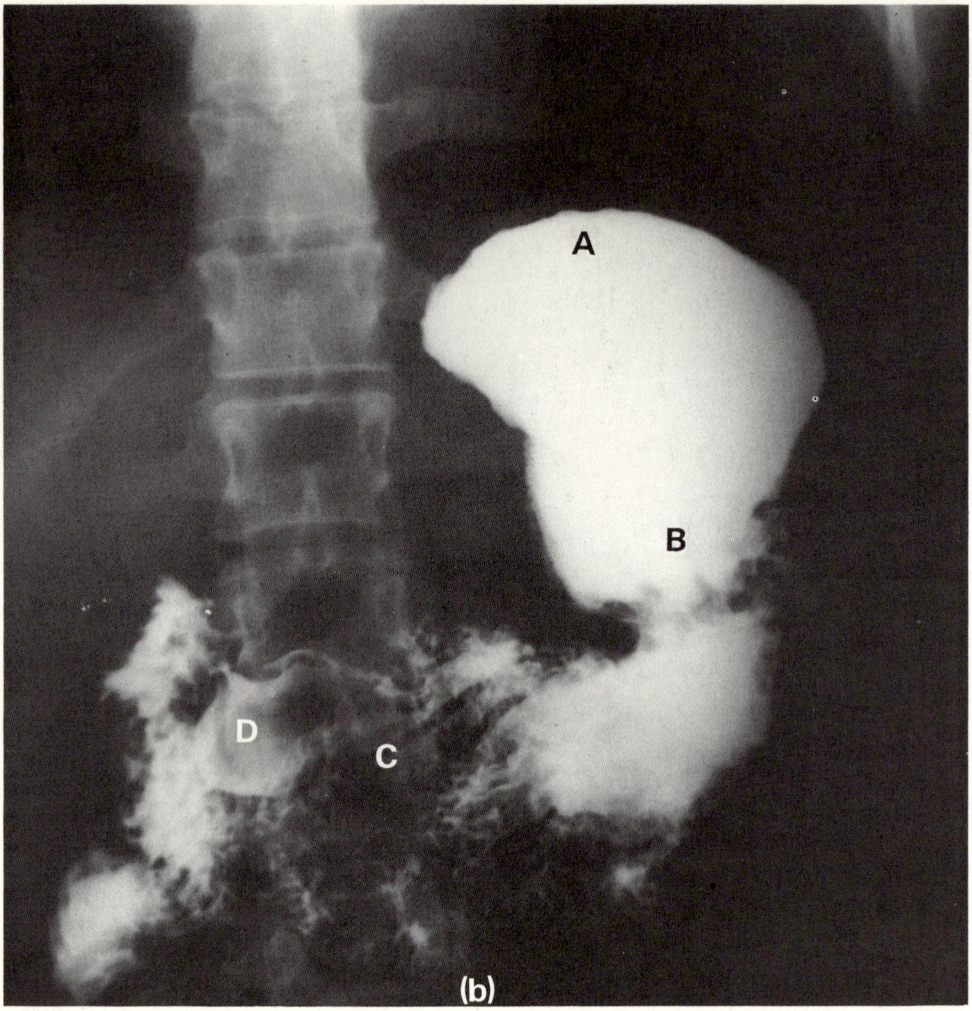

Fig. 6.2b. A supine posteroanterior immediate radiograph after a barium meal.

A Gastric fundus
B Body of the stomach
C Gastric rugae
D Pyloric antrum

distending the distal part of the body of the stomach. The gastric air bubble tends to reappear at the fundus.

Apart from radiographic positioning, factors which significantly influence the stomach's form and position include: (i) the amount of its contents;

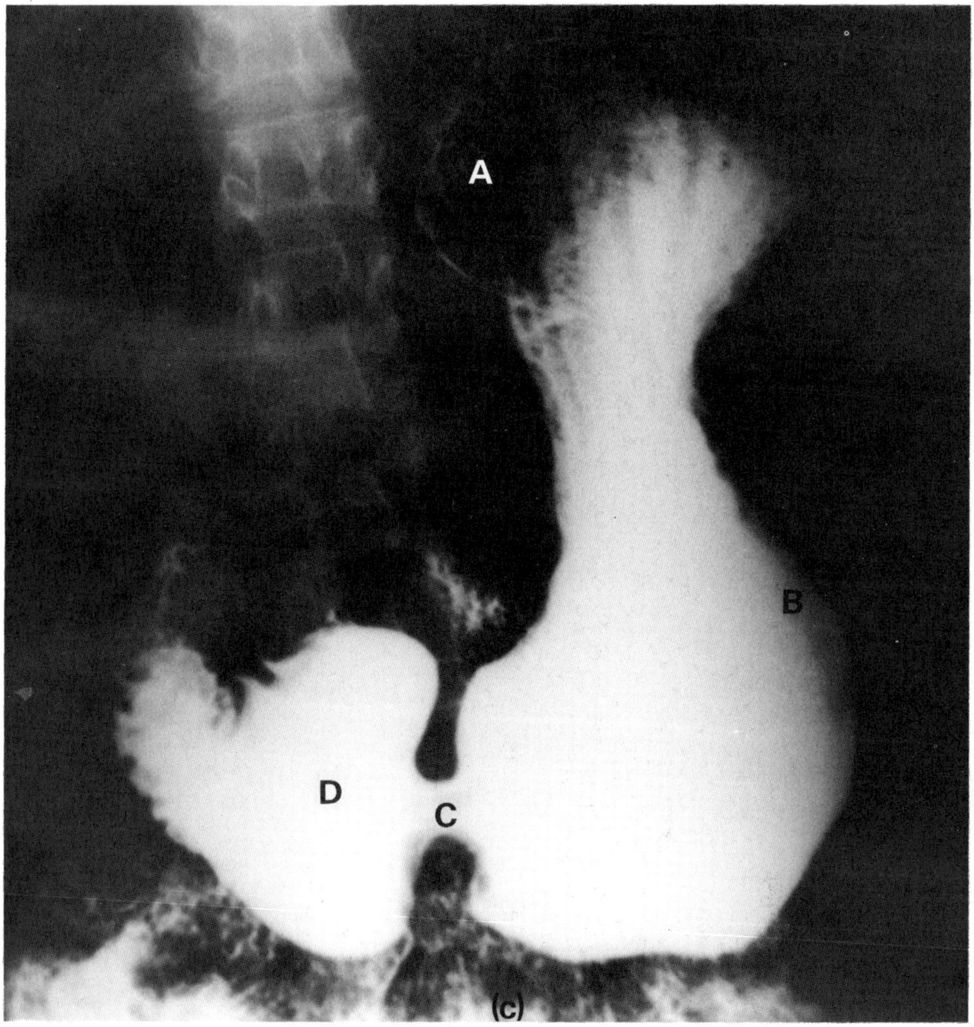

Fig. 6.2c. A prone anteroposterior immediate radiograph after a barium meal. This is the same patient as in Plate 6.2(b).

A Air in the fundus of the stomach

B Greater curvature of the stomach

C A contraction due to a wave of peristalsis

D Pyloric part of the antrum

(ii) the stage of digestion;

(iii) the tone of the abdominal musculature (a lax abdominal wall may be accompanied by a long atonic stomach of the fish-hook shape, as in Fig. 6.3);

(iv) the condition of the adjacent intestines and other organs (for example, the pregnant uterus may displace the stomach upwards).

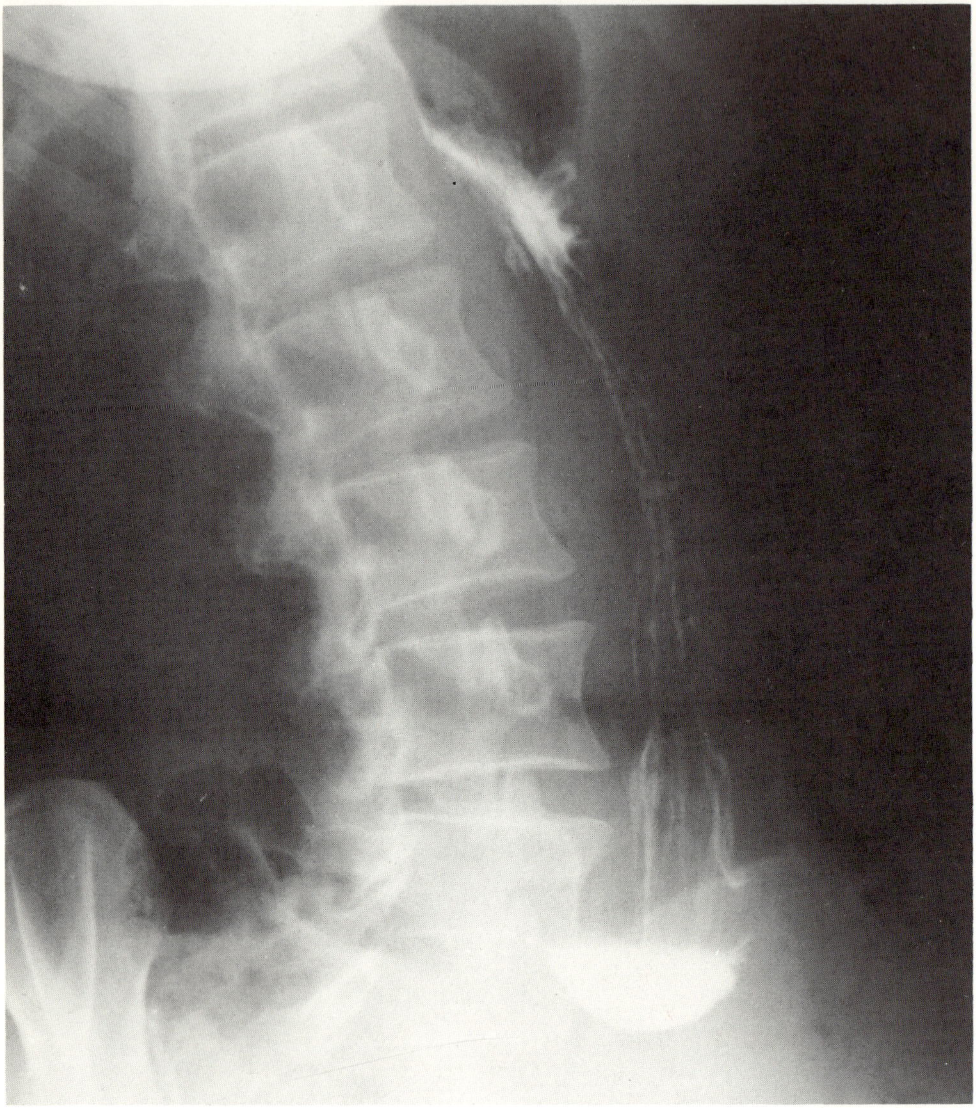

Fig. 6.3. An erect right anterior oblique immediate radiograph after a barium meal. The stomach is of the elongated 'fish hook' type.

THE OPENINGS OF THE STOMACH

The stomach has two openings:
(i) the cardiac orifice at its upper end;
(ii) the pyloric orifice or pylorus, which communicates with the duodenum distally.

The cardiac orifice is the opening through which the oesophagus communicates with the stomach. There is a short abdominal portion of the oesophagus (see Fig. 6.2a), about 2.5 cm long, curving to the left and conical in shape, the base of the cone being continuous with the cardiac orifice. This orifice consequently is to the left of the median plane: it lies behind the seventh left costal cartilage and is at the level of the eleventh thoracic vertebra. The part of the stomach which is above and to the left of the cardiac orifice (see Fig. 6.2a) is called the fundus.

The pyloric orifice is the opening from the stomach to the small bowel, of which the first part is the duodenum. This orifice lies very slightly to the right of the median plane at a level which—depending on the subject and his situation—may range from the lower border of lumbar vertebra 1 to the same reference line on lumbar vertebra 3.

The pyloric orifice is associated with a sphincter, similarly named and composed of an aggregated ring of the circular muscle fibres of the stomach (in this region the circular muscle fibres are especially plentiful).

THE CURVATURES OF THE STOMACH

The stomach is considered to possess two curvatures, a lesser curvature and a greater curvature. The lesser curvature of the stomach (see Fig. 6.2a) begins above as a continuation of the right margin of the oesophagus and descends on a line—somewhat convex to the left—to the pyloric orifice. At the lowest part of the curve there is a sharp notch, the incisura (see, for example, Fig. 6.1). The lesser curvature constitutes the right and posterior border of the stomach.

The greater curvature which forms the left and anterior border of the stomach (see Fig. 6.2c and others), is about four times longer than the lesser curvature. It corresponds to a line which may be drawn from the cardiac orifice over the summit of the fundus and then passes downwards and forwards, with some convexity to the left. Opposite the incisura the greater curvature bulges (see Fig. 6.1a); turning to the right it ends, like the lesser curvature, at the pylorus.

THE PARTS OF THE STOMACH

For convenience of description the stomach is considered in three parts (see Fig. 6.4):
(i) the fundus, which lies above a plane through the cardiac orifice;
(ii) the body, a large portion to the left of a line drawn from the incisura to the left limit of the opposed prominence of the greater curvature;
(iii) the pyloric part, a much smaller region to the right of this same line.

The pyloric part of the stomach is subdivided into:
(i) the pyloric antrum, which is the lowest part of the stomach and may bulge considerably when it is distended;
(ii) the pyloric canal, a short, relatively more fixed passage, about 1 cm in length, which is the lumen of the pyloric sphincter.

Radiologically a firm distinction between the pyloric antrum and the body of the stomach often cannot—and perhaps should not—be made, because the shape of the organ varies greatly in different circumstances: for example when a patient is recumbent the incisura tends to disappear as the lesser curvature becomes straighter.

THE COVERINGS OF THE STOMACH

The stomach wall is composed of four coats. These are: (i) serous; (ii) muscular; (iii) submucous; (iv) mucous. They are discussed briefly below.

Serous coat

The serous coat of the stomach is the visceral layer of the peritoneum which covers almost the entire outer surface of the organ. There is a small bare patch near the cardiac orifice

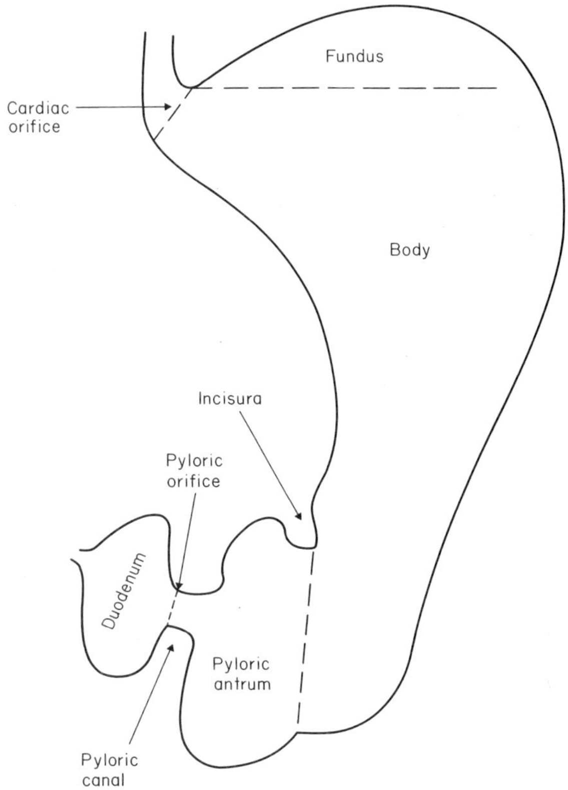

Fig. 6.4. The parts of the stomach.

where the stomach is in contact with the lower surface of the diaphragm. Another narrow space, which contains vessels and nerves, is present along the lines of reflection on the curvatures of the stomach of the greater and lesser peritoneal omenta.

Muscular coat

The muscular coat is connected closely to the serous covering and consists of three layers of fibres. Counting from the superficial to the deep these are: (i) longitudinal fibres; (ii) circular fibres; (iii) oblique fibres. The distribution and thickness of these fibres vary severally in different parts of the stomach.

Submucous coat

The submucous coat of the stomach is composed of loose areolar connective tissue, serving to join the muscular and mucous layers.

Mucous coat

The mucous membrane which lines the stomach is thick, soft and riddled with numerous minute depressions caused by the ducts of gastric glands. These are much too small to be visible on a radiograph.

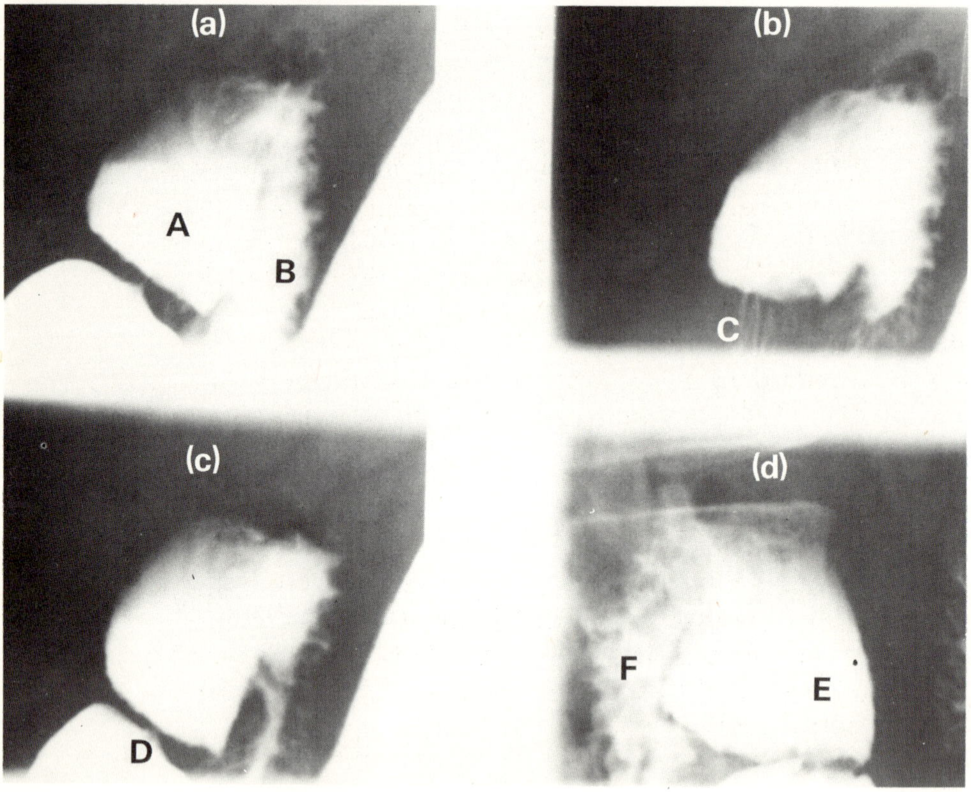

Fig. 6.5. Serial radiographs of the duodenal cap taken during a barium meal. **a**, **b** and **c** are left anterior oblique projections; **d** is a right anterior oblique projection.

A 1st part of the duodenum
B 2nd part of the duodenum
C Rugae in the pyloric canal
D Pylorus
E 1st part of the duodenum
F 2nd part of the duodenum

What is apparent radiologically is that when the stomach is empty and contracted its mucous membrane becomes folded longitudinally in a series of ridges or rugae, particularly on the posterior wall where they are densely convoluted (see Fig. 6.2a). On the lesser curve, a few—three to six—long rugae are seen (for example on Fig. 6.1b) running through the whole body of the stomach to the pyloric antrum. Gastric rugae are seen also on Figs. 6.2a and b, 6.3, 6.5b (in the pyloric canal), 6.6 and 6.7.

GASTRIC PERISTALSIS

Peristalsis is the worm-like movement of tubular organs which is characterised by alternating waves of contraction and relaxation. In the barium-filled stomach peristaltic waves normally occur at the rate of about three a minute and this motor activity much influences the general configuration of the stomach. The wave of movement is initiated in the body and sweeps towards the pylorus: it is most clearly seen in the pyloric antrum. Such a peristaltic wave, affecting the pyloric antrum, and the resultant changes which occur in the shape of the stomach are demonstrated on Fig. 6.2c. It is a further reminder that radiographic anatomy is daily concerned with the living and the lively and seldom with the dead and immutable.

The small bowel

The small intestine is the longest part (about 6·5 m) of the digestive tube. It extends from the gastric pylorus to the ileocaecal valve on the posteromedial wall of the caecum; at this orifice the small bowel enters and becomes continuous with the large. The small intestine is a very convoluted tube, of gradually diminishing calibre, which is coiled in the central and lower parts of the abdominal cavity, mainly within the arch of the large intestine (see for example Fig. 6.6). It has three recognisable parts:

(i) the duodenum;
(ii) the jejunum;
(iii) the ileum.

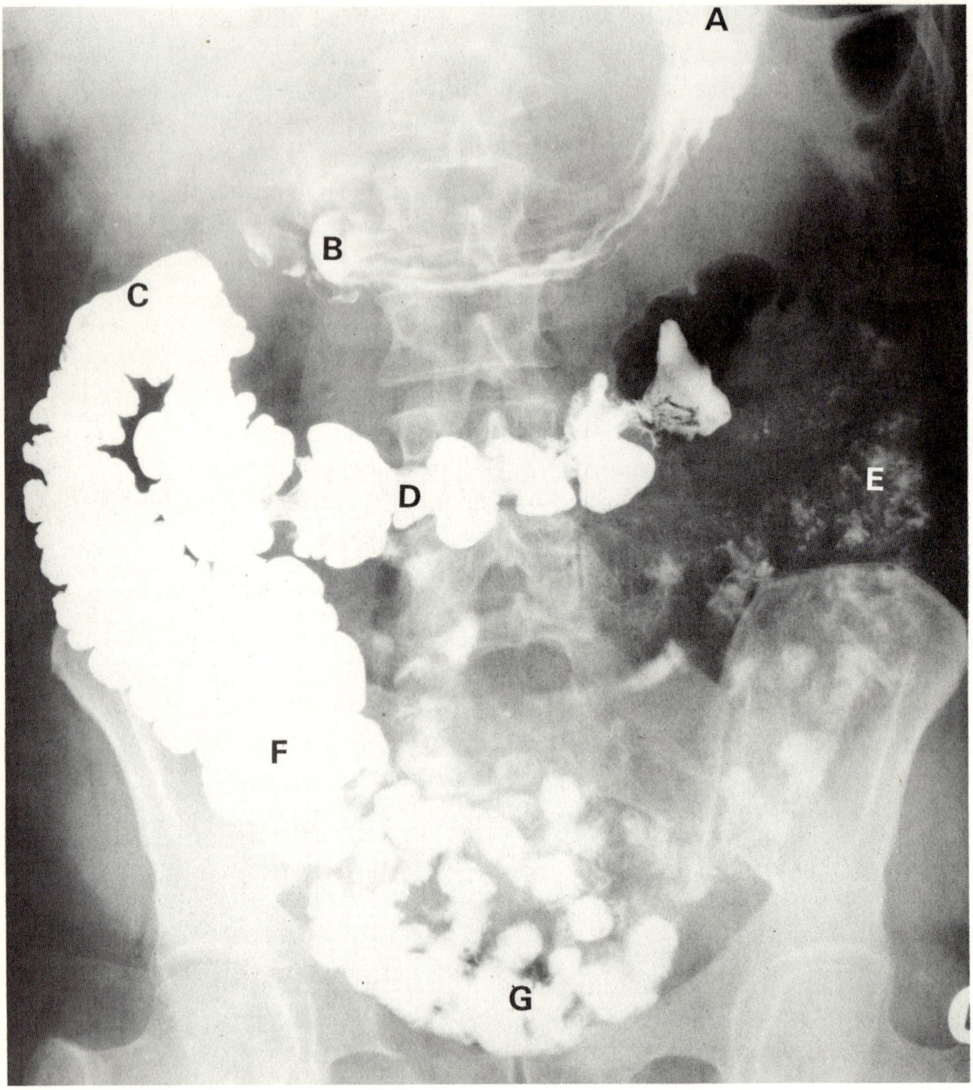

Fig. 6.6. A posteroanterior radiograph of the abdomen, exposed two hours after the administration of a barium meal. It illustrates the relationship of the stomach to parts of the gut, indicating the general arrangement of loops of small bowel within the arch formed by the large bowel.

A Body of the stomach
B Pyloric antrum
C Hepatic flexure of colon
D Transverse colon
E Barium residue in the jejunum
F Ascending colon
G Coils of ileum

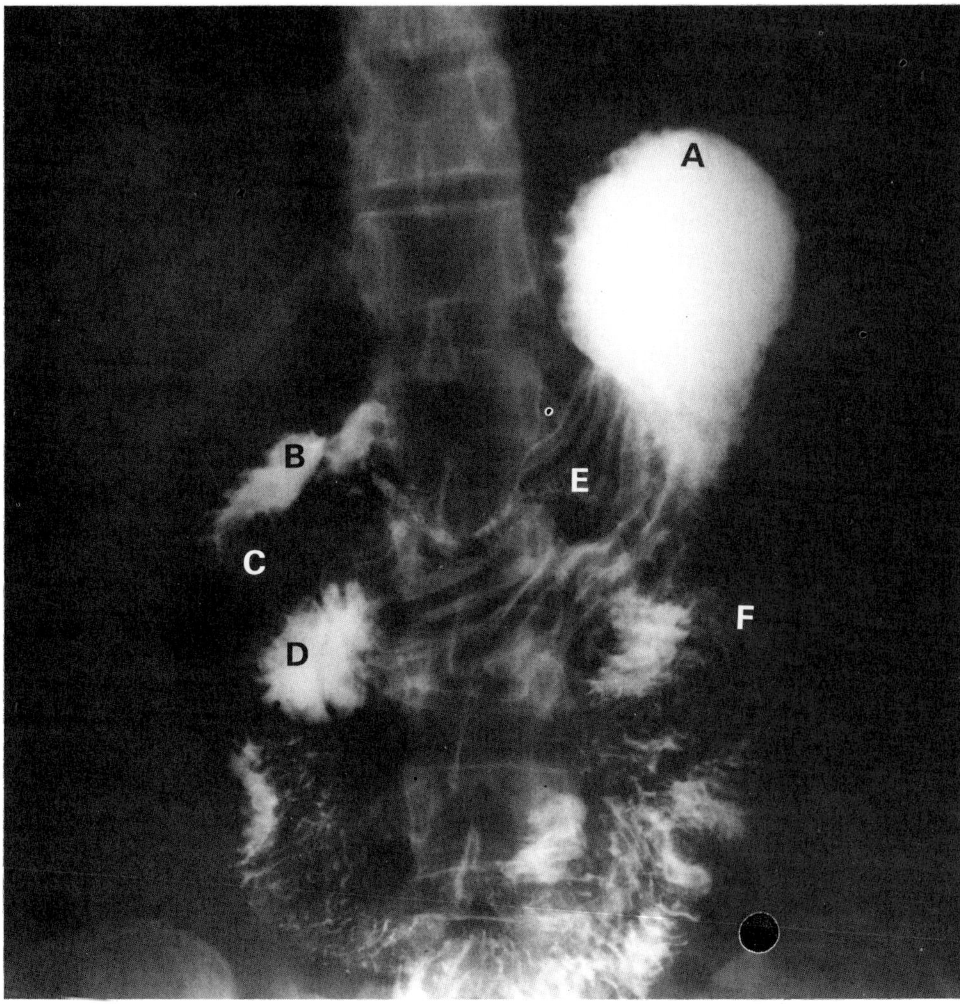

Fig. 6.7. A supine posteroanterior radiograph exposed very shortly after a barium meal.

A Gastric fundus
B Superior duodenal flexure
C 2nd part of the duodenum
D Inferior duodenal flexure
E Duodeno-jejunal flexure, visualised through the linear pattern formed by gastric rugae
F Coils of jejunum

STRUCTURE OF THE SMALL BOWEL

The wall of the small intestine is similar to the wall of the stomach in that it consists of four coats:

(i) a serous coat formed by the peritoneum;
(ii) a muscular coat, composed of external longitudinal fibres and inner circular fibres, which is thicker in the upper part of the small bowel than it is in the lower;
(iii) a submucous coat of areolar tissue containing blood vessels, lymph vessels and nerves;
(iv) a mucous membrane, which is thick and very vascular in the upper part relative to the lower part of the small intestine.

This mucous membrane possesses certain noteworthy structures which vary severally in incidence and to some extent in character, depending on the region of the bowel considered. These features include:
(i) circular folds, which are large transverse folds of the lining projecting into the intestinal lumen and retarding the passage of food, so as to increase absorption during the processes of digestion;
(ii) intestinal villi, which are very small vascular processes projecting from the mucous membrane and increasing its effective surface area, again so that absorption during digestion is aided;
(iii) lymphatic nodules, which may be either solitary or aggregated in groups known as Peyer's patches;
(iv) tubular glands which secrete mucus.

THE DUODENUM

The duodenum is the most proximal, the most fixed in position and the shortest and widest part of the small bowel. It owes its Latin name to an historic measurement which made its length equal to the total breadth of 12 fingers (25 cm). For descriptive purposes the duodenum is considered to have four parts which are explained below.

The first part

The first part of the duodenum arises at the gastric pylorus. The most mobile of the duodenum's four parts, it passes backwards, upwards and to the right, at an angle which—viewed from the anteroposterior direction—may have any value between the two extremes of vertical and horizontal.

This first part of the duodenum shows a characteristic X-ray appearance which differs from the form in which it presents itself to either the abdominal surgeon at operation or the pathologist in the post-mortem room. To these investigators it is tubular and similar to the remainder of the duodenum. To the radiologist the first part of the duodenum is a bulb or cone—more accurately a triangle, as the image is two dimensional—fed at its base by the pyloric canal, which normally appears as a narrow short channel. These features are demonstrated in Figs. 6.1a, 6.5 and others. The reasons for such a discrepancy are to be found in the fact that the radiologist sees exclusively the internal contours of the tract, whilst to the surgeon the presenting aspect is external; on a surgical approach it may even be difficult to distinguish accurately the first part of the duodenum from the pyloric canal.

On the radiograph the straightness of the pyloric canal is thought to be due to muscular development and activity in this part of the stomach. The cone-shape of the duodenal bulb or 'cap' is attributed, perhaps uncertainly, to two features: (a) the flexure which occurs between the first and second parts of

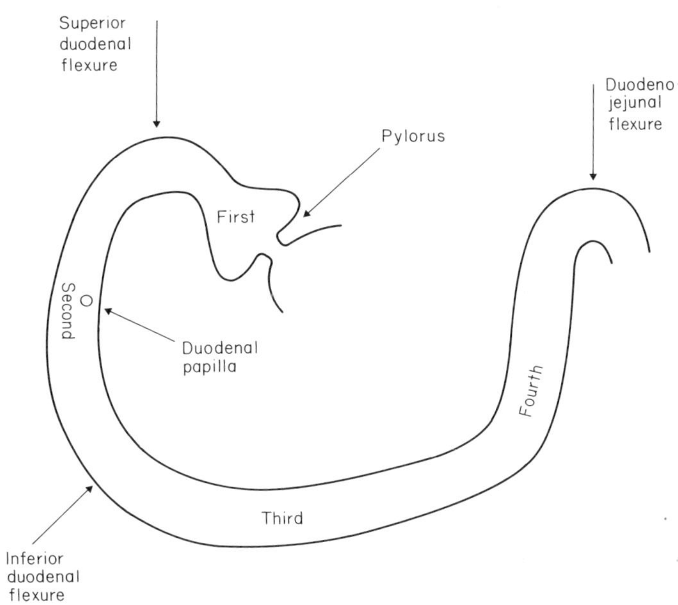

Fig. 6.8. The parts of the duodenum.

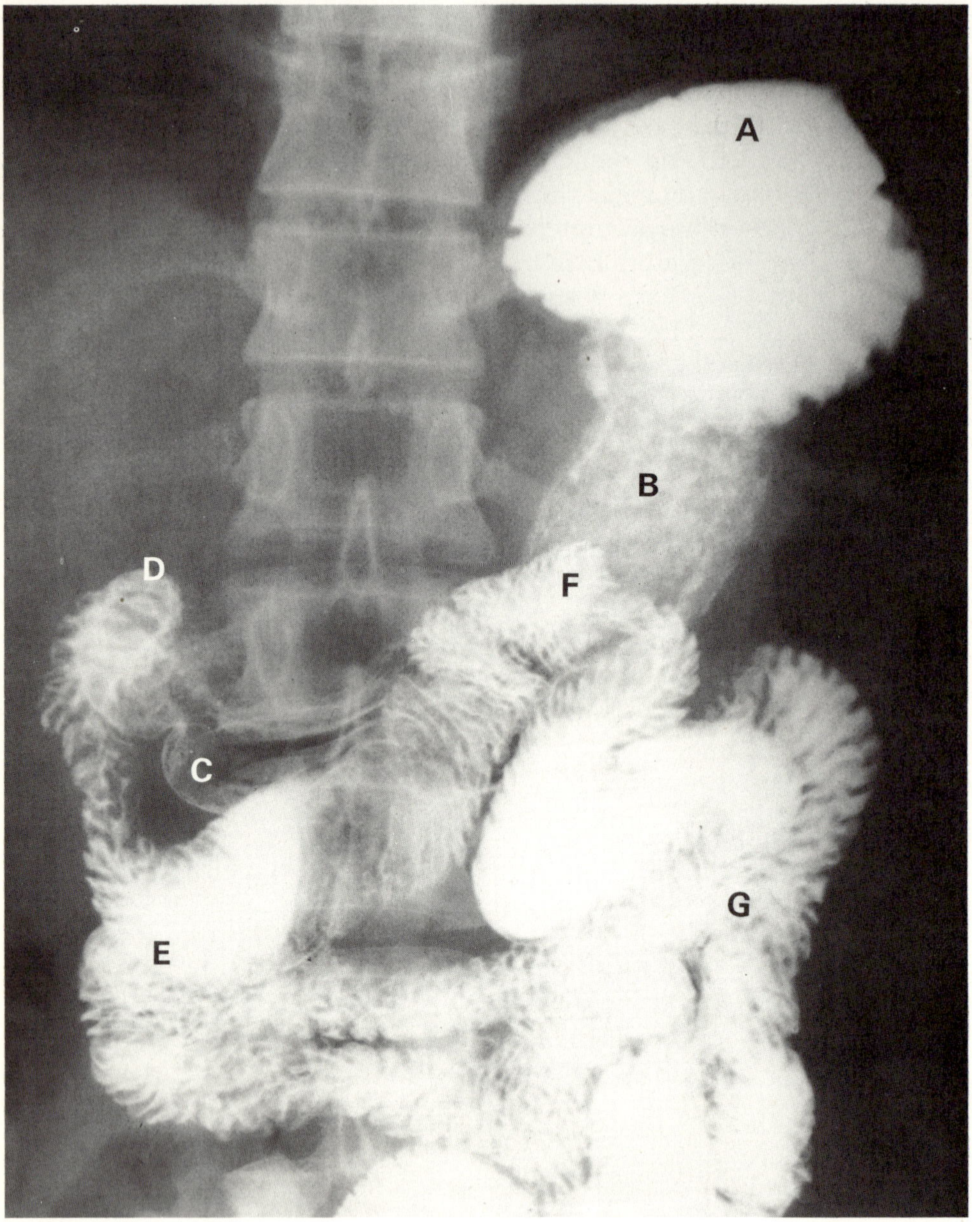

Fig. 6.9a. A supine posteroanterior radiograph exposed during a barium meal series.

A Fundus of the stomach
B Body of the stomach
C Pyloric part of the stomach
D Superior duodenal flexure
E Inferior duodenal flexure
F Duodeno-jejunal flexure
G Jejunum

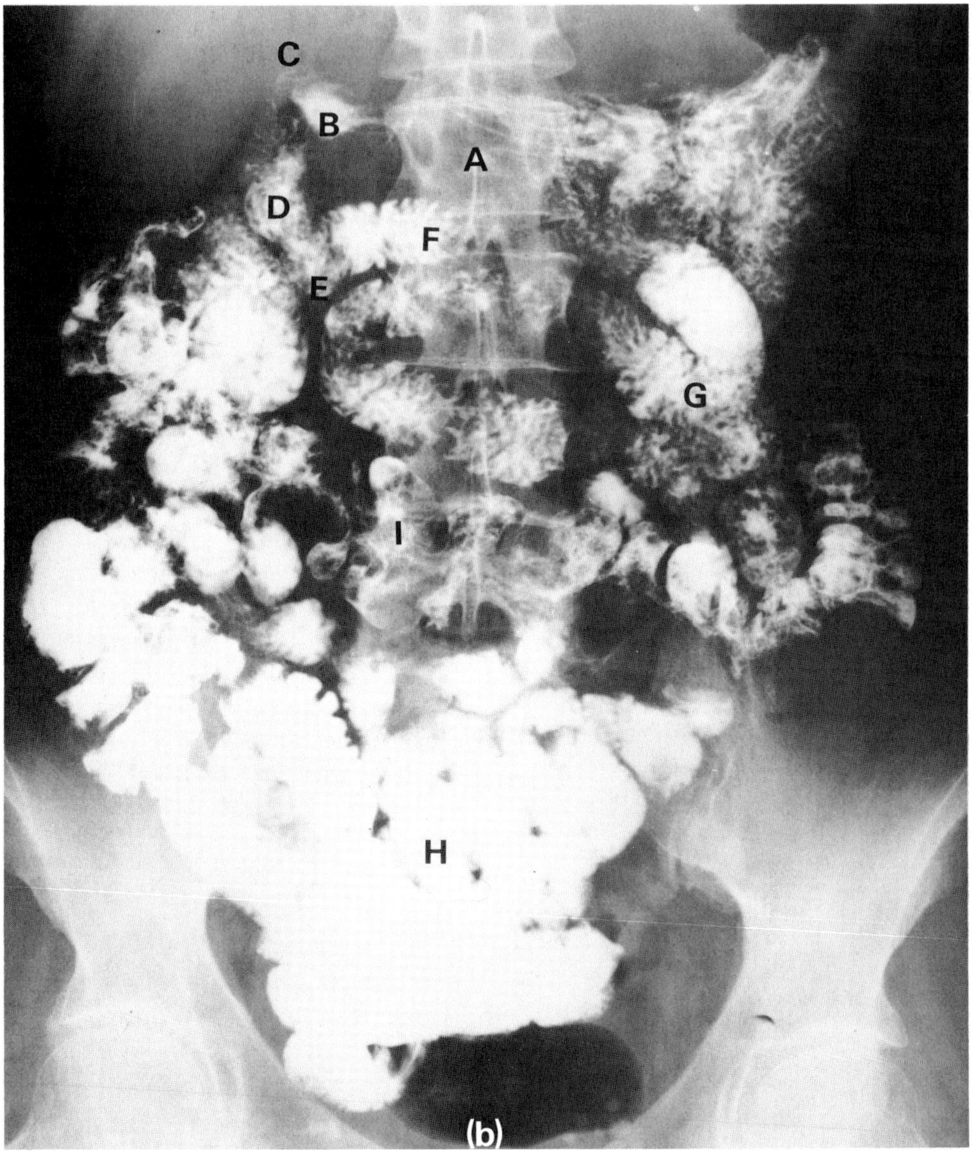

Fig. 6.9b. One of a follow-through series after a barium meal (postero-anterior projection).

A Gastric rugae
B 1st part of the duodenum
C Superior duodenal flexure
D 2nd part of the duodenum
E Inferior duodenal flexure
F 3rd part of the duodenum
G Loops of jejunum
H Loops of ileum
I Transverse colon

the duodenum; (b) the sphincter-like function which this region of the alimentary tube seems to exercise. Observation on a fluoroscopic screen during an X-ray examination usually shows barium entering the duodenum as the pylorus relaxes within a few minutes of the patient having taken the drink; sometimes a delay occurs which is not necessarily significant of organic obstruction. When filled, the duodenal bulb seems to become dilated by the accumulation within it of a small reservoir of barium, which is released to the next part of the duodenum in successive 'filling' and 'emptying' phases.

The second part

The second part of the duodenum is considered as beginning at the superior duodenal flexure, where the duodenum makes a sharp downward curve in front of the medial part of the right kidney. Its downward run may take it as far as the lower border of lumbar vertebra 2 or lumbar vertebra 3 (see Figs. 6.8 and 6.9). The duodenal loop is neither freely movable nor totally fixed and certain normal variations in its form are recognised. Typically it may be U-shaped or C-shaped.

About half-way along the second part of the duodenum the common bile duct and the pancreatic duct enter on the posteromedial wall through the duodenal papilla (see Chapter 9, p. 226–227).

The third part

The third part of the duodenum begins at the inferior duodenal flexure where the duodenum makes a second sharp bend, to traverse the abdomen from right to left almost horizontally (see Fig. 6.9b). It is about 10 cm in length and at the level of the umbilicus.

The fourth part

The fourth part of the duodenum is ascendant in direction. It passes upwards and to the left for about 2·5 cm, either in front or to the left of the abdominal aorta. At about the level of lumbar vertebra 2 this part of the duodenum turns forwards at the duodeno-jejunal flexure and terminates. A swallowed foreign body—especially if it is long, such as a hair-grip—may fail to negotiate this acute bend and become lodged at the duodeno-jejunal flexure (see Fig. 6.8, p. 159).

THE JEJUNUM

From the duodeno-jejunal flexure the rest of the small intestine presents a sinuous arrangement of coils which are attached to the posterior abdominal wall by the mesentery, a broad, fan-shaped fold of peritoneum. The jejunum and the ileum together are about 6 metres long and no formal line of demarcation exists between them. Nevertheless, the character of the bowel changes gradually from the beginning of the jejunum to the termination of the ileum at the ileocaecal valve. Thus the supposition of two distinct parts is not unreasonable, the jejunum being designated as the proximal two-fifths of the total. Radiology may accurately locate the beginning of the jejunum (from its relationship to the duodenum) and the terminal coils of the ileum (as they approach the ileocaecal orifice), but is no more able than the anatomist to say where the one region of the bowel becomes the other. However, there is no doubt that there are anatomical, physiological and radiological differences between them.

The jejunum, as opposed to the ileum, normally has the following characteristics:

(i) relatively greater calibre;

(ii) more prominent, densely set circular folds, which give the jejunum a complex 'feathery' radiological pattern because barium is retained in the small spaces between the folds;

(iii) large villi (not a radiological sign);

(iv) high motor activity which results in the rapid transit of barium during X-ray examination and is accompanied by some variability in the bore of this part of the digestive tube;

(v) fewer and smaller lymphatic nodes (not radiological evidence during barium study).

As may be seen from Figs. 6.9 and 6.10, the first jejunal coils tend to occupy the left upper abdominal quadrant. For reasons already described, the distal loops cannot be accurately located but much of the jejunum is found in the umbilical

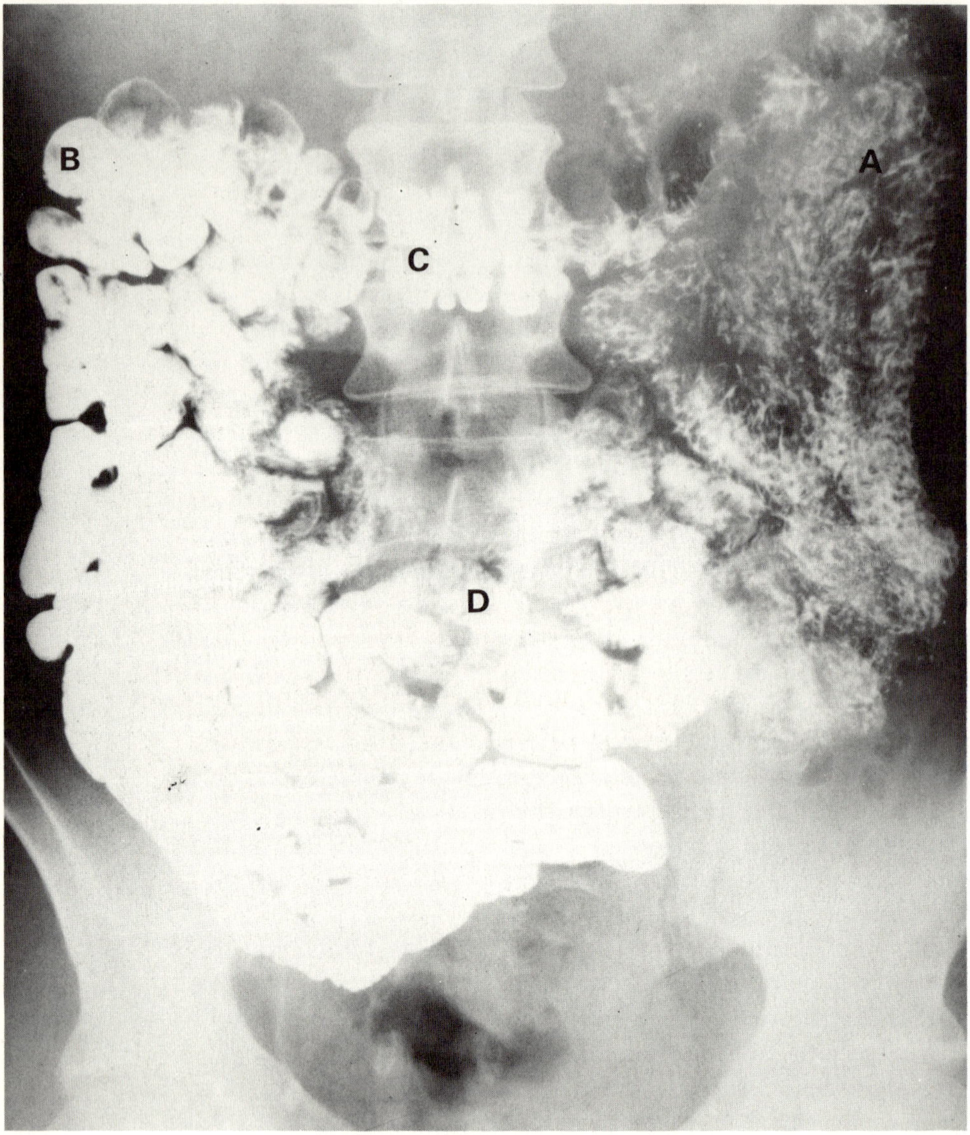

Fig. 6.10. One of a follow-through series (posteroanterior projection) which was exposed an hour after the administration of a barium meal.

A Jejunum
B Hepatic flexure of colon
C Transverse colon
D Ileum

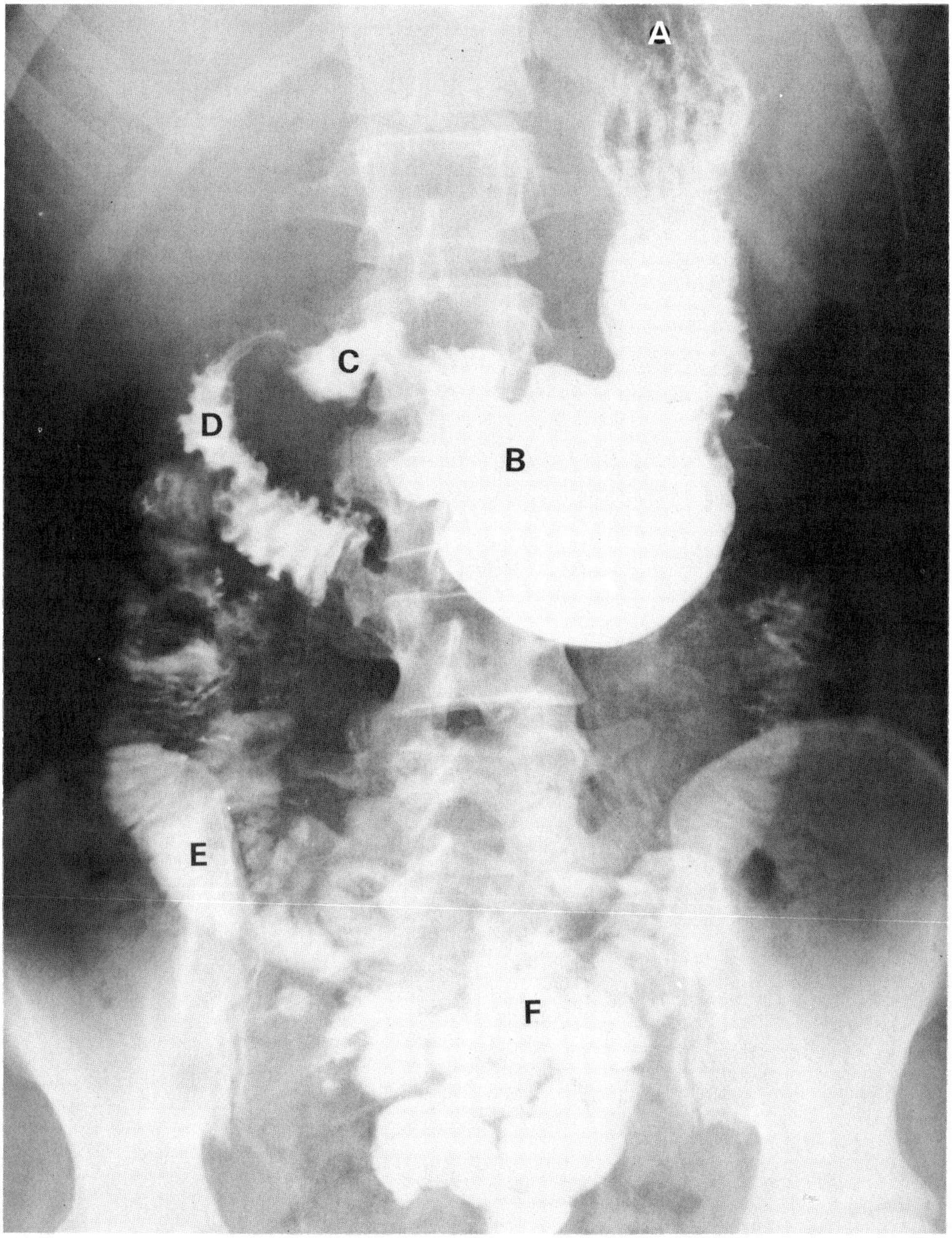

Fig. 6.11. One of a follow-through series. This posteroanterior radiograph was exposed 15 minutes after the administration of a barium meal; the patient is erect.

A Rugae in gastric fundus
B Pyloric part of the stomach
C 1st part of the duodenum
D 2nd part of the duodenum
E Coils of jejunum
F Coils of ileum

region of the abdomen, with extension in surrounding areas, and rarely is any seen in the pelvis.

THE ILEUM

The ileum constitutes the distal three-fifths of the small intestine. Our discussion has shown that anatomically and radiologically the ileum differs from the jejunum without a recognisable boundary between them. Relative to the jejunum, the ileum has the following characteristics:

(i) a lumen which is a little smaller;

(ii) thinner coverings (not shown radiologically);

(iii) only a few circular folds, which are situated in the upper part of the ileum and almost absent from the lower part;

(iv) a less complex radiological mucosal pattern when coated with barium;

(v) much less motor activity, resulting in a slower and more intermittent transit of barium;

(vi) larger and more numerous lymphatic nodules (not apparent radiologically during barium study).

The situation of the ileum (see Figs. 6.10 and 6.11) is mainly hypogastric and in the right iliac fossa of the pelvis. The terminal loops ascend over the right psoas major muscle and end at the ileocaecal orifice (see Chapter 7, p. 171). The direction from which the ileum approaches the caecum is variable. Usually the junction is made on the medial wall of the caecum but sometimes it occurs posteriorly.

Chapter 7
Contrast Examinations: The Large Bowel

The large bowel is the most distal part of the alimentary canal and is usually examined radiologically by means of a barium enema. In this procedure, a solution of barium sulphate—a salt which is opaque to X-rays—is introduced at the anus and allowed to flow in sufficient quantity to fill the large bowel. The passage of the barium enema is controlled by fluoroscopic observation and normally the whole of this part of the digestive tract may be delineated on a series of radiographs.

Like other sections of the alimentary canal, the large bowel is a tube. It is about 1·5 m long and extends from the termination of the ileum to the anus. Certain characteristics of the large bowel distinguish it radiologically and anatomically from the small intestine. These include the following features:

(i) it has a greater calibre than the small intestine;
(ii) its position tends to be more fixed;
(iii) although in a continuous layer over the surface, the longitudinal muscular fibres of the large intestine thicken at three situations on the circumference of the tube and form prominent longitudinal bands, the taenia coli;
(iv) as the taenia coli are shorter than the other coats of the intestine, the surface of the bowel over which they extend is gathered in a series of bulges or haustrations. These give to this part of the tract a particular sacculated form and

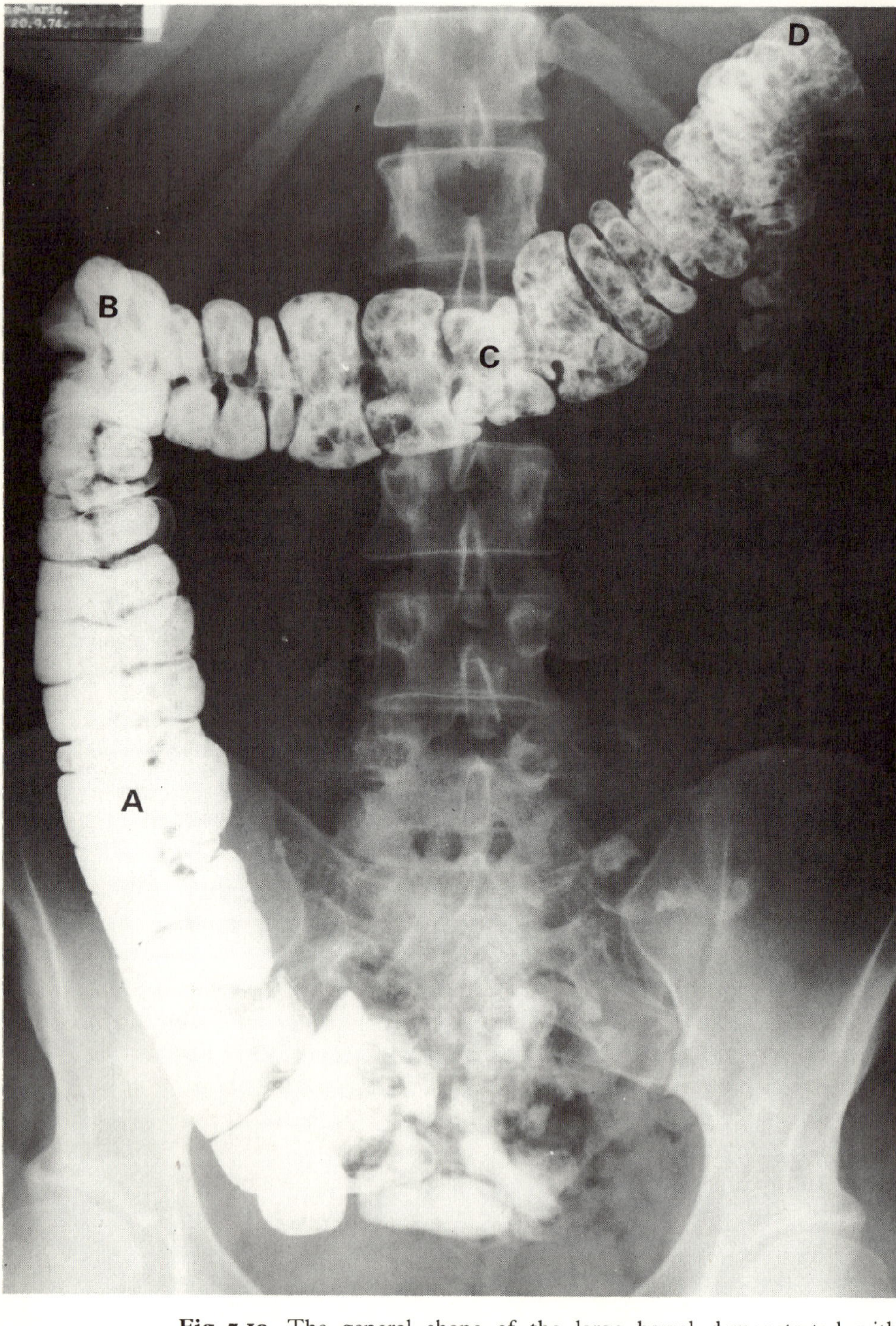

Fig. 7.1a. The general shape of the large bowel demonstrated with barium sulphate; a posteroanterior projection of the abdomen exposed after partial evacuation of a barium enema.

A Ascending colon
B Hepatic flexure of colon
C Transverse colon
D Splenic flexure of colon

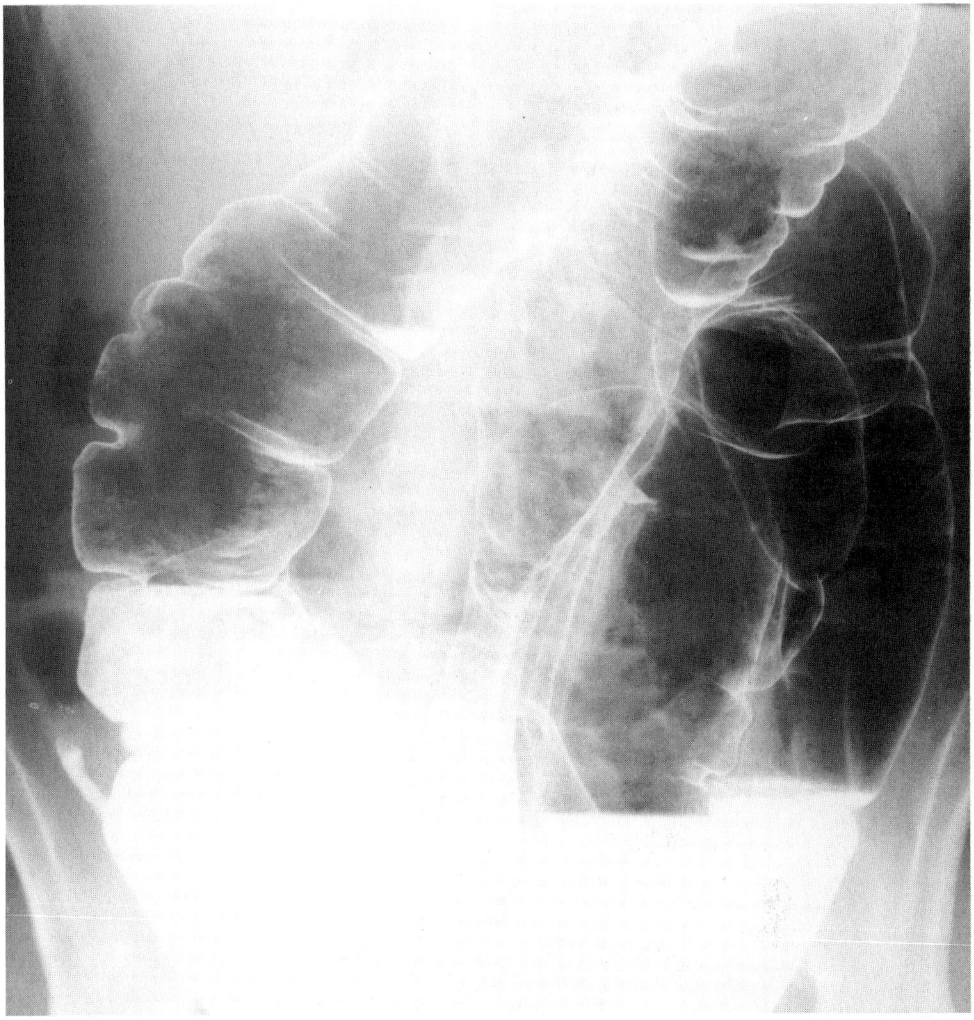

Fig. 7.1b. A posteroanterior radiograph of the large bowel taken during the air-replacement phase of a barium enema: a double contrast is provided where air is outlining the barium-coated walls of the gut. The taenia coli are well demonstrated.

appearance (see Fig. 7.1a). The general configuration of the large bowel (see, for example Fig. 7.2) provides an arch which encloses coils of the small bowel.

The large bowel is considered as having several parts:
(i) the caecum;
(ii) the colon;

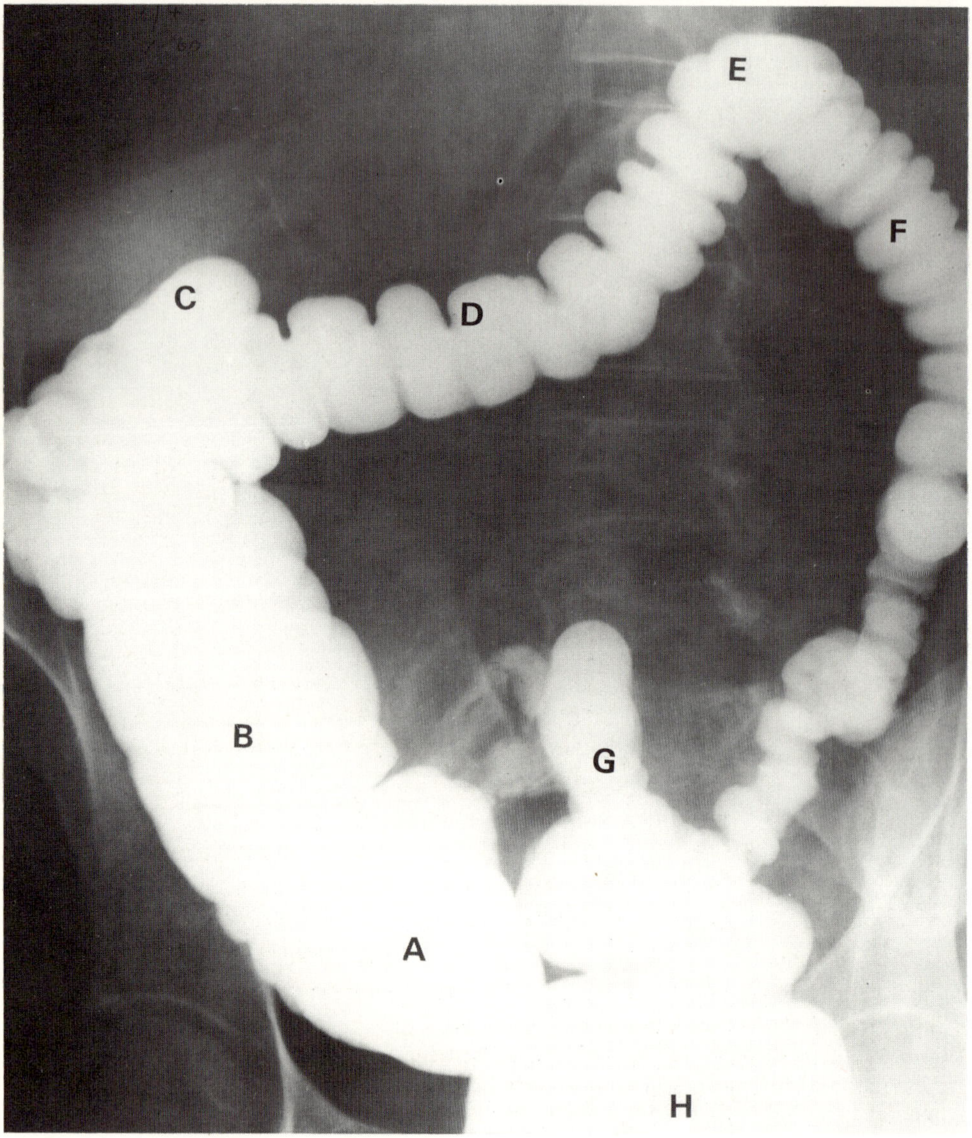

Fig. 7.2. The large bowel after the administration of a barium enema; a left anterior oblique projection.

A	The caecum	E	The splenic flexure
B	The ascending colon	F	The descending colon
C	The hepatic flexure	G	The sigmoid colon
D	The transverse colon	H	The rectum

(iii) the rectum;
(iv) the anal canal.

The caecum

The caecum, which is about 6 cm long, is the beginning of the large bowel. Its diameter is greater than that of the colon, which gradually diminishes in calibre and with the first part of which the caecum is continuous. The caecum is a mobile structure, situated normally in the right iliac fossa and presenting some variations in shape. Essentially it is a sac, the lower end of the tube being closed and the open, upper end becoming the colon.

At the junction of the caecum with the colon, the ileum enters the large bowel through the ileocaecal orifice on the posteromedial aspect of the tube; the orifice is associated with a valve of the same name.

About 2 cm below the ileocaecal orifice, on the posteromedial wall of the caecum, another blind tube is found: this is the vermiform appendix. It is a narrow tube, which varies in length from 2 cm to 20 cm and owes its name to its worm-like characteristics. In the language of anatomy, the term appendix may properly be used of any accessory part attached to a main organ. However, members of the general public and the medical community who speak of 'the appendix' are usually referring familiarly to the vermiform appendix of the caecum. Fig. 7.3 shows the caecum, part of the colon and a rather long vermiform appendix, filled with barium. The translucencies present in the appendix are probably due to faecoliths (inspissated faeces) which have accumulated there slowly over a period of time. During adult life, the lumen of the appendix may become obliterated. The organ is neither certain of radiological demonstration, nor to be suspected of pathology if a contrast agent fails to enter it.

Within limits, the position occupied by the appendix is variable. Each of five possibilities is recognised:
(i) it may lie behind the caecum and colon;
(ii) it may hang down past the brim of the pelvis (close to the right ovary and uterine tube if the subject is female);
(iii) it may lie beneath the caecum;

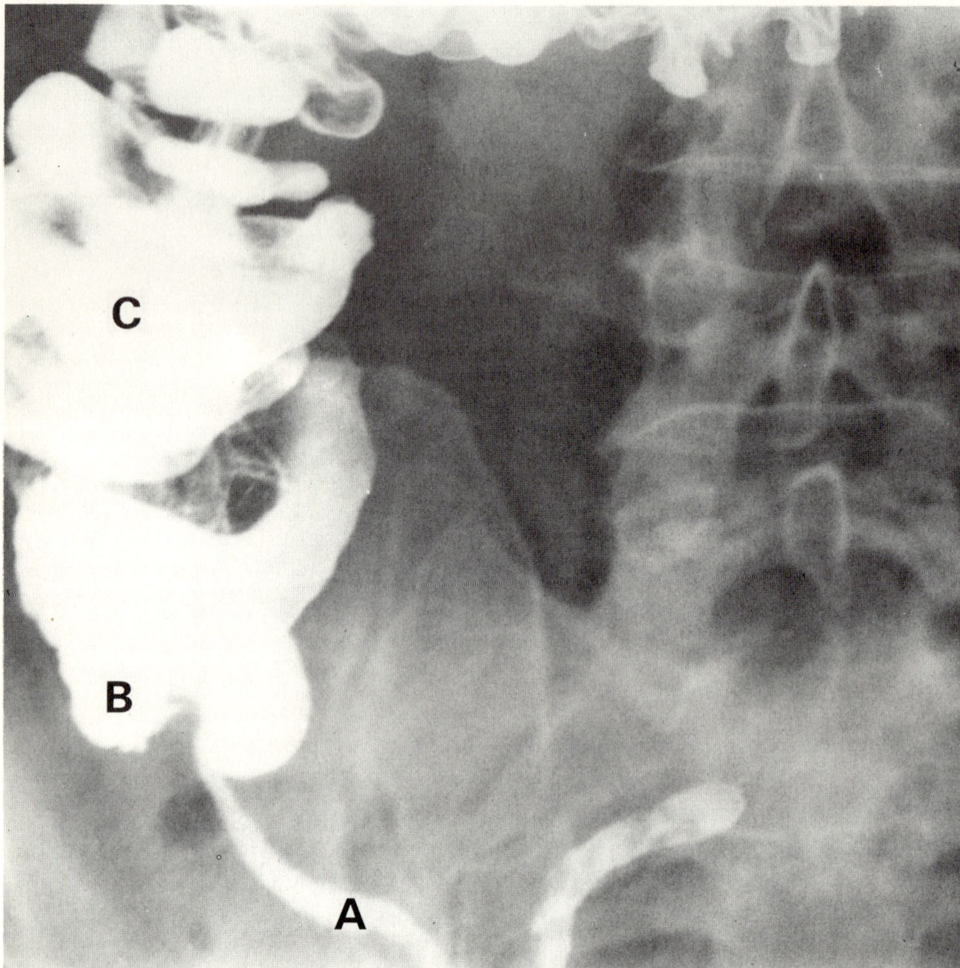

Fig. 7.3. Part of the large bowel shown by barium sulphate.
A The vermiform appendix C The ascending colon
B The caecum

(iv) it may lie in front of the terminal ileum in contact with the anterior abdominal wall;
(v) it may lie behind the terminal ileum.

This potential variety of situation is perhaps more significant for the surgeon than for the student of radiographic anatomy. However, such a variety may exert an influence on the radiographic projection of the organ and thus on its radiographic appearance. It is for these reasons that its several likely sites have been enumerated here. The commonest is the first, the retrocaecal and retrocolic appendix.

The appendix possesses similar coats to those of other parts of the intestine. These coats are: (i) serous; (ii) muscular; (iii) submucous; (iv) mucous. As we can see from Fig. 7.3, the taenia coli and the haustrations which they produce are absent from the appendix. The submucous coat is particularly well developed and contains many masses of lymphoid tissue which reduce and make irregular the lumen of the appendix.

The colon

For descriptive purposes the colon is considered to have four parts: the ascending colon; the transverse colon; the descending colon; the pelvic or sigmoid colon.

THE ASCENDING COLON

The ascending colon begins at the caecum, with which it is continuous and in comparison a little smaller in calibre. It passes upwards on the right side of the abdominal cavity (see Figs. 7.1a and 7.2), reaching a small depression (the colic impression) on the undersurface of the right lobe of the liver. Here the ascending colon turns sharply to the left and forwards. This bend is known as the right colic flexure or—more succinctly and informatively—as the hepatic flexure.

THE TRANSVERSE COLON

The transverse colon, as we might suppose, traverses the abdomen from right to left, being suspended from the posterior abdominal wall by a fold of peritoneum, the mesocolon. Beginning at the hepatic flexure, in the right lumbar region or the right hypochondrium, the transverse colon curves on itself downwards and backwards and then loops upwards in a swag formation beneath the lower (medial) end of the spleen (see Fig. 7.1a and 7.4a and b). The left colic flexure, which is

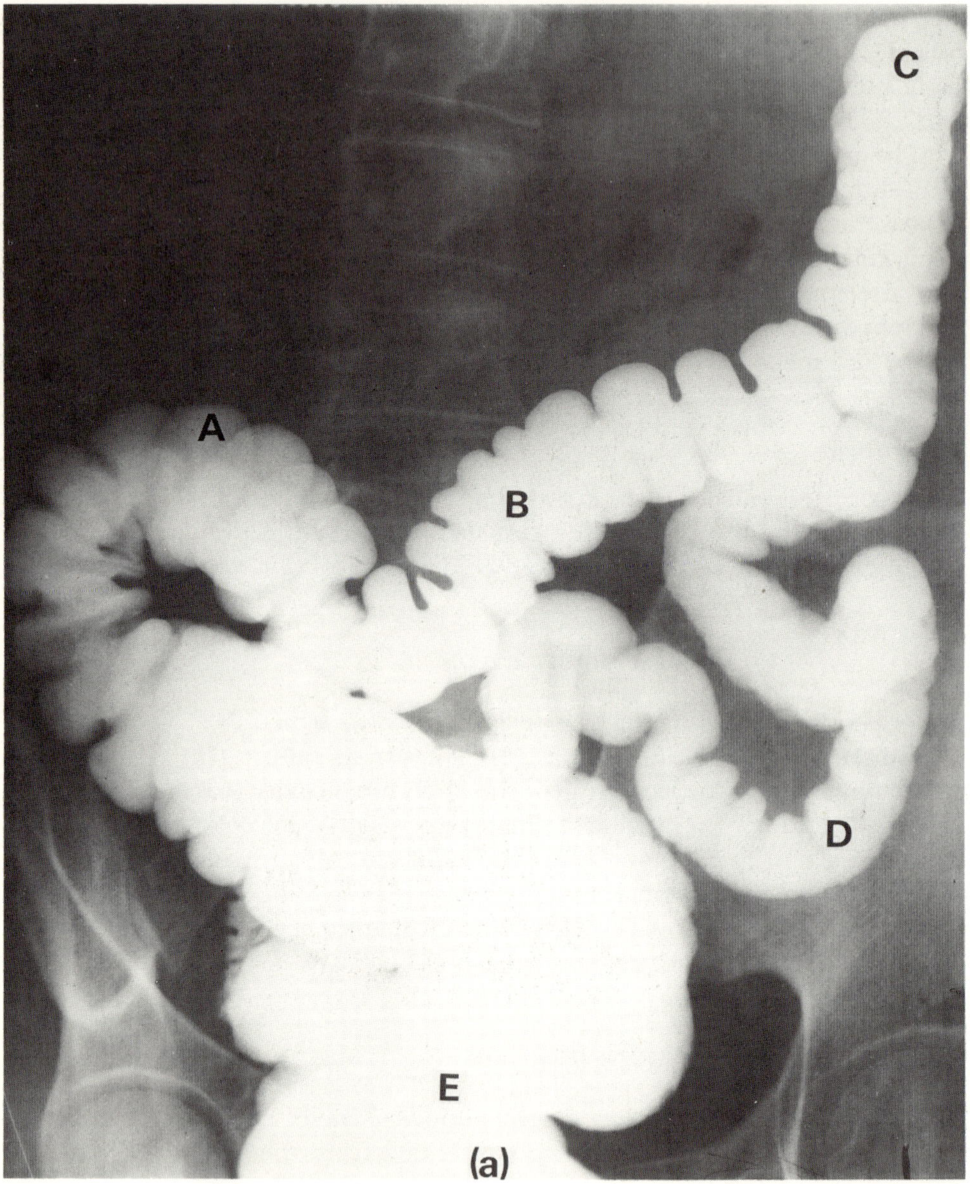

Fig. 7.4a. A slightly oblique (right anterior) projection of the large bowel during a barium enema.

A Hepatic flexure of the colon
B Transverse colon
C Splenic flexure of the colon
D The sigmoid loop
E The rectum

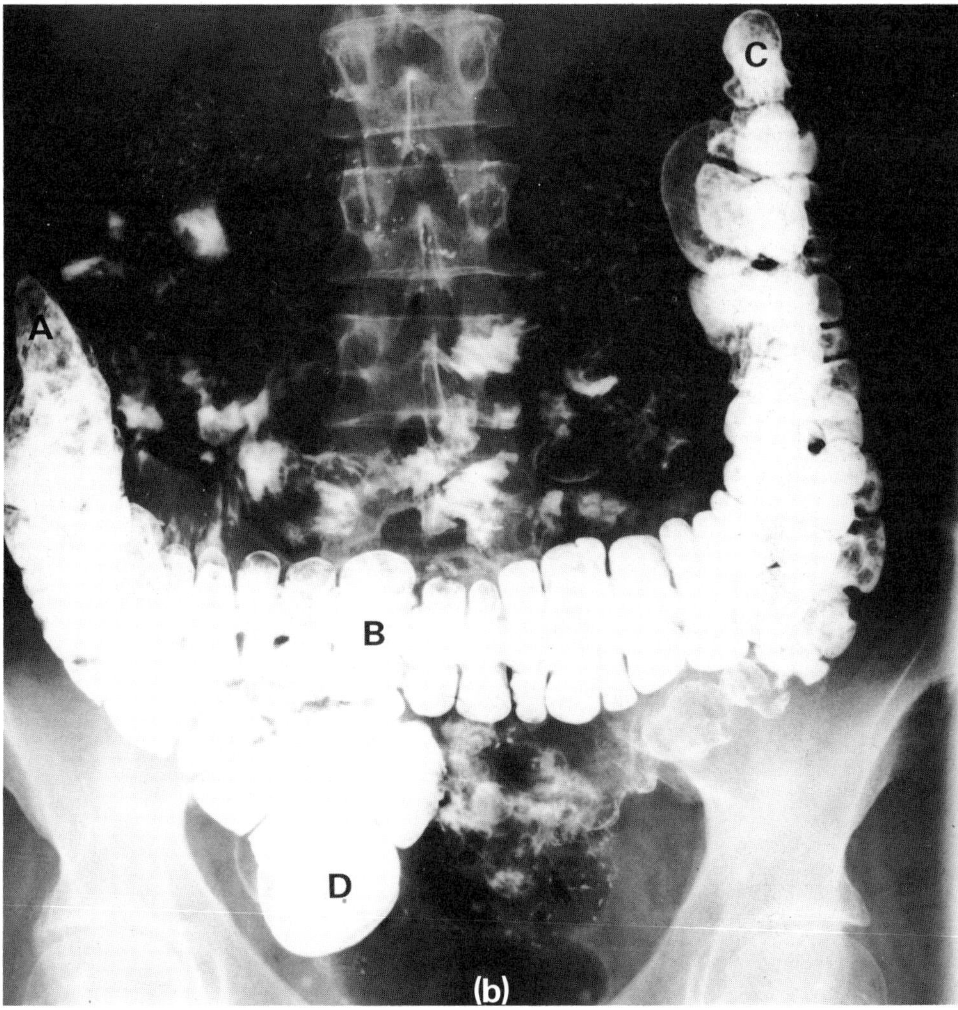

Fig. 7.4b. A posteroanterior radiograph exposed 105 minutes after a barium meal. Parts of the small and large bowels are seen.

A	Hepatic flexure of the colon	C	Splenic flexure of the colon
B	Transverse colon	D	The rectum

the terminus of the transverse colon, is a sharp bend of the colon in the left hypochondrium behind the stomach.

The left colic flexure has the lateral end of the spleen as one of its superior relations and for this reason has been called —more memorably—the splenic flexure. Towards the splenic end of the transverse colon there is sometimes a U-shaped

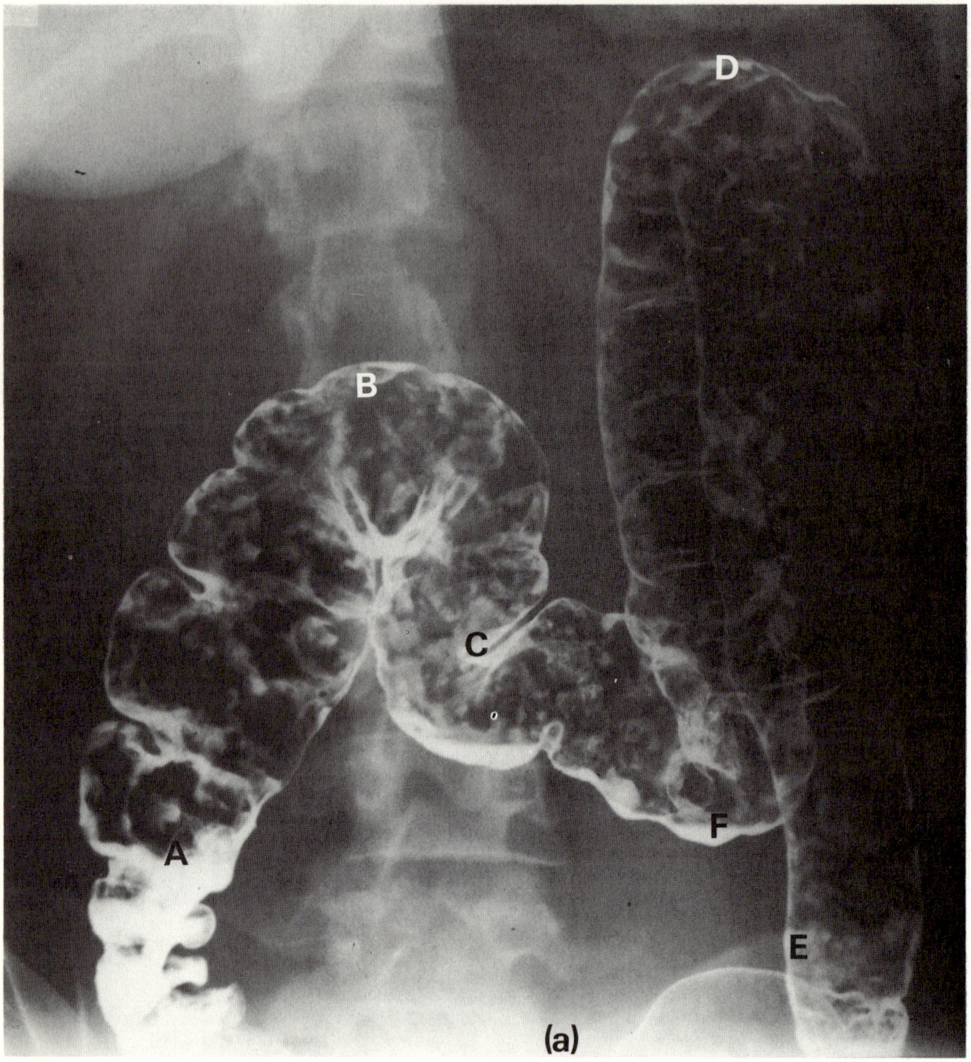

Fig. 7.5a. A radiograph taken during the air-replacement phase of a barium enema. The formation of fluid levels shows that this film was exposed by means of a horizontal X-ray beam while the patient was upright.

A Ascending colon
B Hepatic flexure of the colon
C Transverse colon
D Splenic flexure of the colon
E Descending colon
F Barium residue forming a fluid level

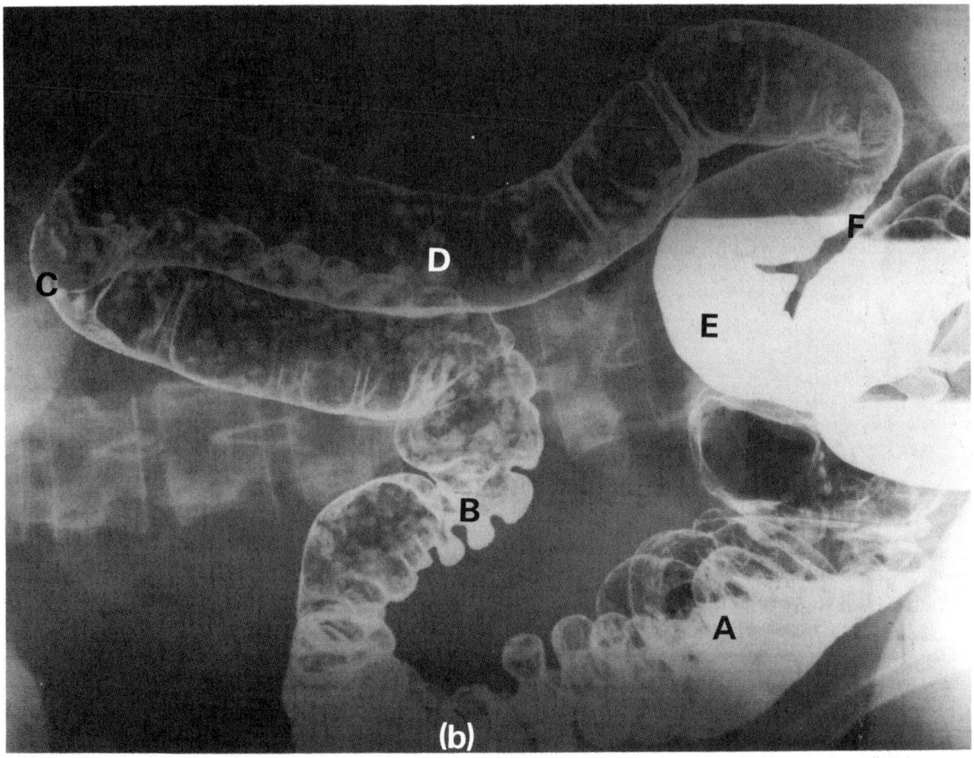

Fig. 7.5b. A radiograph taken during the air-replacement phase of a barium enema. The formation of fluid levels shows that this film was exposed by means of a horizontal beam while the patient occupied the right lateral decubitus.

A Ascending colon
B Transverse colon
C Splenic flexure of the colon
D Descending colon
E Sigmoid loop
F Fluid levels in barium sulphate

curve dependent below the level of the main loop (see, for example, Fig. 7.5a).

The position occupied by the transverse colon frequently varies between individuals and in the same individual at different times. As illustration of this point, we may compare the appearances of the transverse colon on Fig. 7.2 with that of the subject depicted on Fig. 7.1a (this radiograph was taken after partial evacuation of the barium enema): the transverse colon is seen to cross the spine at the level of lumbar vertebrae 3 and 2 in the first instance and at the level of lumbar vertebrae 2 and 1 in the second instance. Figs. 7.5a and 7.5b are two

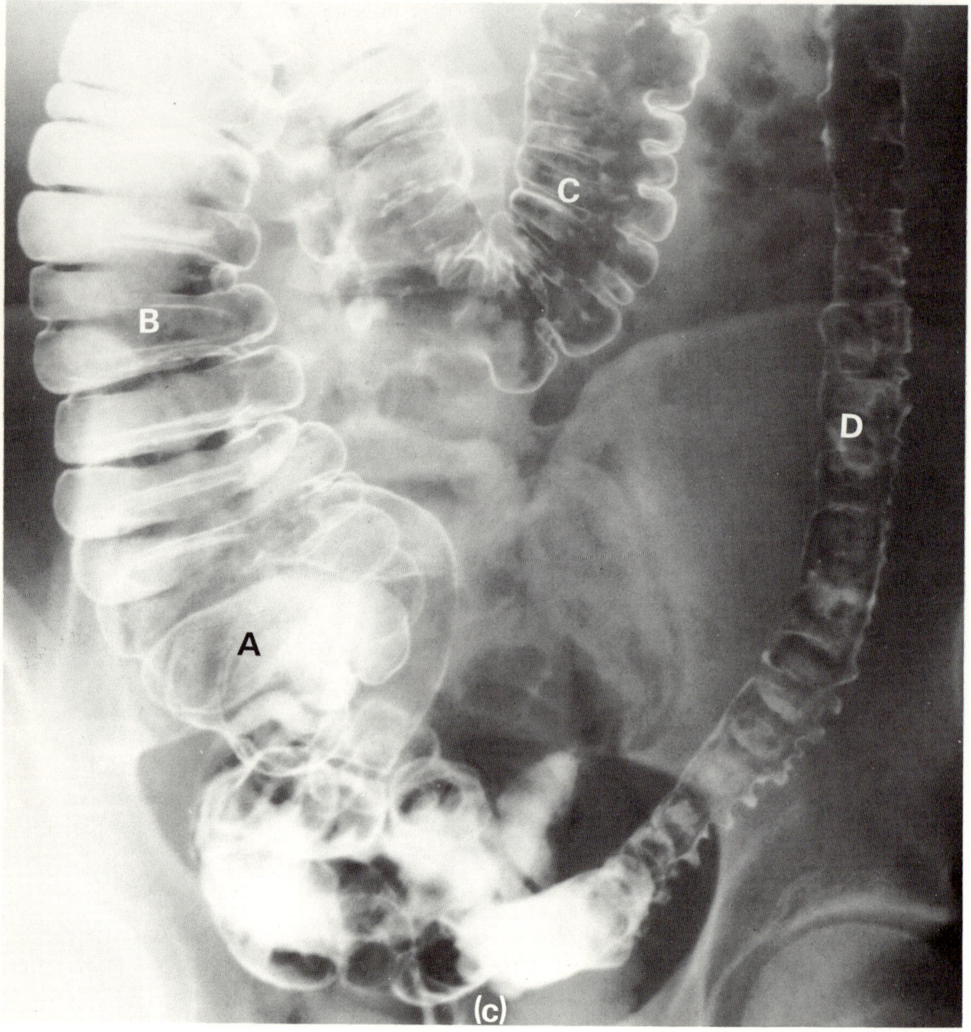

Fig. 7.5c. Another air-replacement study of a barium enema: a right anterior oblique radiograph, exposed when the patient was recumbent. The taenia coli and colonic mucosa are well seen.

A The caecum
B Ascending colon
C Transverse colon
D Descending colon

radiographs of the same patient which—like Figs. 7.1b and 7.6—were taken during the air-replacement phase of a barium enema: that is, after evacuation of the barium, air has been introduced for the purpose of obtaining a double contrast and resultant delineation of the bowel mucosa. (See Fig. 7.5c for another example of this.) When Fig. 7.5a was exposed the patient was on her feet, but for Fig. 7.5b she lay on her right side. Relative to its position in (a), the transverse colon is a little higher in (b) and much of the colon has moved to the right with the change of position.

In this book we can include no more than a few examples of the radiographic appearances of the large bowel. Film-viewing rooms in diagnostic X-ray departments offer opportunities not only to see many others but to recognise that human anatomy is not always as static as textbooks and the post-mortem room may show. In some ways at least it is a dynamic subject! The extremes of the position occupied by the transverse colon are greater than our radiographic examples so far have indicated. Sometimes its most dependent part may reach a level well below the transtubercular plane (see Fig. 7.4b); or it may—see for example Fig. 7.1a—lie in the upper umbilical region almost on a level with the transpyloric plane.

The splenic flexure of the colon is more acute than the hepatic flexure and it is higher in the abdomen (see Fig. 7.5 and others). It is also further back in the abdominal cavity but this is not apparent from posteroanterior and anteroposterior radiographs. The splenic flexure is attached to the diaphragm opposite the tenth and eleventh ribs by a fold of peritoneum, the phrenicolic ligament, below the lateral end of the spleen.

THE DESCENDING COLON

Beginning at the splenic flexure, the descending colon passes downwards (see Fig. 7.5a) on the left side of the abdomen, through the left hypochondrium and left lumbar region. At the crest of the ilium the descending colon curves, still in a downwards direction but now slightly medially (see Fig. 7.6), becoming continuous with the pelvic colon at the brim of the true pelvis.

The descending colon is smaller in calibre and more deeply placed in the abdominal cavity than is the ascending colon. Many vessels and nerves pass behind the descending colon; anteriorly its relationship is mainly with coils of the jejunum.

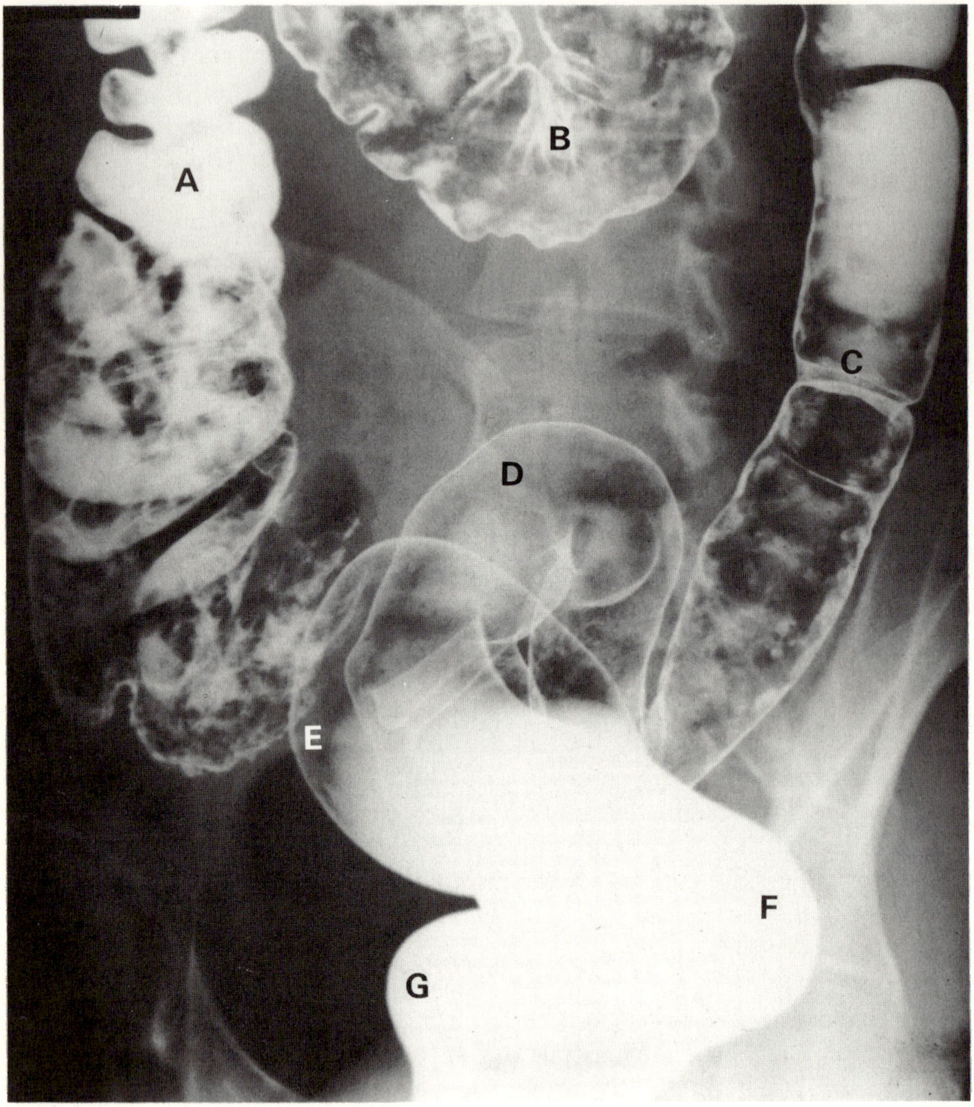

Fig. 7.6. An air-replacement study of a barium enema: a left anterior oblique projection, exposed when the patient was recumbent. Most of the residual barium is in the rectum.

A Ascending colon
B Transverse colon
C Descending colon
D Sigmoid colon
E Upper sacral curve of rectum
F Middle sacral curve of rectum
G Lower sacral curve of rectum

However the lower part of the descending colon approaches the anterior abdominal wall, through which it may sometimes be felt.

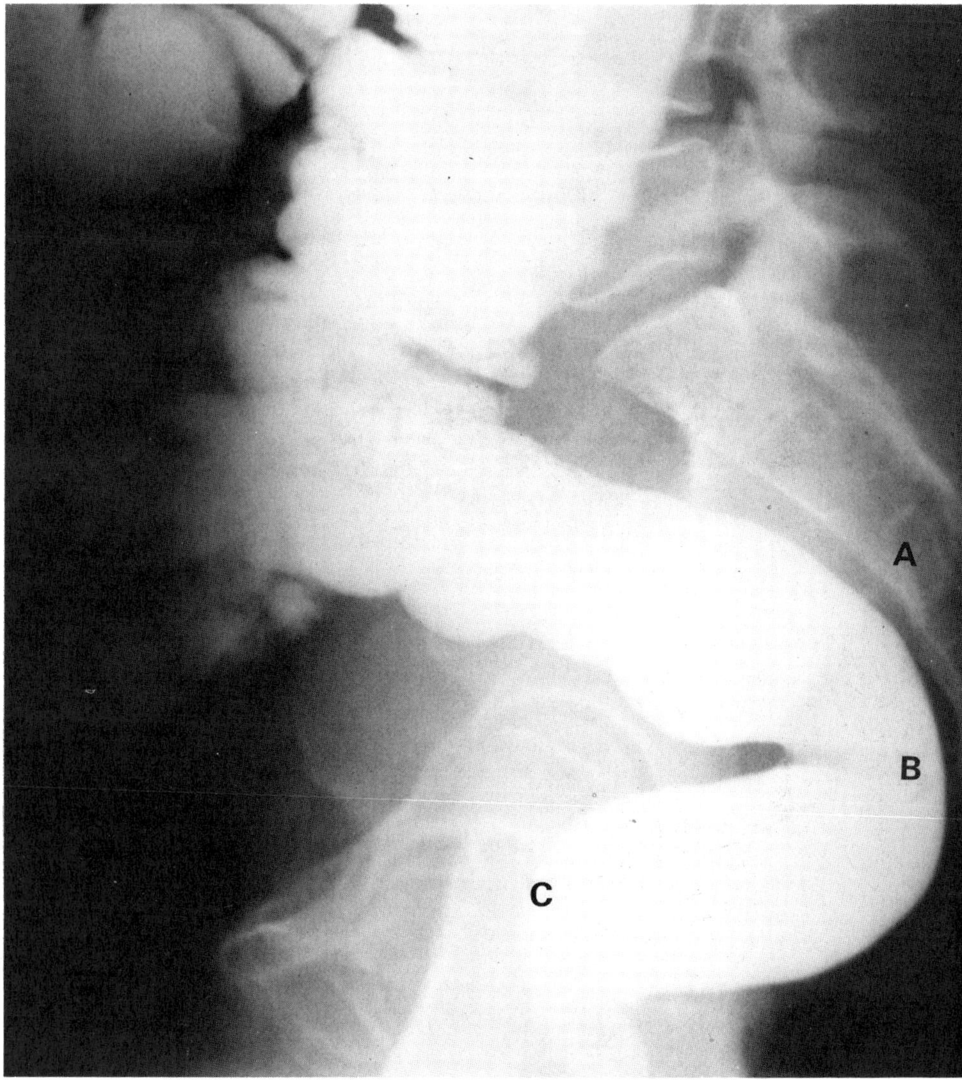

Fig. 7.7. A lateral radiograph of the pelvic colon and rectum taken during the administration of a barium enema.

A 3rd sacral segment

B Upper anteroposterior curve (sacral flexure) of the rectum

C Lower anteroposterior curve (perineal flexure) of the rectum

THE PELVIC (SIGMOID) COLON

The pelvic colon begins at the pelvic brim as the continuation of the descending colon. In the pelvis it forms a loop, from which the name sigmoid (S-shaped) is derived (see Figs. 7.6, 7.5b and 7.4a). The length of this loop varies greatly between individuals.

The sigmoid colon is described in three parts:
(i) a part which descends in contact with the left pelvic wall;
(ii) a part which crosses the pelvic cavity and may come in contact with the right pelvic wall;
(iii) a part which takes first a backward arch, reaching the median plane at the level of sacral segments 2 to 3, and then a downward arch to the terminus of the colon at the recto-sigmoid junction (see Fig. 7.7).

The sigmoid loop is fixed at its junctions with the descending colon and rectum but otherwise is free to move—and does move—quite considerably. The shape and position of the loop depend on several features:
(i) the length and mobility of its mesocolon (the fold of peritoneum attaching it to the posterior abdominal wall);
(ii) the degree of distension of this part of the bowel (when empty the loop is in the pelvic cavity and will rise to the abdominal cavity when distended);
(iii) the extents to which the bladder and rectum are distended (distension of these organs lifts the sigmoid loop).

The variability of the pelvic colon's position results in some variation in its relations. These relations include:
(i) the terminal coil of the ileum above and to the right;
(ii) the male bladder, or the uterus and female bladder, below;
(iii) the left ureter posteriorly;
(iv) the left ovary if the subject is female, the vas deferens in the male and the left pelvic wall laterally.

The rectum

THE RECTAL CURVES

The rectum is continuous with the pelvic colon above and the anal canal below. It has two anteroposterior curves.
(i) From its origin at the level of the third sacral segment, the

rectum passes downwards, following the sacrococcygeal bend (see Fig. 7.7).
(ii) Some few centimetres from the tip of the coccyx, the rectum turns backwards into the anal canal. The upper curve is called the sacral flexure and it is convex backwards. The lower curve is the perineal flexure and it is convex forwards.

The rectum has three lateral curves (see Fig. 7.6):
(i) an upper curve which is opposite sacral segments 3 to 4 and convex to the right;
(ii) a middle curve which is opposite the sacrococcygeal articulation and convex to the left;
(iii) a lower curve which is in front of the coccygeal tip and convex to the right.
As a result of these curves, the rectum is not truly a midline structure except at its extremities: the middle part of the rectum protrudes to the left.

THE RECTAL STRUCTURE

The rectum is about 12 cm in length and generally similar in calibre to the pelvic colon. However, a dilated portion of the rectum, the rectal ampulla, is to be noticed near its distal end.

The sacculations which characterise the caecum and colon are not present in the rectum but a permanent transverse fold may occur at any or all of certain sites, most usually at two or three of them. These folds are situated each as follows:
(i) on the right wall of the rectum near its beginning;
(ii) on the left wall slightly below the first fold;
(iii) on the anterior wall, opposite the fundus of the bladder and projecting backwards;
(iv) on the left and posterior walls, close to the lower end of the rectum.
These folds contain some circular muscle fibres.

The longitudinal muscle fibres, which form the external muscular coat of the large bowel and are rather scattered in the pelvic colon, become in the rectum a layer which encircles it thickly on the anterior and posterior surfaces.

The anal canal

The anal canal is the most distal part of the large bowel and only a few centimetres in length. It makes an angle with the rectum and is directed downwards and backwards to its terminus at the anal orifice in the natal cleft. When it is empty, the anal canal is merely a longitudinal slit. The upper part of the anal canal has a lining of mucous membrane similar to other areas of the bowel, but its lower half is lined with skin.

In the muscular coat of the anal canal, circular fibres are very numerous and constitute the internal anal sphincter. The external anal sphincter is a band of voluntary muscle, normally in a state of contraction but capable of increased contraction by an exercise of the will. A radiographer attempting to insert a rectal catheter for the administration of a barium enema will find it very difficult to do so when the subject of the procedure is tense and uneasy in advance; and then in acute pain if any force is employed. The sufferer, although he may not be fully aware of his action, will have tightened the external anal sphincter and more firmly occluded the anal orifice. It is very efficient protection. In these circumstances, increasing the quantity of lubricant on the catheter may appear to offer a way through the difficulty—or rather the orifice—but actually gives very little help. The only effective ploy is a polite request to the patient that he try to relax, as if he does so he should not be hurt.

Chapter 8
Contrast Examinations: The Urinary Tract

In Chapter 5 of this book some account was given of the appearances of the urinary tract which plain radiographs may offer. The information to be obtained from such an examination of the renal system is relatively limited and may be negative in character (for instance, a report might read 'There is no evidence of an opaque urinary calculus'). Because of this and because there are safe and reliable radiological procedures available, many contrast examinations of the kidneys, ureters, bladder and urethra are performed. The most common of these is the intravenous urogram.

Intravenous urography

During intravenous urography a number of radiographs—perhaps four or five—are exposed at various times over a period of about half an hour, following the administration to the patient of an appropriate radiological contrast agent. When such a contrast agent—which will have been one of several suitable organic iodine compounds—is injected intravenously, the kidneys should normally rapidly excrete it by way of natural physiological processes and anatomical pathways. Radiographs may be taken which demonstrate renal architecture and function. At a later stage of the urogram it should be possible to visualise the ureters and bladder as well.

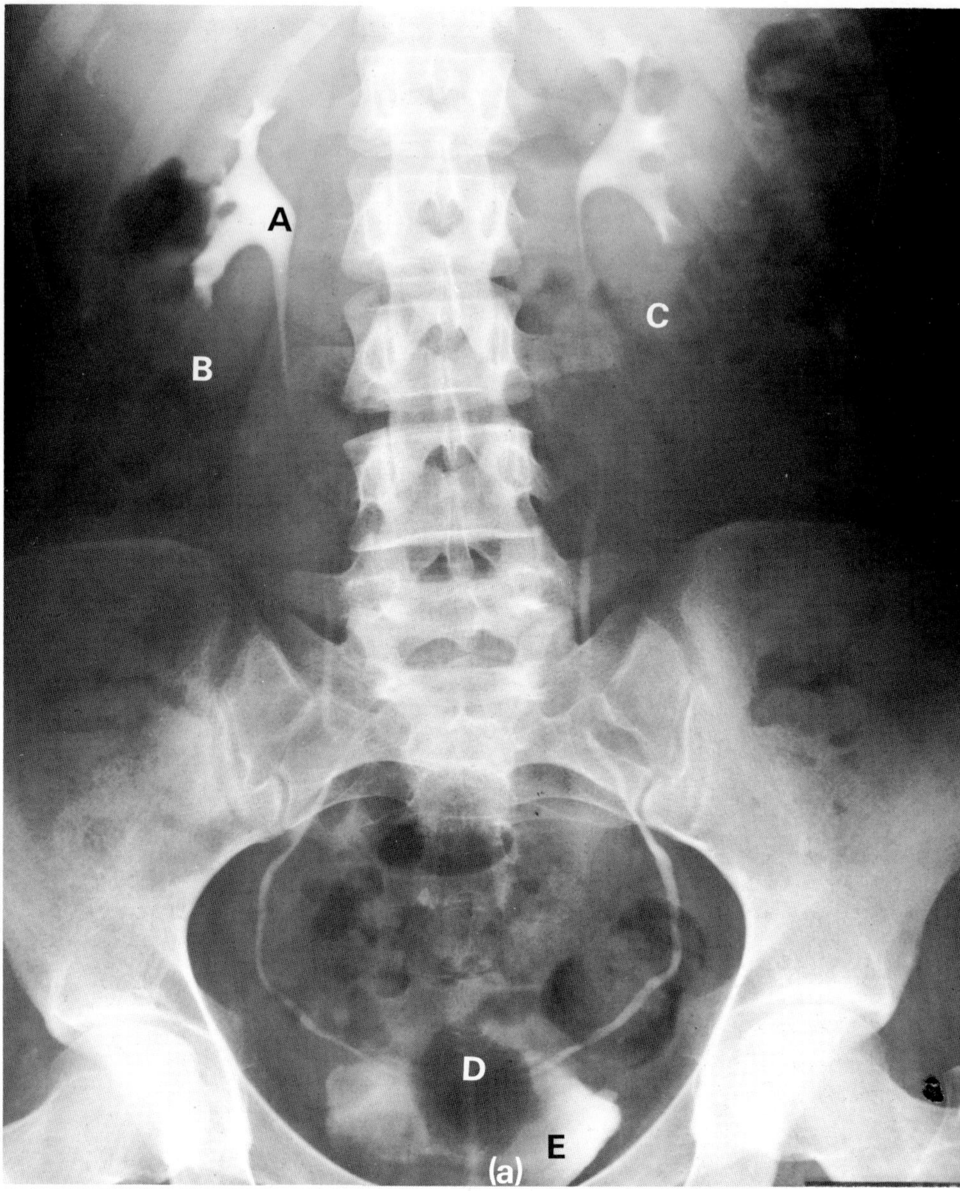

Fig. 8.1a. An intravenous urogram exposed 15 minutes after injection. Both renal pelvicalyceal systems, both ureters and the bladder are delineated by the contrast agent.

A Pelvis of the right kidney
B Lower pole of the right kidney
C Lower pole of the left kidney
D Radioparency due to gas contained in the rectum
E Bladder partially filled

Fig. 8.1a shows intravenous urography fifteen minutes after the contrast agent was given. The kidneys and ureters are well outlined and a little of the contrast substance has reached the bladder.

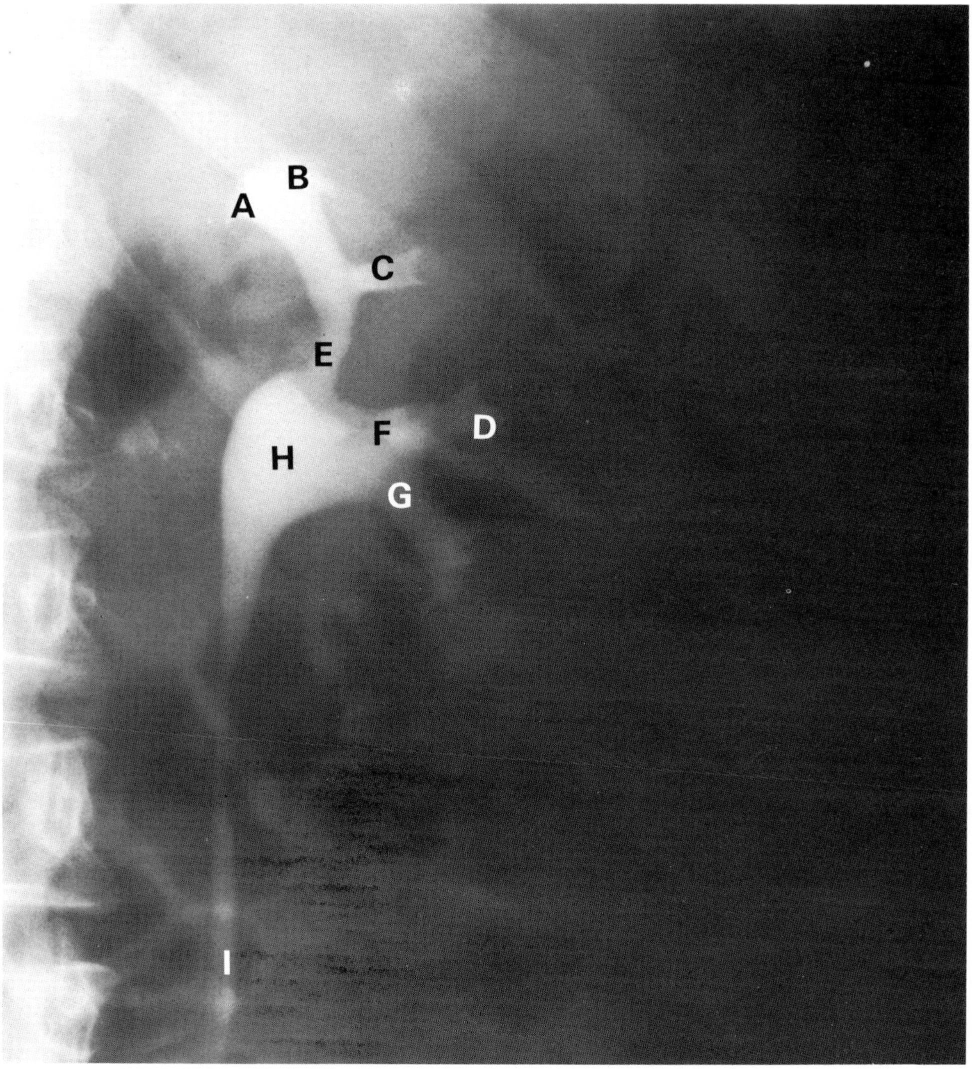

Fig. 8.1b. A coned view of a left kidney exposed during intravenous urography.

A, B, C, D Minor calyces
E, F, G Major calyces
H Pelvis of the kidney
I The left ureter

THE KIDNEYS

Size, shape and position

The radiograph illustrated in Fig. 8.1a confirms the description of renal topography which appears on page 190 and may be summarised as follows:
(i) the kidneys are symmetrical paired organs, situated to either side of the twelfth thoracic and upper lumbar vertebrae, and are about 11 cm in length and 6 cm in width;
(ii) the left kidney is a little higher and longer than the right and more oblique in direction;
(iii) the upper pole of each kidney is more pointed than the lower and each has a smooth, convex outer border.

Fig. 8.2 is not an intravenous urogram but a retrograde pyelogram and demonstrates a similar anatomy; in this case the contrast agent has been introduced directly through a catheter placed in either ureter from the bladder by means of a cystoscope (the lower part of each catheter is seen curled within the bladder).

An opaque residue of some kind is present in this patient's large bowel and we may notice that the lower part of the anterior surface of the right kidney is in relation to the hepatic flexure of the colon (actually they are in contact with each other) and that a lateral part of the left kidney has a corresponding relationship with the splenic flexure. Fortunately for the anatomist reader of the radiograph, this patient has swallowed air which is delineating much of the body of the stomach, on the greater curve of which we can see the impression of the spleen. Both these organs are in relation to the lateral part of the anterior surface of the left kidney. For completeness' sake, the relations of each kidney are listed below.

Right kidney	**Left kidney**
Right suprarenal gland	Left suprarenal gland
Right lobe of the liver	The spleen
Hepatic flexure of colon	The stomach
Second part of duodenum	The splenic vessels and pancreas
	The jejunum
	Splenic flexure of colon

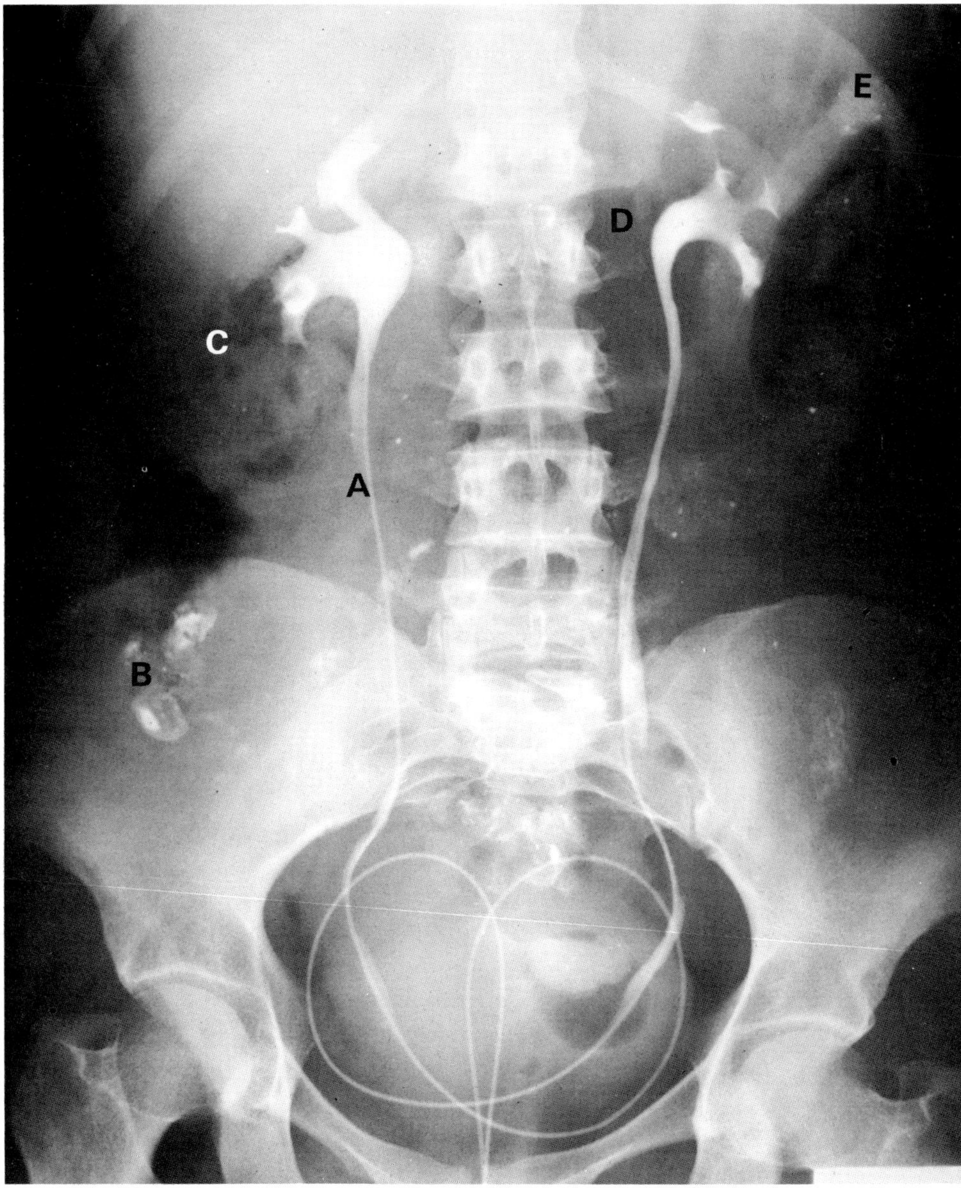

Fig. 8.2. Retrograde pyelography. A contrast agent has been introduced to each renal pelvicalyceal system by means of a catheter inserted in the appropriate ureter from the bladder. Some ingested opaque material is present in the large bowel. The coiled catheters and dilute contrast agent are seen in the bladder. Swallowed air has demonstrated part of the body of the stomach.

A Catheter in the right ureter
B The caecum delineated by a radiopaque residue.
C Hepatic flexure of the colon
D Air in the stomach
E Splenic flexure of the colon

The structure of the kidney

Each kidney is characterised by a deep, open, vertical indentation on its medial border which is called the renal hilum. Through this fissure, within a cavity known as the renal sinus, three important structures pass:
(i) the renal vein anteriorly;
(ii) the renal artery in the middle;
(iii) the funnel-shaped upper end of the ureter (the ureteric pelvis) behind.

Of the three, only the pelvis of the ureter is demonstrable by intravenous urography and is easily recognised in Fig. 8.1a and on the localised view of the left kidney depicted in Fig. 8.1b. (See Fig. 8.10a for an illustration of the renal artery.)

Within the renal sinus the pelvis of the ureter divides into either two or three main branches, the major calyces; these subdivide to form minor calyces (see Fig. 8.1b), of which there are some seven to thirteen in all. Figs. 8.1a and 8.1b show that the ends of the minor calyces are cupped. They are moulded around renal papillae, which are the apices of the renal pyramids composing the medullary substance—the inner layer—of the kidney. The outer layer or cortex of the kidney contains the many thousands of its functional unit, the nephron. Enclosing the kidney is a thin, fibrous capsule.

Radiologically no difference is apparent between the renal capsule, cortex and medulla, but the distinction is readily visible to any student radiographer who is also a cook and may sometimes provide kidneys on the menu: the capsule is smooth, glistening and is easily stripped from the kidney; the medullary substance is pale; the cortex is red-brown in colour and soft and granular in consistency (these appearances are before cooking!).

Whilst it is not possible to say from a radiograph which part of the kidney is medullary and which cortical, measurements of the thickness of the total renal substance are significant to determinations of renal assymetry which may accompany disease. Such a measurement should be made between an imaginary line joining the papillae of the outermost calyces and the nearest point of the renal outline; this is a reason why it is important that these radiographs should demonstrate the renal silhouette as well as the filled pelvicalyceal system.

The minute anatomy of the functioning kidney is not visualised on radiographs.

THE URETERS

The ureters are two muscular tubes which employ peristalsis to take urine from the kidneys to the bladder. Each has a narrow bore, relatively thick walls and a length of 25–30 cm. Anatomically the ureter is usually described in three parts:
(i) the pelvis of the ureter;

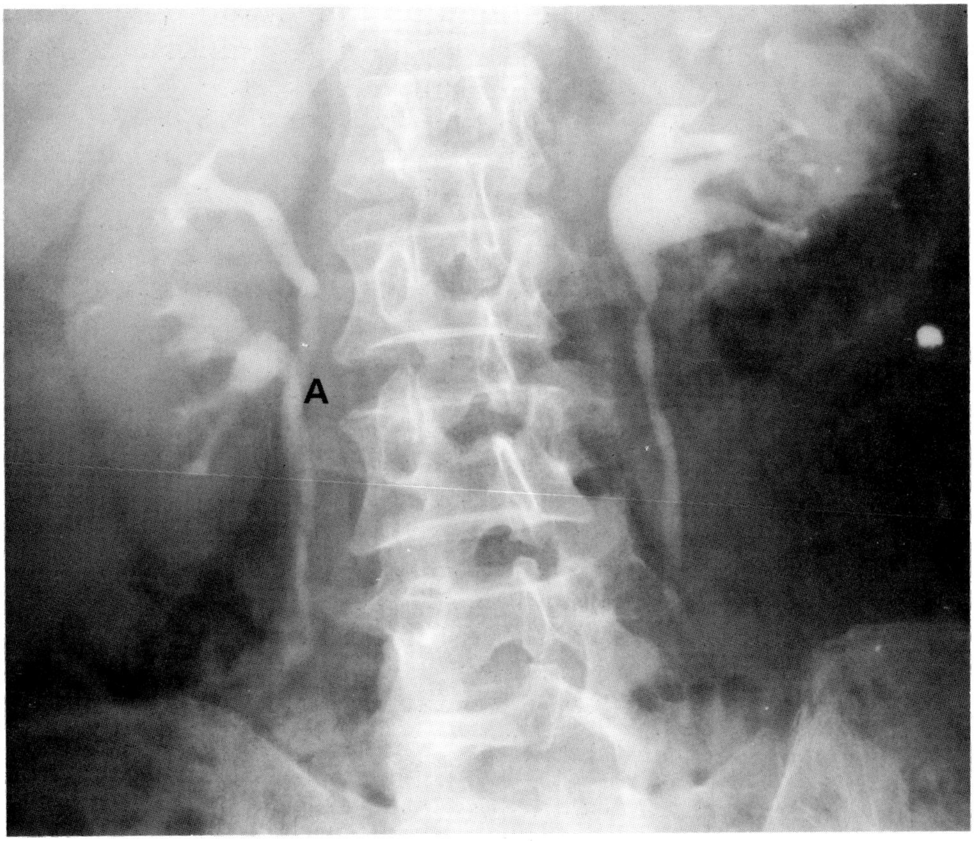

Fig. 8.3. An intravenous urogram showing a duplicated right ureter (A). Some ingested radiopaque material is present in the gut in the left lumbar region.

(ii) an abdominal portion on the surface of the psoas major muscle, which separates it from the lumbar vertebral transverse processes;
(iii) a pelvic portion, the course of which is described elsewhere in this book (see p. 125).
Radiographers accustomed to visualisations of the ureter as a whole (see Fig. 8.1a) may find such divisions arbitrary.

Structurally the ureter has three coats:
(i) a fibrous coat which is continuous with the capsule of the kidney;
(ii) a muscular coat in two layers, one of circular and another of longitudinal fibres;
(iii) an innermost mucous coat which is continuous with the mucous membrane of the bladder.

None of these features may be appreciated from radiographs since the contrast agent fills—and therefore delineates—only the lumen of the ureter. Such filling is not necessarily complete during intravenous urography and, depending on this, the calibre of the normal ureter may appear rather smaller than is really the case.

Some people have a duplicated ureter on one or both sides (for example see Fig. 8.3). The double configuration may continue as far distally as the bladder and when it does so the two tubes may enter the bladder either together or separately.

From the appearance of the left ureter on Fig. 8.4 an interpreter of the radiograph might believe that a non-obstructing calcific calculus was present in the ureter at the level of the disc between lumbar vertebrae 2 and 3. However, this is not so. The increased opacity of the ureter at this point is due to a kink, such that the observer is looking through the lumen of the ureter for a short way. (See Fig. 9.7b, page 229, for a similar effect in the neck of the gall bladder.) On Fig. 8.3, in the upper of the duplicated right ureters the same illusion is seen over the tip of the right transverse process of lumbar vertebra 2.

THE BLADDER

The bladder fills and is visualised during the later stages of an intravenous urogram. Such filling is rarely to capacity unless

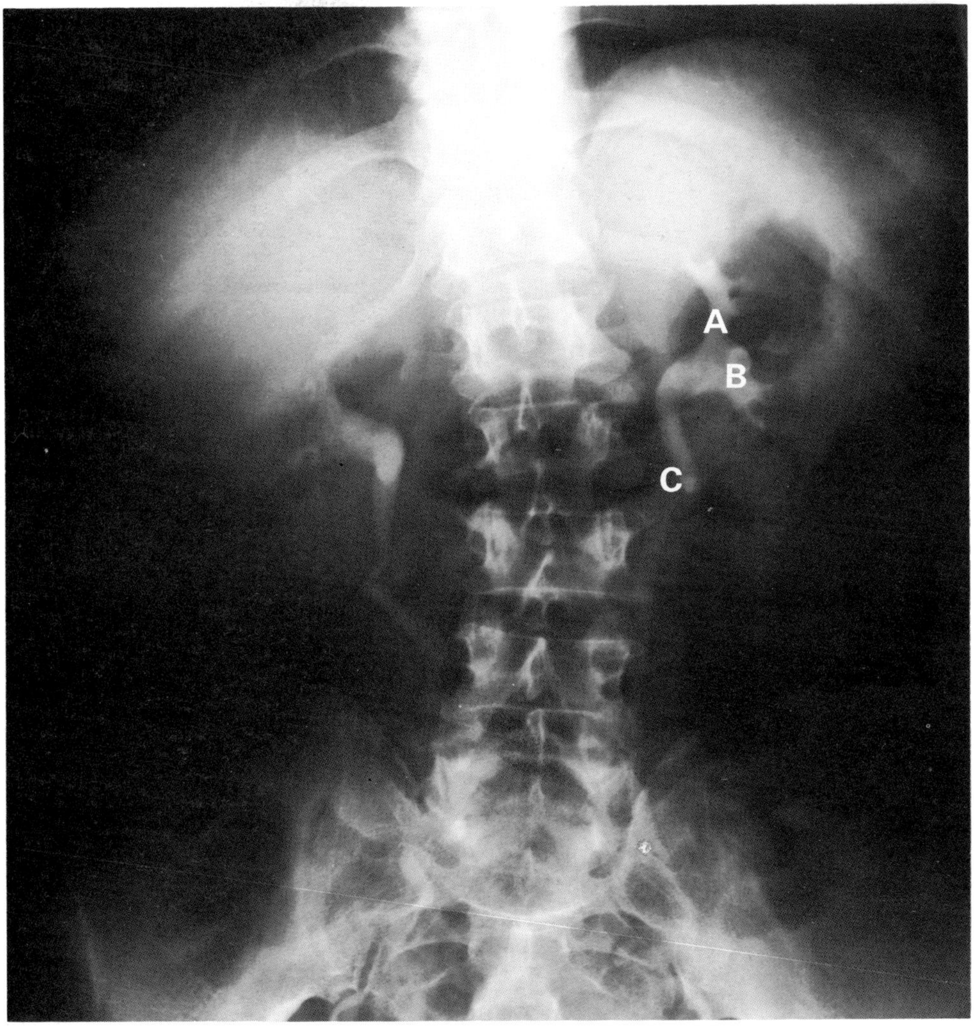

Fig. 8.4. An intravenous urogram exposed 5 minutes after injection. Contrast agent is present in each renal pelvicalyceal system and ureter.

A, B Major calyces of the left kidney

C A 'kink' in the left ureter

an obstruction prevents emptying of the bladder. Fig. 8.5a is an intravenous urogram exposed about 30 minutes after injection of the contrast agent and the appearances of the bladder are characteristic. We may compare this physiological demonstration with Fig. 8.5b which is a typical cystogram; that is,

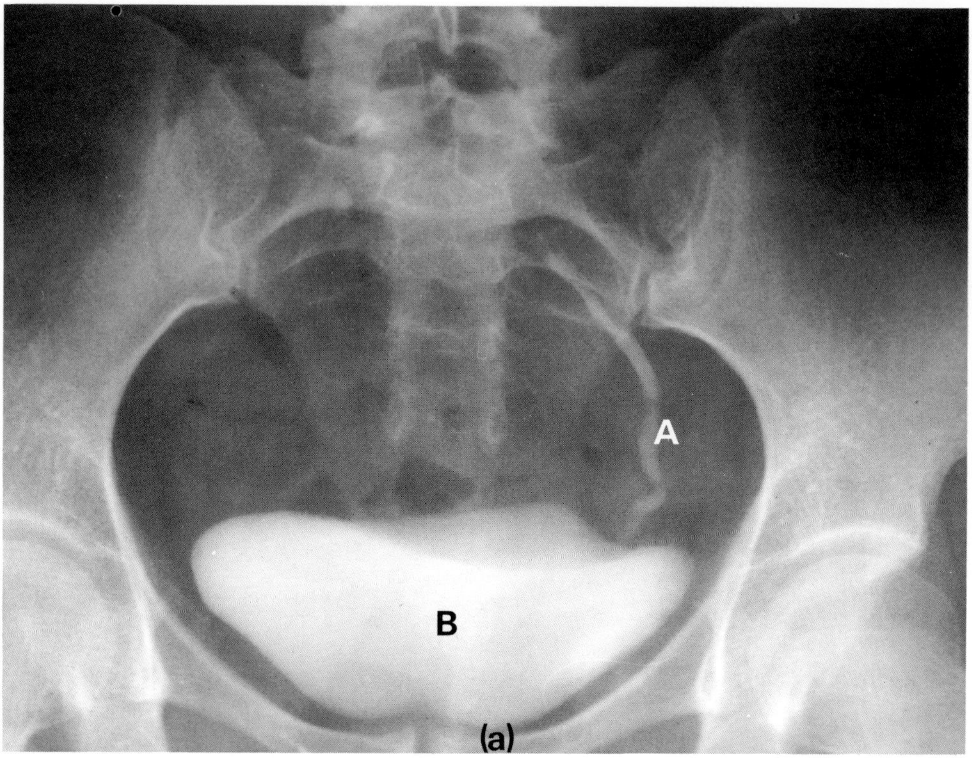

Fig. 8.5a. The bladder as seen during intravenous urography, about 20–30 minutes after injection. The lower left ureter is delineated by the contrast agent.

A Left ureter

B The bladder partly filled with contrast agent

the bladder was first emptied and then filled to its physical capacity with the contrast agent through an urethral catheter.

The bladder is faintly visualised in Fig. 8.2, a retrograde pyelogram. In this case a small quantity of contrast agent is seen to have flowed—and to be in the process of flowing—from the filled renal pelvicalyceal systems by way of both ureters to the bladder; the contrast agent is diluted with urine.

Fig. 8.1a is another intravenous urogram (not the same patient as in Fig. 8.5a) which shows the bladder containing only a little contrast agent. This exposure was made 15 minutes after the intravenous injection and again the appearance is typical of the particular phase of the procedure.

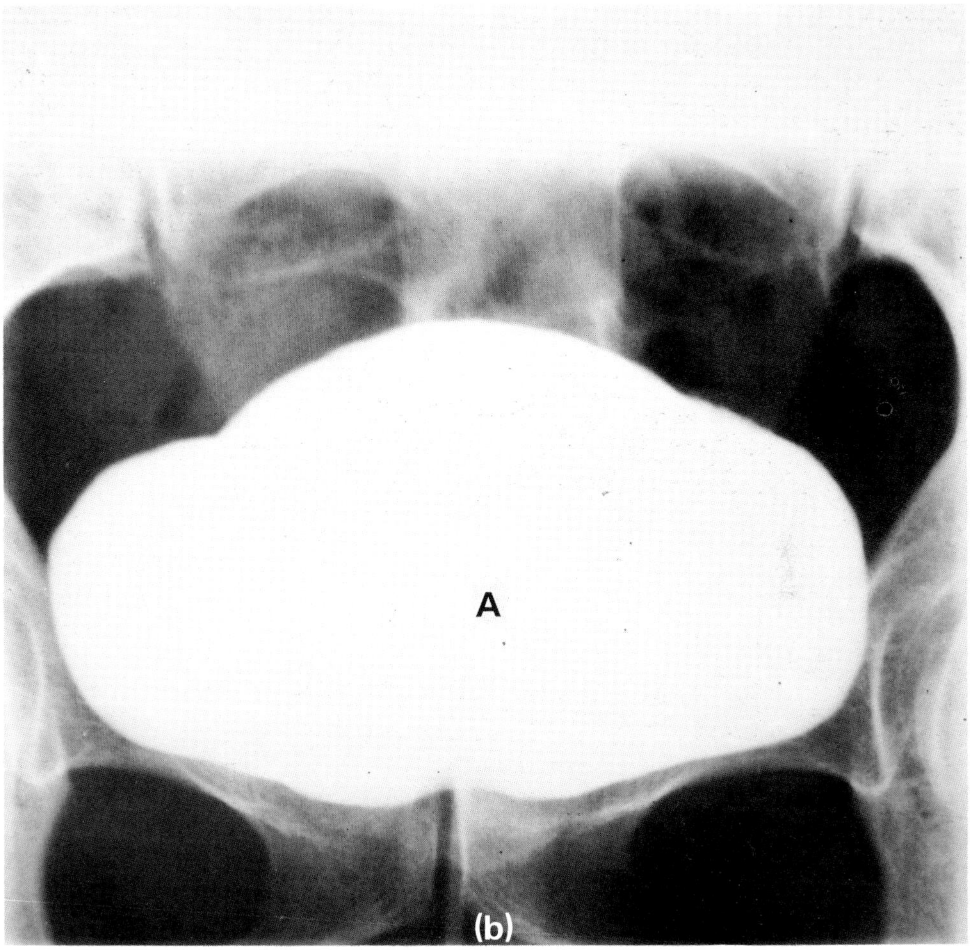

Fig. 8.5b. The bladder filled with a radiological contrast agent during cystography.
A The bladder, filled to near capacity

Since the urinary bladder is a distensible sac, the function of which is to provide a reservoir for urine, the size, position and even shape of the organ frequently change depending upon (a) the quantity of urine within the organ, (b) the condition of neighbouring viscera and other structures which themselves may enlarge: examples are a loaded rectum or hypertrophied prostate. By comparing the appearances of the bladder in Figs. 8.1a, 8.2, 8.5a and 8.5b, we obtain some evidence of the alterations in size of the bladder as the result of a varying quantity in its contents.

Empty, the bladder of an adult is wholly a pelvic organ. In an infant the bladder is relatively at a higher level, but even so only about half the organ is above the plane of the pelvic inlet. When empty and contracted, the bladder is described as a four-faced structure, which has a base, two inferolateral surfaces, a superior surface and an apex. As it fills, the superior surface of the bladder rises gradually into the

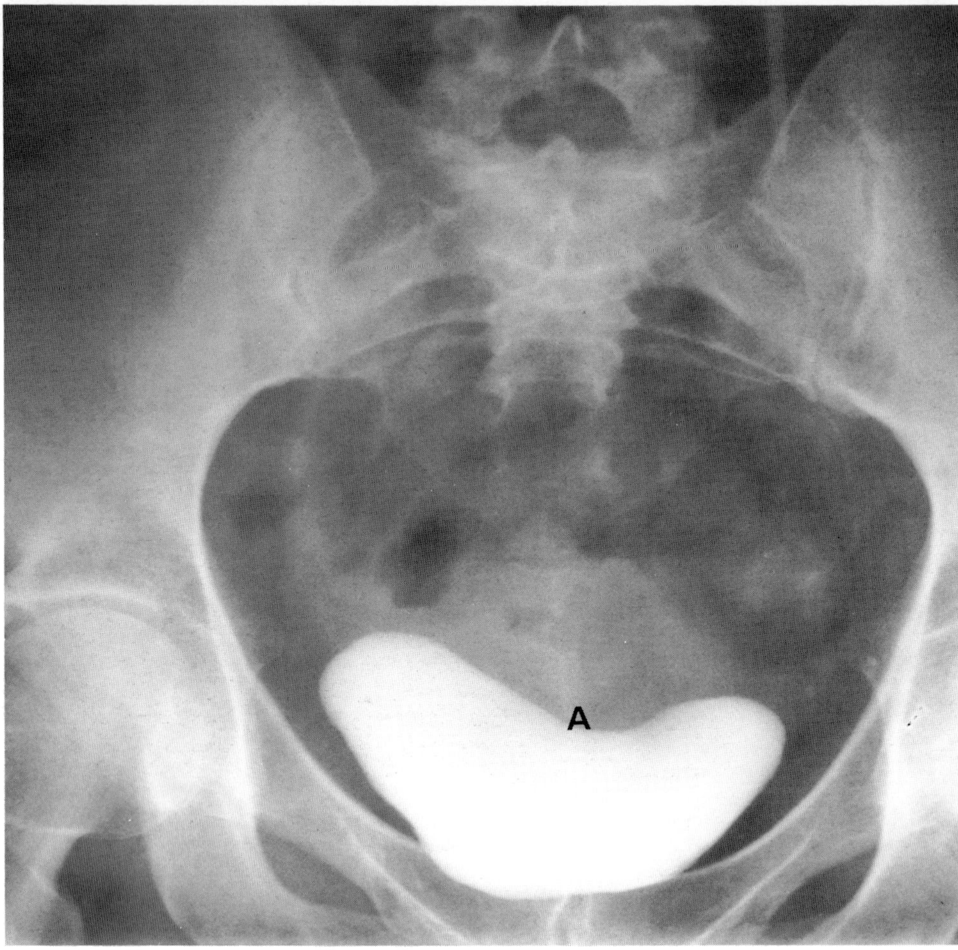

Fig. 8.6. The bladder seen during intravenous urography. It is well filled with contrast agent: the indentation (A) on its superior surface is caused probably by the uterus.

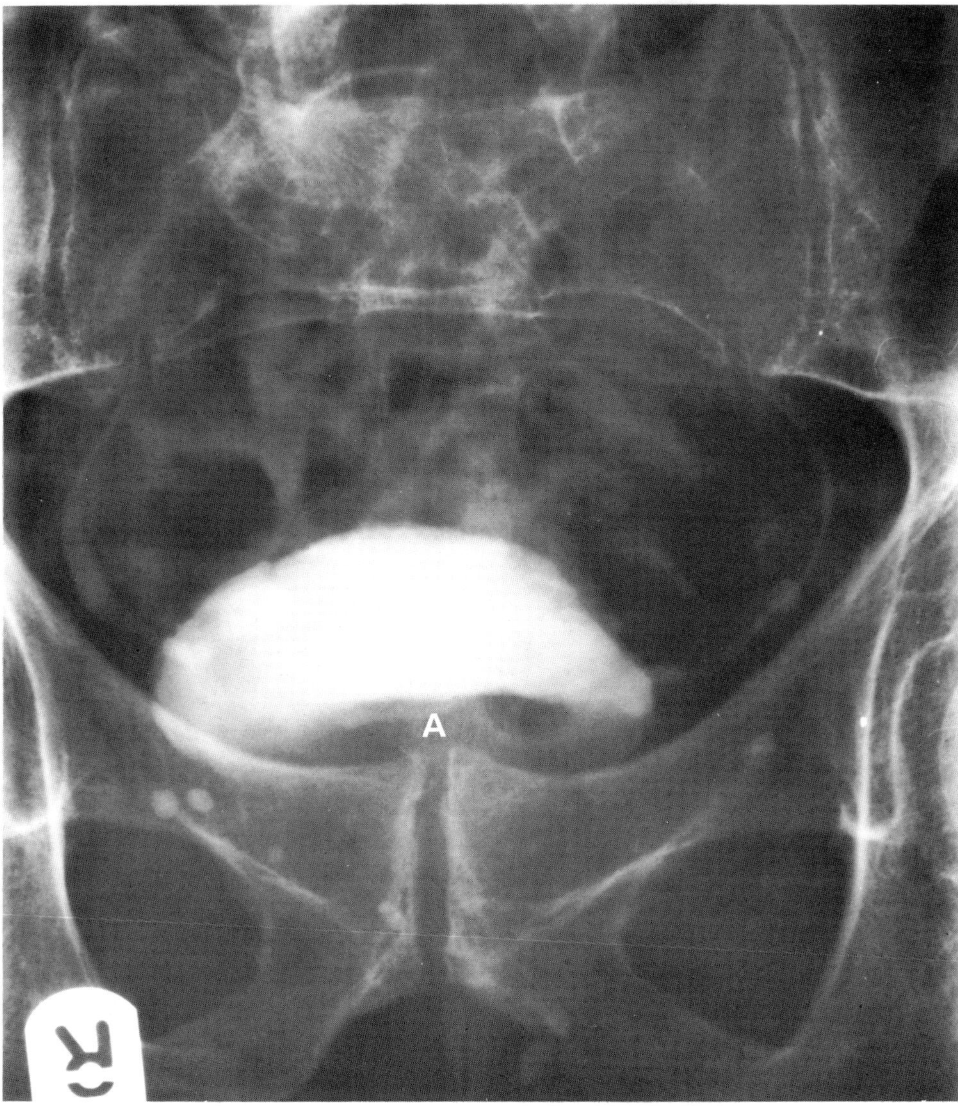

Fig. 8.7. The bladder filled with contrast agent during intravenous urography. The radiolucency—or 'filling defect'—(A) which is impressing the base of the bladder is due to an enlarged prostate. This is a post-micturition radiograph which has demonstrated that pressure from the hypertrophied prostate is obstructing the outflow of urine.

abdomen and the organ becomes more ovoid in shape with increasing distension. Since the empty bladder is not visualised on a radiograph, radiographers do not usually observe it, but they can hardly avoid the awareness of its rounded contours as a contrast agent delineates these during the process of filling.

Fig. 8.6 shows a result of extrinsic pressure on the bladder by another organ, in this case by the uterus. The appearance here is not necessarily indicative of a uterine lesion: the radiograph might be of a patient who was menstruating, at which time the uterus normally becomes more vascular, enlarged and rounded.

In Fig. 8.7 external pressure from the prostate has made an impression on the base of the bladder. In many men after the age of 45–50 the prostate gradually enlarges. Such hypertrophy, whilst often benign in nature, may advance in late life to a stage when projection of a large prostate into the bladder causes obstruction and urinary retention. The condition then requires surgery.

In the school of radiography and in the X-ray department students usually have many more opportunities to see and notice the effects on the bladder of volumetric content, age and abdomino-pelvic environment than can be shown within the limits of this book.

The last, that is most distal, of the urinary organs is the urethra, through which urine is discharged from the bladder. The anatomy of the urethra is considered below.

Cystourethrography

In both males and females the urethra is a tube which is merely a slit unless fluid is flowing along it. Like the bladder itself when empty, the urethra is not normally seen on a plain radiograph but its lumen will be demonstrated when it is made radiopaque. Cystourethrography is such an examination of the bladder and urethra by means of a radiological contrast agent; this enters the bladder through a catheter placed in the urethra, as distinct from the physiological processes which participate in intravenous urography. Fig. 8.5b shows the bladder filled in this way.

THE MALE URETHRA

In the male, the urinary and reproductive systems share the urethra. It is an outflow tube for both urine and seminal fluid and is some 18–20 cm long. It is described as having three parts.

(i) The prostatic portion of the urethra is the widest and runs vertically through the prostate gland from base to apex, for a distance of about 3 cm.

(ii) The membranous portion is the shortest and—except for the external orifice—the narrowest part of the urethra; and it is the least dilatable. Its length is about 2 cm and its course curves downwards and forwards from the prostate to the penis. The membranous part of the urethra is surrounded by the fibres of the urethral sphincter muscle.

(iii) The spongy portion of the male urethra is contained within the correspondingly named part (corpus spongiosum) of the penis, through which it runs to the external urethral orifice. When the penis is dependent, this portion of the urethra makes another downward and forward curve; it is about 15 cm long.

Fig. 8.8a—a cystourethrogram in an oblique projection—demonstrates the penile part of the urethra filled with a radiological contrast agent. There is some contrast agent in the bladder above and a sufficient delineation of other parts of the urethra for the reader to appreciate the relatively vertical course of the prostatic and membranous portions.

The radiograph (Fig. 8.8a) visualises the soft tissues of part of the body of the penis, which is composed of three columns of erectile tissue. Two of these (the corpora cavernosa) are anterior; the third is the corpus spongiosum which encloses the urethra and lies posteriorly. This topography may be followed from the appearance of the penis in Fig. 8.8a.

The male urethra is much longer than the female and in consequence more prone to obstruction. A stricture is present on Fig. 8.8a. The cause of this is seen on Fig. 8.8b, a plain radiograph. It shows the presence of two small calcific calculi which the contrast agent almost obliterates on Fig. 8.8a.

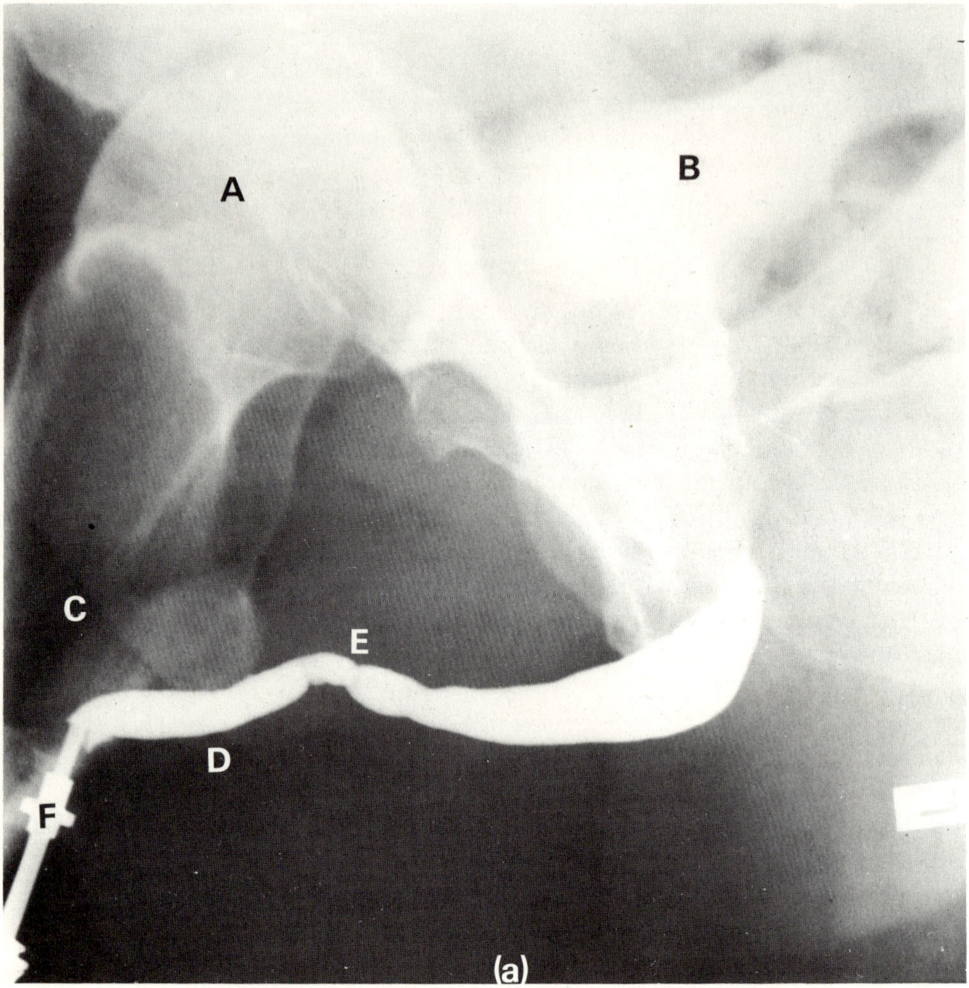

Fig. 8.8a. An oblique radiograph of the male urethra which has been filled with a radiological contrast agent during cystourethrography.

A Head of the right femur
B Contrast agent in the bladder
C Anterior aspect of the body of the penis
D Posterior part of the body of the penis
E Stricture of the urethra
F The cannula used for injection of the contrast agent

THE FEMALE URETHRA

The female urethra—unlike the male's—is associated exclusively with the urinary tract and perhaps gives the

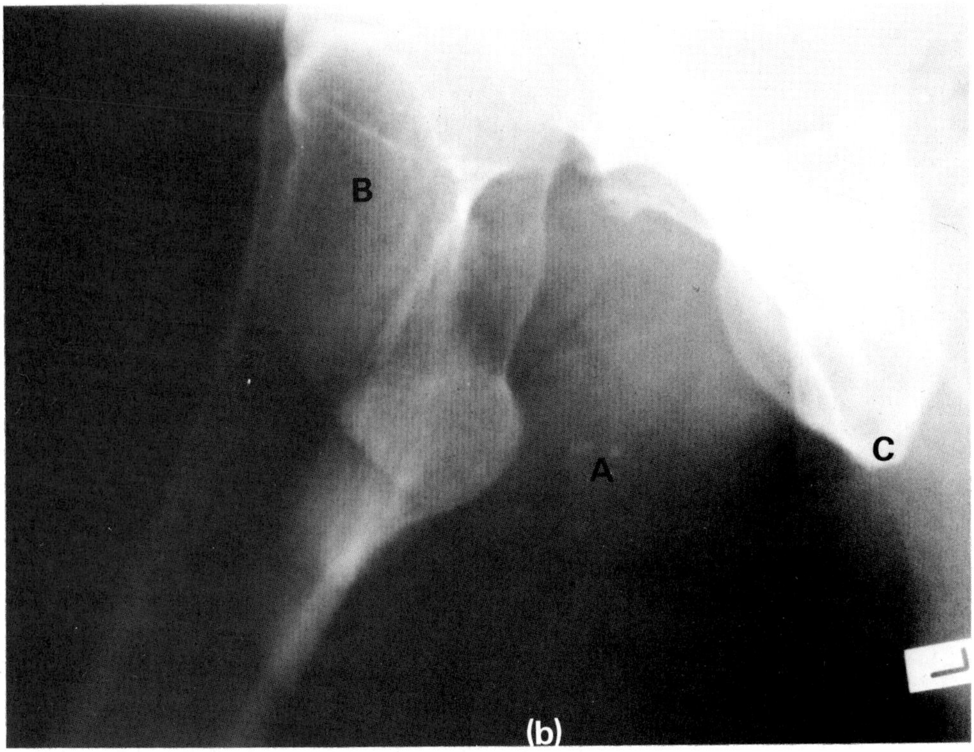

Fig. 8.8b. An oblique plain radiograph of the same patient as on Fig. 8.8a. Calcific calculi are seen which are responsible for the urethral obstruction shown previously.

A Calculi in the urethra
B Femoral neck
C Ischial tuberosity of the hip bone

impression of being better designed. Although no greater in diameter (6 mm) than the penile portion of the male urethra, the female urethra is very much shorter and more readily dilatable and consequently is less easily obstructed. Embedded in the anterior wall of the vagina, it has a safer situation in the event of crush injuries to the pelvis, which sometimes result in rupture of the male urethra between the prostatic and membranous parts.

The course of the female urethra is downwards and forwards behind the pubic symphysis and is about 4 cm in length.

Radiologically, during cystourethrography, an angle is

formed between the opacified silhouettes of the bladder and the urethra; more correctly, we may recognise that there is an anterior and a posterior urethrovesical angle. Such an appearance can be seen on Fig. 8.9a which is a lateral projection of the filled bladder; the catheter, by means of which the contrast agent was introduced, is still in place and is indicating the direction of the urethra.

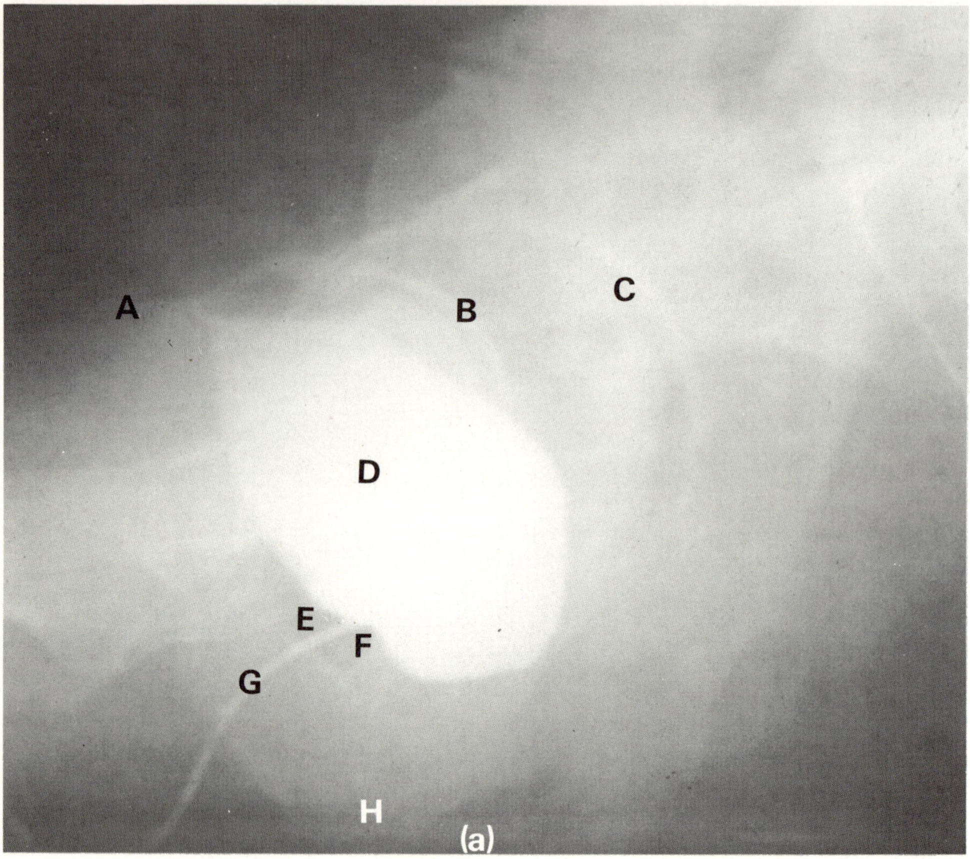

Fig. 8.9a. A cystourethrogram of a female patient. The radiograph is a lateral projection exposed by means of a horizontal beam while the patient was seated.

A Pubic symphysis
B, C Margin of each acetabulum of the hip bone
D The bladder
E Anterior urethrovesical angle
F Posterior urethrovesical angle
G Catheter in the urethra
H Superimposed images of the ischial tuberosities

The urethrovesical angle is a radiological sign of the competence of the internal sphincter muscle which surrounds the internal urethral orifice in the base of the bladder. The competence of this muscle is maintained normally except during the act of micturition. Fig. 8.9b illustrates some of the changes which then occur and of which the most significant for successful emptying of the bladder is the loss of the posterior urethrovesical angle. The control of this angle is

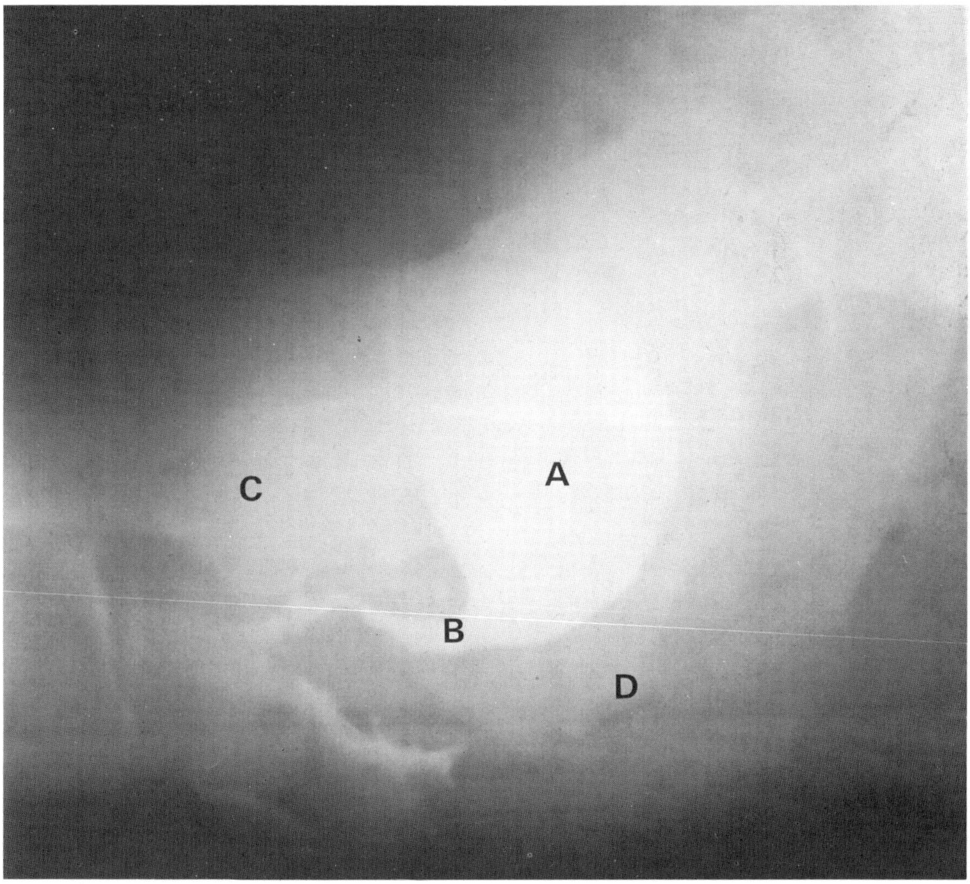

Fig. 8.9b. A similar radiograph of the same patient as on Fig. 8.9a, exposed during micturition.

A The bladder
B The urethra
C The femoral necks and upper part of the shafts
D The ischia of the hip bones

dependent upon involuntary muscles at the urethrovesical junction.

Urinary incontinence sometimes occurs in women when intra-abdominal pressure is raised during such actions as laughing, coughing or the expulsive effort described as 'bearing down'. This form of incontinence is known as stress incontinence and in such cases the most frequent radiographic finding is a loss—or poor formation—of the posterior urethrovesical angle, when intra-abdominal pressure is increased and even sometimes when the patient is at rest.

Renal aortography (arteriography)

The renal arteries may be demonstrated by a direct injection of a suitable radiological contrast agent, during either abdominal aortography or selective catheterisation of the renal artery itself. Fig. 8.10a is an example of abdominal aortography.

In this procedure a catheter is introduced to the femoral artery at a point where the vessel is relatively superficial in the groin, its pulsations are tangible and a needle and cannula may be easily inserted as a rule. In Fig. 8.10a the intra-arterial catheter is seen to have entered the aorta from the right femoral artery by way of the right external iliac artery and the right common iliac artery, part of which is included in the radiograph.

The film, which was exposed during the first second or two following injection of the contrast agent, shows most of the course of the abdominal aorta from the aortic opening in the diaphragm to its bifurcation on the body of lumbar vertebra 4 (to form the common iliac artery on each side). From the aorta, the contrast agent has entered a number of other major arteries and subdivisions of these. The large vessels which have been delineated are described below.

(i) The hepatic artery is a branch of the coeliac axis, a short arterial trunk which is not itself readily identifiable from a supine radiograph since it arises from the front of the aorta, just below the diaphragm, and passes forwards almost horizontally. The direction of the hepatic artery is first forwards and then to the right and upwards, in front of the portal vein and to the left of the common bile duct. The hepatic artery divides into right and left branches which supply the corresponding lobes of the liver and gives off other vessels which feed (a) parts of the stomach and duodenum, (b) the gall bladder, (c) the pancreas.

(ii) The splenic artery is the largest branch of the coeliac axis (the third and smallest is the gastric artery). The splenic artery, surrounded by a plexus of nerves and accompanied by the splenic vein, takes a tortuous course horizontally to the left behind the stomach, along the upper border of the pancreas and in front of the upper part of the left kidney. Close to the spleen the artery divides into five or six branches which enter the splenic hilum.

(iii) The superior mesenteric artery arises from the front of the aorta about 1 cm below the coeliac axis. It is a large vessel which supplies (a) all the small intestine except for the first part of the duodenum, (b) the caecum, the ascending colon and most of the transverse colon. Near the origin of the artery the left renal vein lies between it and the aorta. Its downward and forward course then takes the artery between layers of the mesentery, in front of the inferior vena cava, the right ureter and the psoas major muscle; the artery is accompanied by the superior mesenteric vein. In the right iliac fossa the superior mesenteric artery diminishes in size and terminates by anastomosis with one of its own branches.

(iv) The renal arteries are two large vessels which arise one on either side of the aorta immediately below the superior mesenteric artery. Because the aorta lies a little to the left of the midline, the right renal artery is longer than its fellow; it is also slightly lower in origin. Each takes a course nearly at right angles to the aorta: the right renal artery passes behind the inferior vena cava, the right renal vein and the head of the pancreas; the left renal artery passes behind the left renal vein, the body of the pancreas and the splenic vein. Each artery divides into branches just before reaching the hilum of the kidney.

In the case shown on Fig. 8.10a there is an accessory renal artery supplying the lower pole of the left kidney. One or even two accessory renal arteries are often found. Such an artery most commonly occurs on the left—as here—but arises from the aorta rather more often above the main artery than

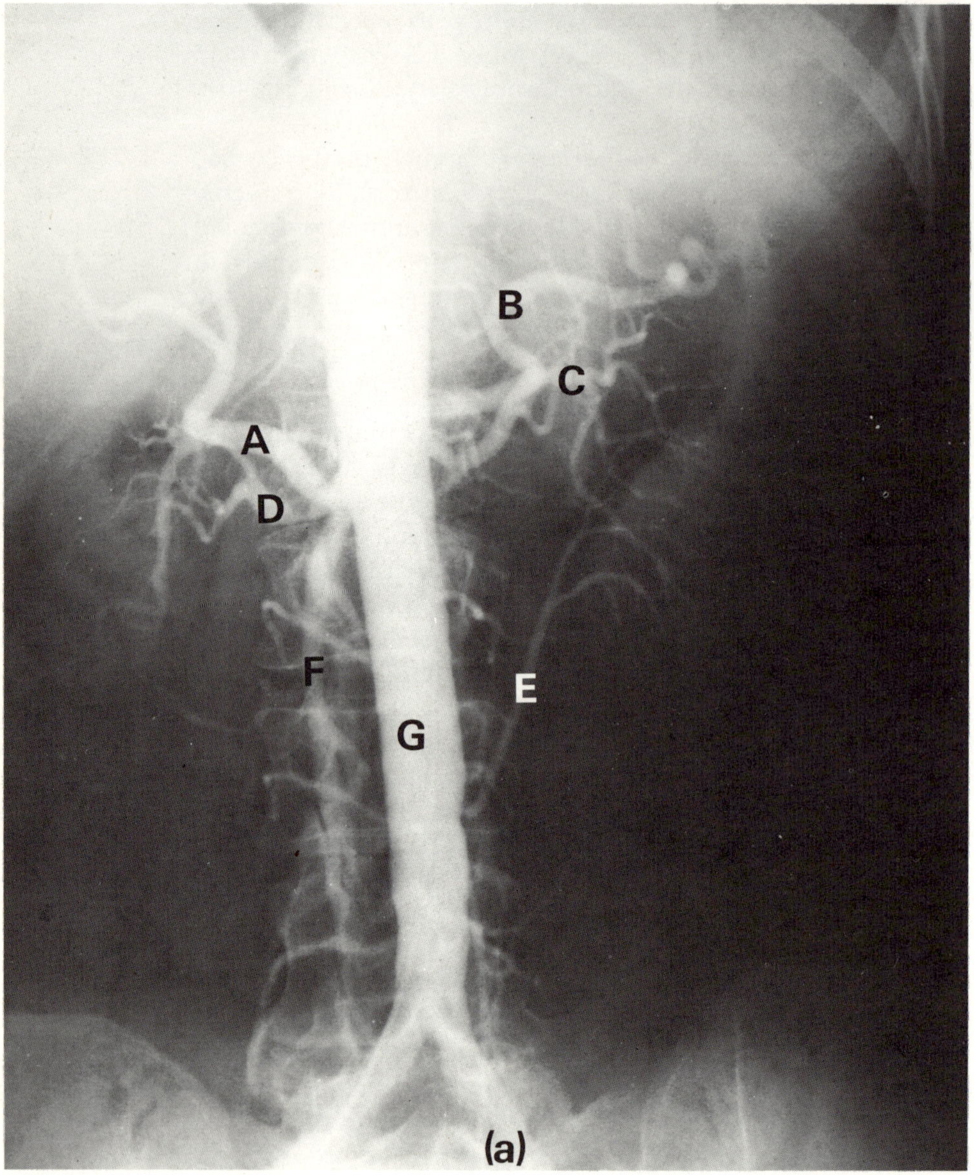

Fig. 8.10a. An immediate radiograph taken during abdominal aortography. The aorta and some principal branches are filled with contrast agent (see also Fig. 10.3a).

A The hepatic artery
B The splenic artery
C The left renal artery
D The right renal artery
E An accessory left renal artery
F The superior mesenteric artery
G The abdominal aorta

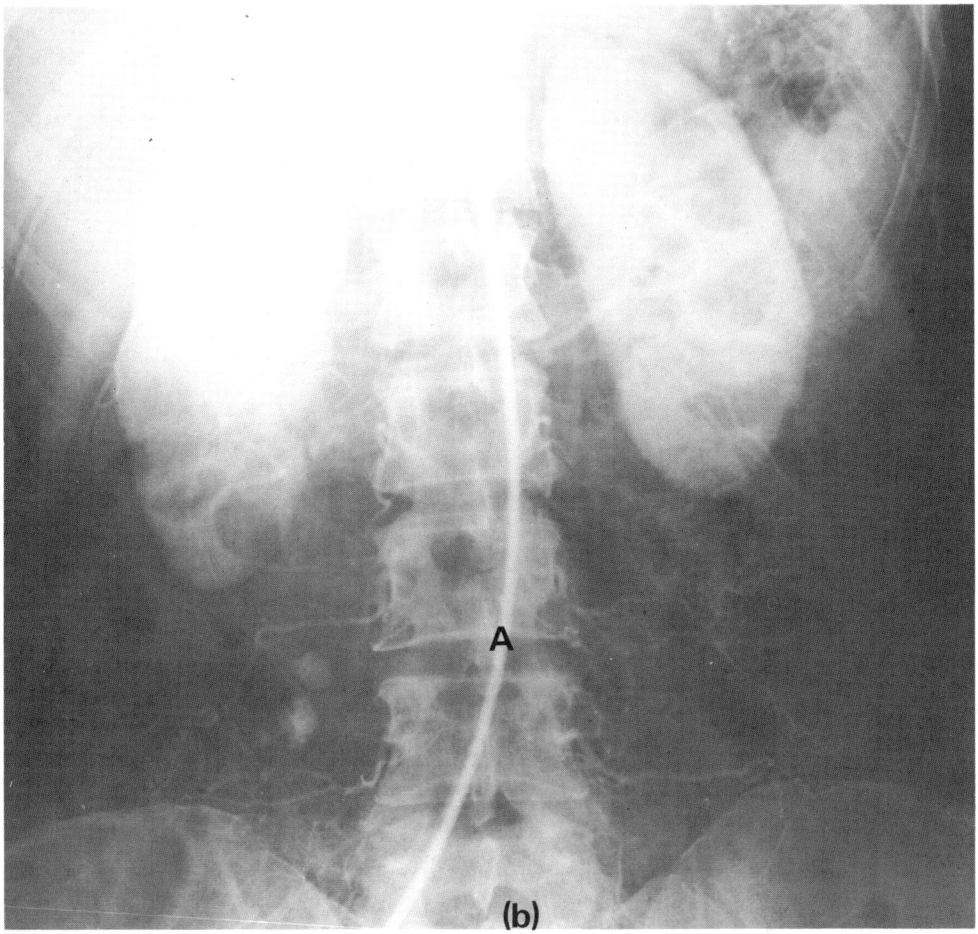

Fig. 8.10b. A later radiograph in a series taken during abdominal aortography. Contrast agent has opacified the renal tissues.
A Intra-arterial catheter in the abdominal aorta

below it: in that case the vessel supplies the upper part of the kidney.

Fig. 8.10b illustrates the appearance of the kidneys and abdominal vasculature during a late phase of aortography. The radiograph was exposed perhaps five to six seconds after the introduction of a contrast agent, through the intra-arterial catheter which is lying in the abdominal aorta and has its tip opposite the body of thoracic vertebra 12. At this stage of the procedure many minor blood vessels have filled. The contrast agent has entered the small arteries and capillaries of the kidney and has opacified the renal substance in an effect which is described as nephrography or as a flushing of the organ. The appearance of the kidneys on Fig. 8.10b confirms the account of their size, shape and position which is given on pages 123 and 188.

Chapter 9
Contrast Examinations: The Gall Bladder and Extrahepatic Ducts

Anatomically and physiologically the gall bladder is less important than the liver, being merely a part of the liver's excretory apparatus (and a dispensable part, at that, without which we can all easily survive if this necessity occurs). In radiological practice, however, the gall bladder is arguably the more significant organ. Diseases of the gall bladder are usually capable of radiological diagnosis by means of safe and relatively simple procedures. Consequently the gall bladder and its ducts are frequently the subject of X-ray examination; in the course of their training, students are likely to see these parts of the biliary system on the relevant radiographs possibly hundreds of times. For these reasons the gall bladder and the extrahepatic ducts are to be described before and separately from the liver.

Oral cholecystography

On a plain radiograph of the abdomen the gall bladder is not apparent. The gall bladder becomes visible on an X-ray film in either of two circumstances:

(a) if it is filled with stones which contain calcium and therefore are radiopaque;

(b) alternatively, if a suitable radiological contrast has been correctly administered to the patient at some appropriate time before the X-ray exposure is made.

In Chapter 5 of this book some description is given of the organs visualised on a plain abdominal radiograph, the necessary preliminary to any contrast examination. On Fig. 5.11 the gall bladder has been demonstrated in the right lumbar region because it is virtually full of radiopaque stones. The anatomist's classic description of the gall bladder that it is 'a . . . conical or pear-shaped sac lodged in a fossa on the under-surface of the liver' (*Gray's Anatomy*) is seen to be well justified.

Among several available radiological examinations which are applicable to the gall bladder and the extrahepatic ducts the most commonly performed is the oral cholecystogram. In this procedure a suitable contrast agent (containing iodine, a substance of high atomic number) is given to the patient by mouth, its administration being followed by overnight starvation. The period of fasting is to ensure that the gall bladder is not required to release bile for the digestive process and may therefore store and sufficiently concentrate a quantity of bile, which the contrast substance has rendered radiologically opaque.

The gall bladder is seen thus demonstrated on Fig. 9.1a, b and c on three radiographs of different patients, exposed about 12 hours after the administration of an oral cholecystographic agent. In all cases the radiographic projection was a left anterior oblique view while the patient lay prone.

THE GALL BLADDER'S POSITION

The position of the gall bladder as classically given is described in the statement that its tip projects beneath the anterior border of the liver in the angle between the ends of the ninth and tenth costal cartilages and the outer border of the right rectus abdominis muscle. (This is a long flat muscle on the front of the abdomen: it arises from the crest of the pubis, extends over the full length of the abdomen and is inserted in the cartilages of the fifth, sixth and seventh ribs.)

However, students of radiographic anatomy soon recognise that the position of the gall bladder—as depicted radiographically—is very variable in different subjects. Fig. 9.1 illustrates this difference between individuals: in

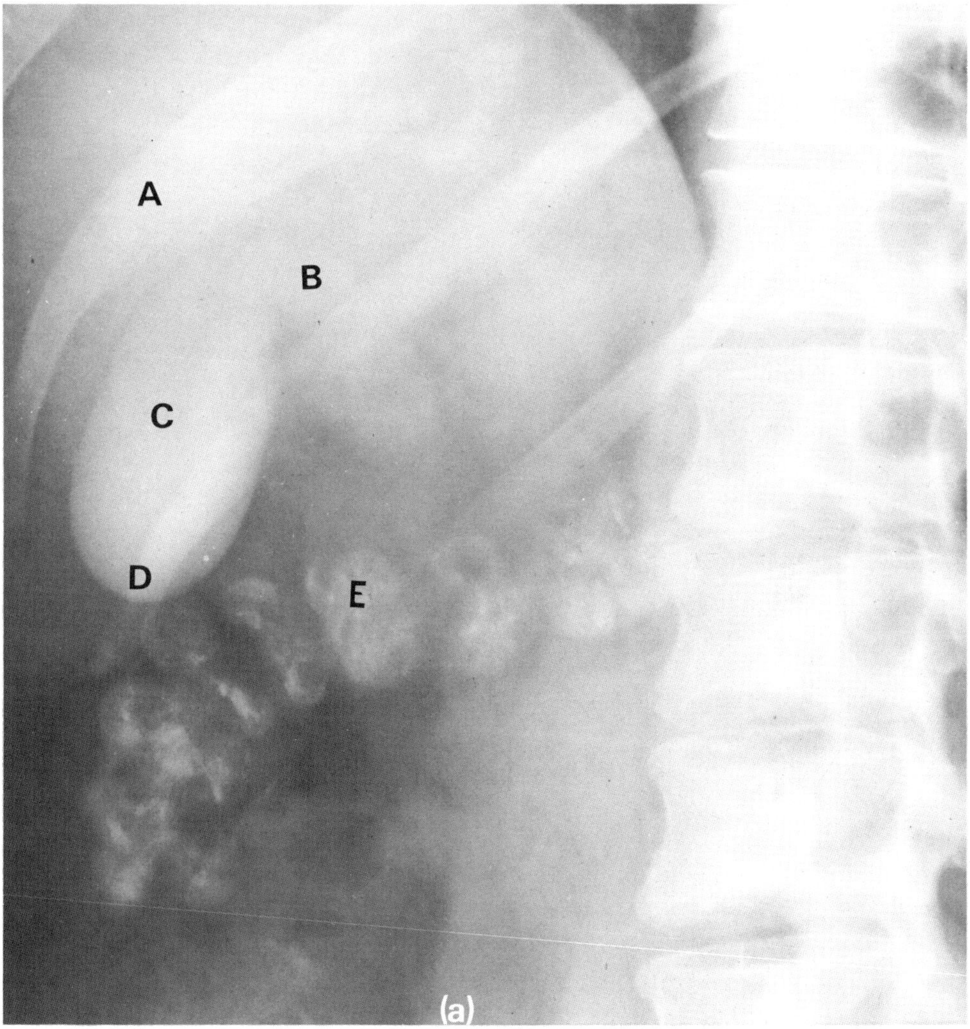

Fig. 9.1a. An oral cholecystogram (left anterior oblique projection) exposed about 12 hours after the contrast agent was taken. The patient was prone during the exposure.

A 10th right rib
B Neck of the gall bladder
C Body of the gall bladder
D Fundus of the gall bladder
E Contrast agent in the large bowel (transverse colon)

Fig. 9.1a the gall bladder is higher and more laterally situated than in Fig. 9.1b; and 9.1c shows a yet more extreme position. This type of variation is influenced significantly by body build. The position of the gall bladder on Fig. 9.1c—high and lateral in the right hypochondrium—is characteristic of the obese subject, although often in such individuals the gall bladder appears more circular than it does on this particular radiograph. This is because in these people the long axis of the

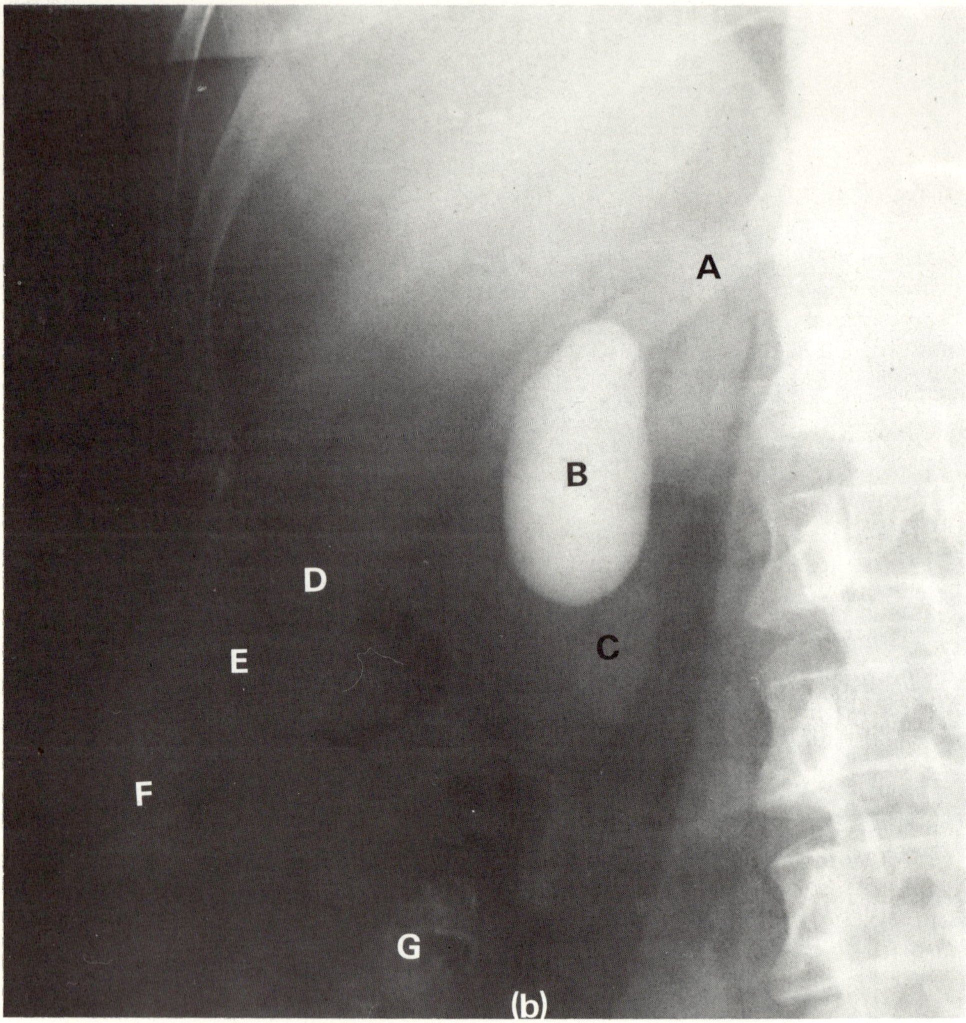

Fig. 9.1b. A similar radiograph to Fig. 9.1a but the gall bladder occupies a different position.

A 12th right rib
B Body of the gall bladder
C Right kidney
D Right lobe of the liver
E Extraperitoneal flank stripe
F Other flank stripes (fat planes)
G Contrast lying in the large bowel

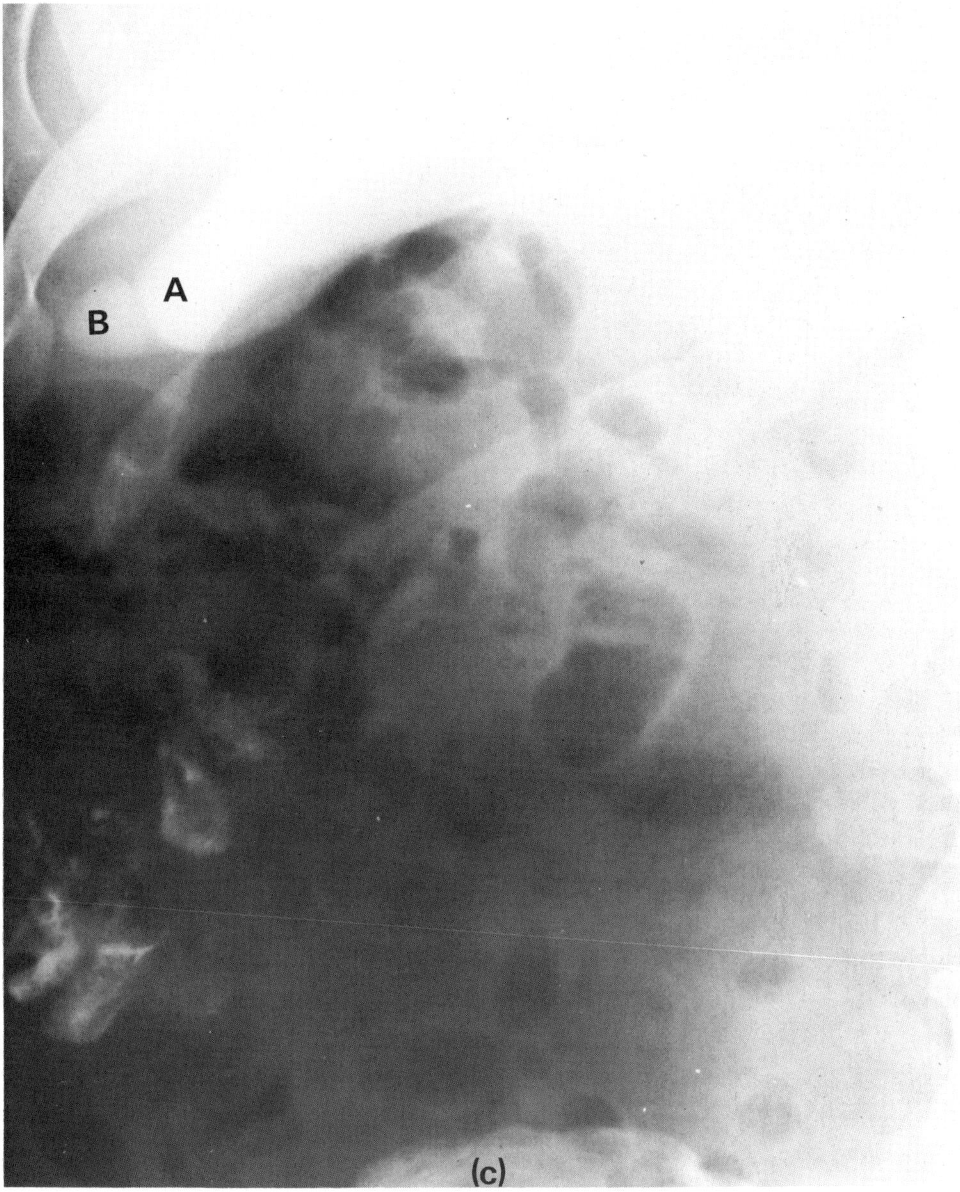

Fig. 9.1c. An oral cholecystogram exposed similarly to Figs. 9.1a and 9.1b.

A Fundus of the gall bladder B Phrygian cap (see p. 221)

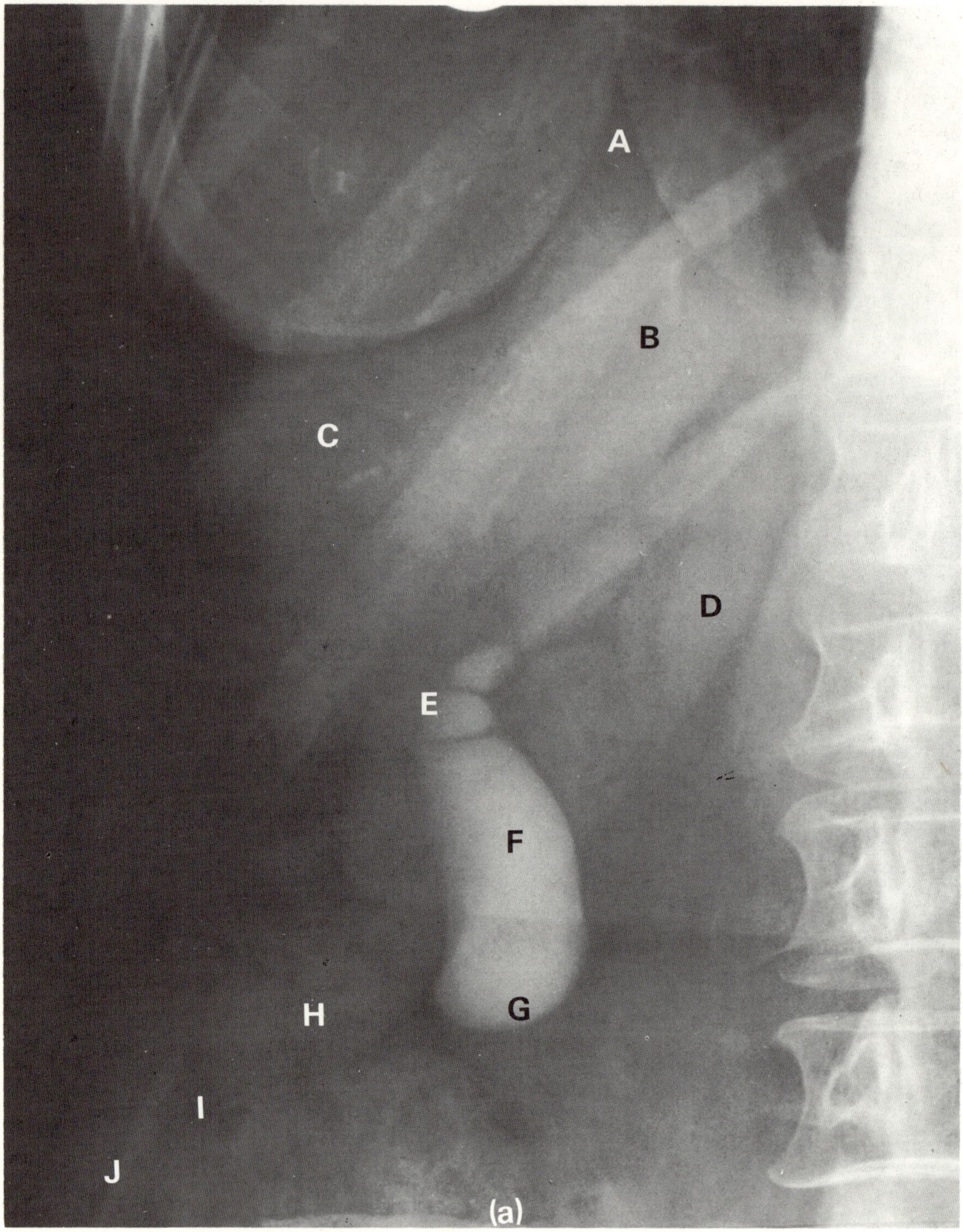

Fig. 9.2a. An oral cholecystogram exposed when the patient was prone.

A Breast shadows (female patient)
B, C Calcification in costal cartilages
D Right kidney
E Neck of the gall bladder, showing Heister's valves
F Body of the gall bladder
G Fundus of the gall bladder
H Right lobe of the liver
I, J Flank stripes (fat planes)

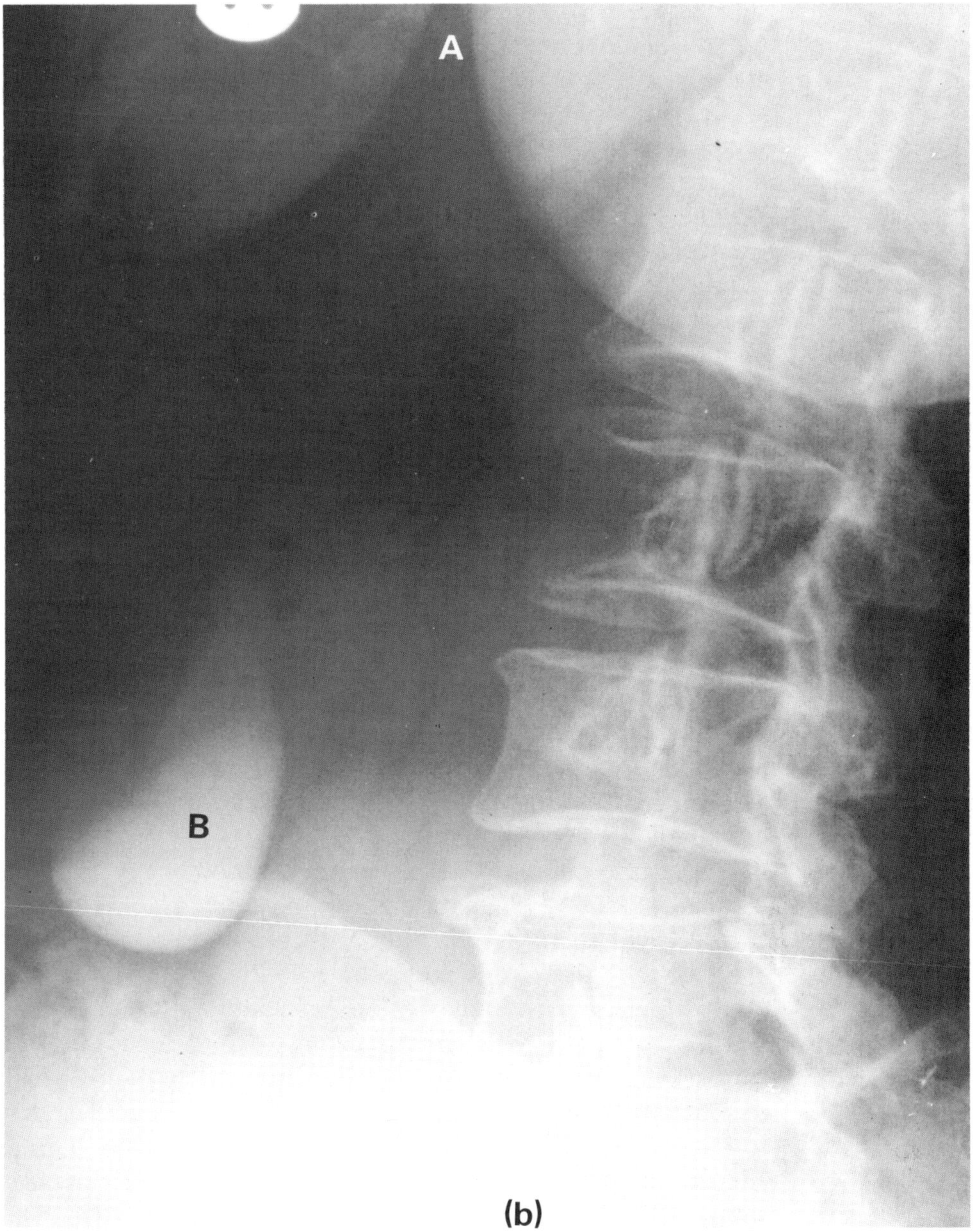

Fig. 9.2b. The same patient as in Fig. 9.2a but the exposure was made while the patient stood upright.

A Female breast shadows B Body of the gall bladder

gall bladder is directed more sharply forwards. In Fig. 9.1b the gall bladder lies nearer to the midline and the vertical: in the case of a lanky, atonic body build its image may even be superimposed on parts of the lower lumbar or even sacral vertebrae and the gall bladder may appear as elongated and thin as its owner. This in no way influences its physiological effectiveness.

There are other factors, as well as body type, in the mobility of the gall bladder as the organ is visualised on radiographs. One of these is the position which the patient occupies during the exposure. Not unexpectedly, the gall bladder obeys the law of gravity and will drop when the patient is erect, compared with its level when he is recumbent. Fig. 9.2 shows a downward swing of the gall bladder of about 10 cm between the prone position (Fig. 9.2a) and the erect position (Fig. 9.2b); Figs. 9.3a and 9.3c also should be compared.

Changing from the prone to the supine decubitus again moves the gall bladder, although as a rule much less so: it tips backwards and a little laterally and upwards (see Fig. 9.3a and b). It may appear more rounded in this position owing to a tendency to an end-on projection. The gall bladder is sensitive to respiration. It lies a little lower and nearer to the midline during the inspiratory phase, when intra-abdominal pressure is greater than in expiration.

These alterations in its projected position are significant features of the gall bladder for the radiographer since knowledge of them may be employed to secure a clear view of the organ, free from confusion or obliteration of detail by the superimposed images of other structures: for example, calcification in the costal cartilages may simulate opaque gall stones in the right hypochondrium and collections of intestinal gas look like cholesterol calculi. Three radioparent cholesterol stones are demonstrated in Fig. 9.4 and should be compared with the radiopaque variety seen in Fig. 5.11. Just below the gall bladder in Fig. 9.4 and following the line of the last rib, intestinal gas patterns are seen.

On Fig. 9.5a small transradiant gall stones both are obscured by the overlying opaque contrast agent in the functioning gall bladder and may be confused with nearby

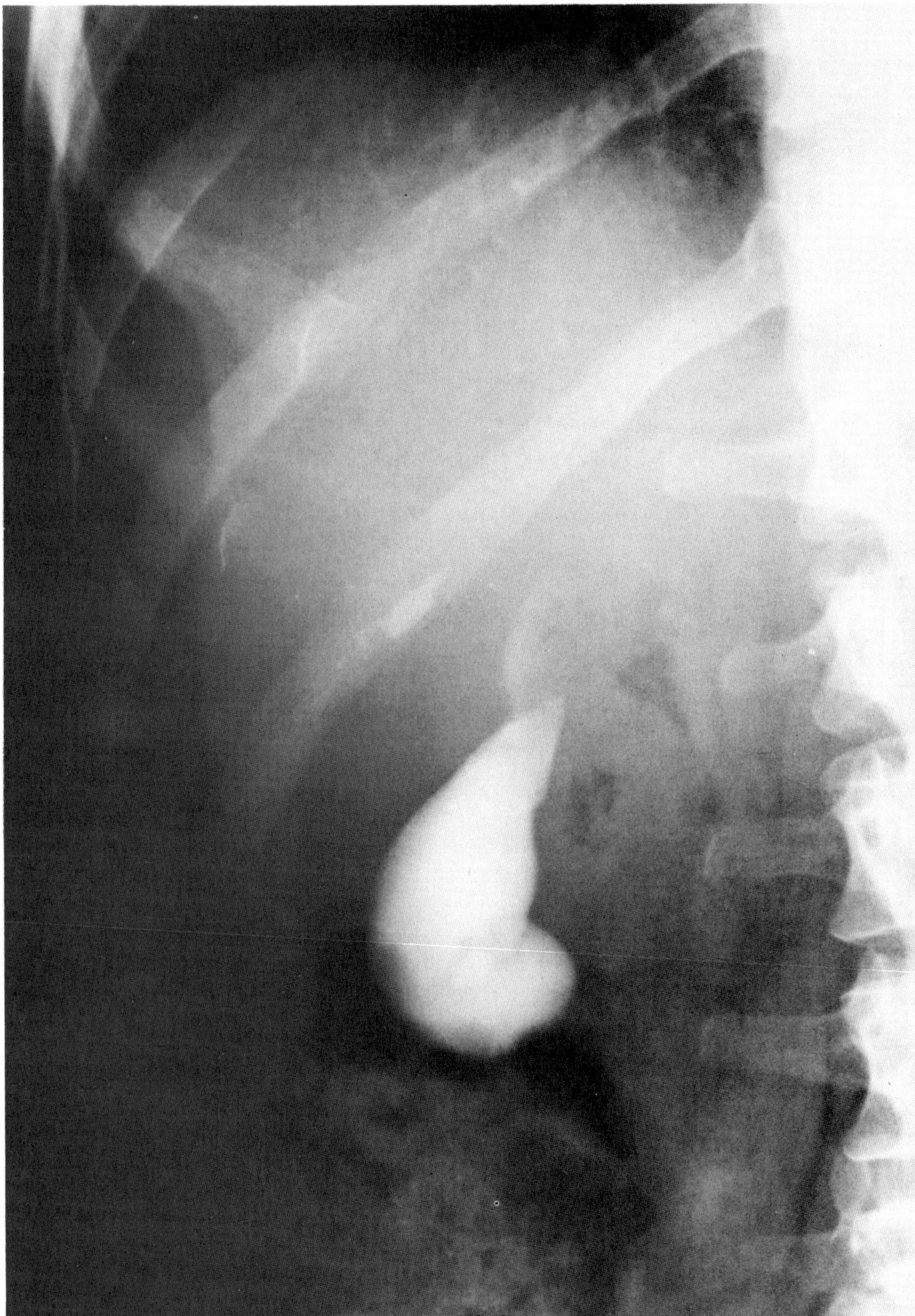

Fig. 9.3. An oral cholecystogram at 12 hours after ingestion of the contrast agent.
Fig. 9.3a. Posteroanterior projection exposed while the patient was prone.

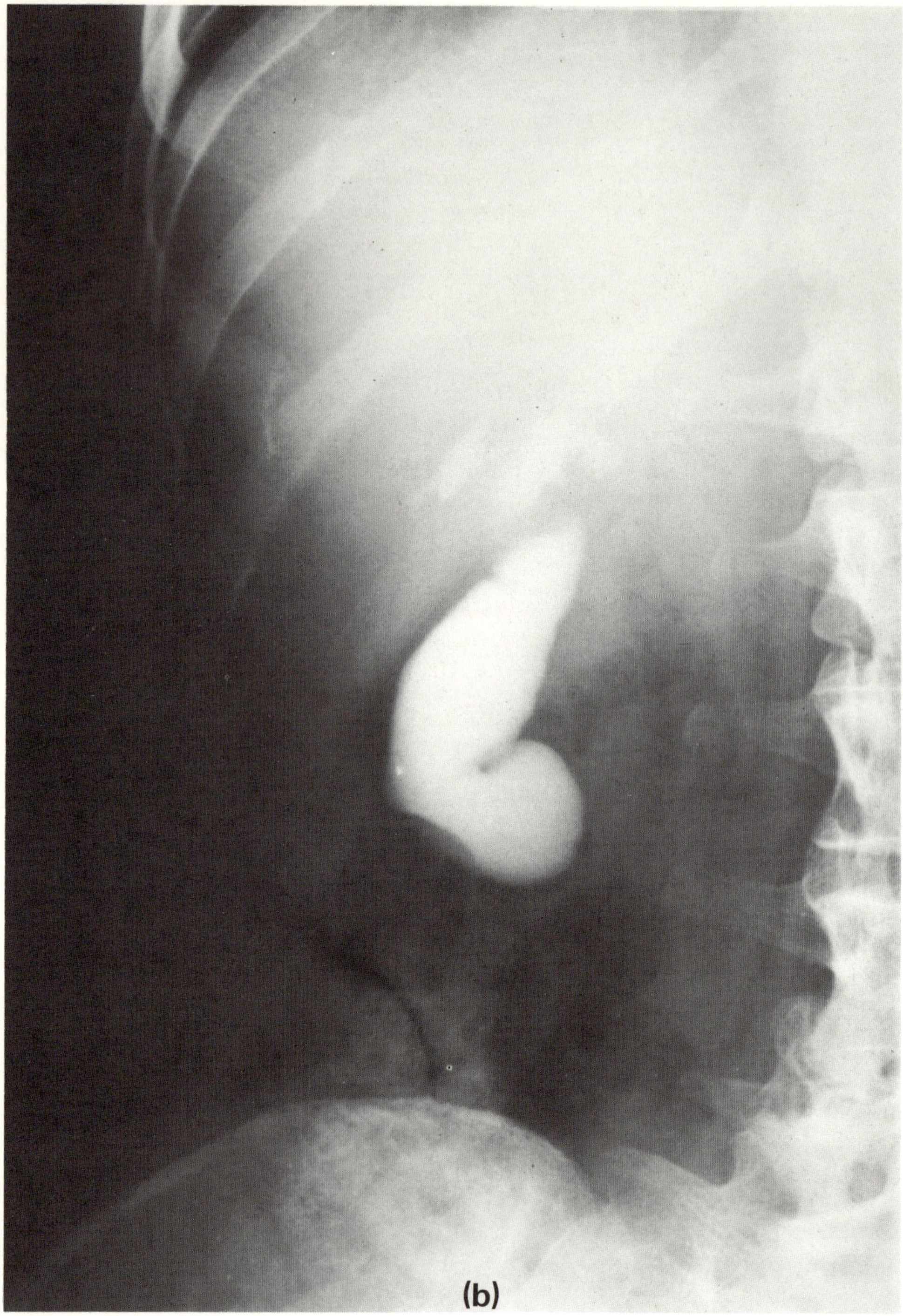

Fig. 9.3b. Anteroposterior projection exposed while the patient was supine.

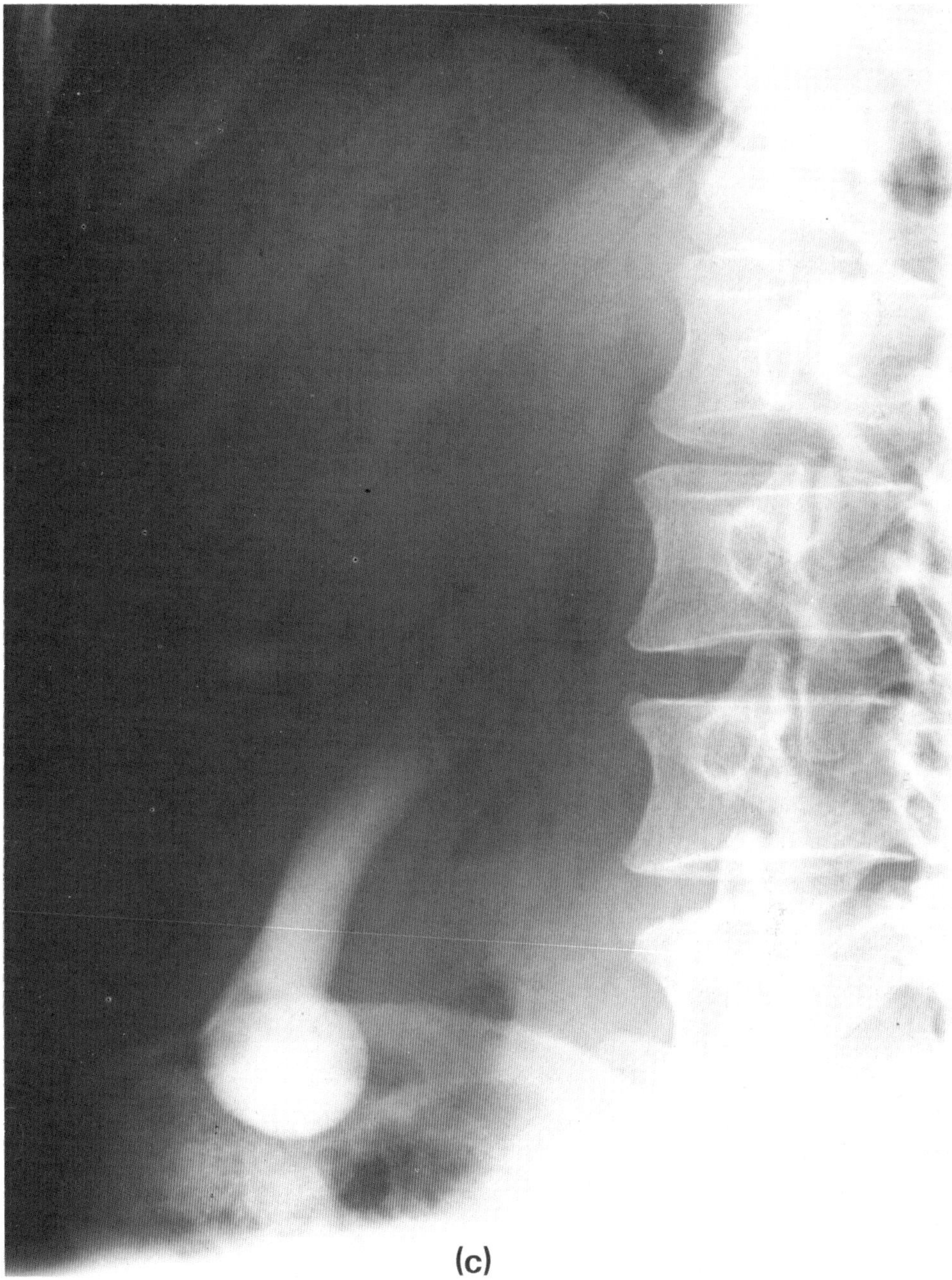

Fig. 9.3c. Left anterior oblique projection exposed while the patient was upright.

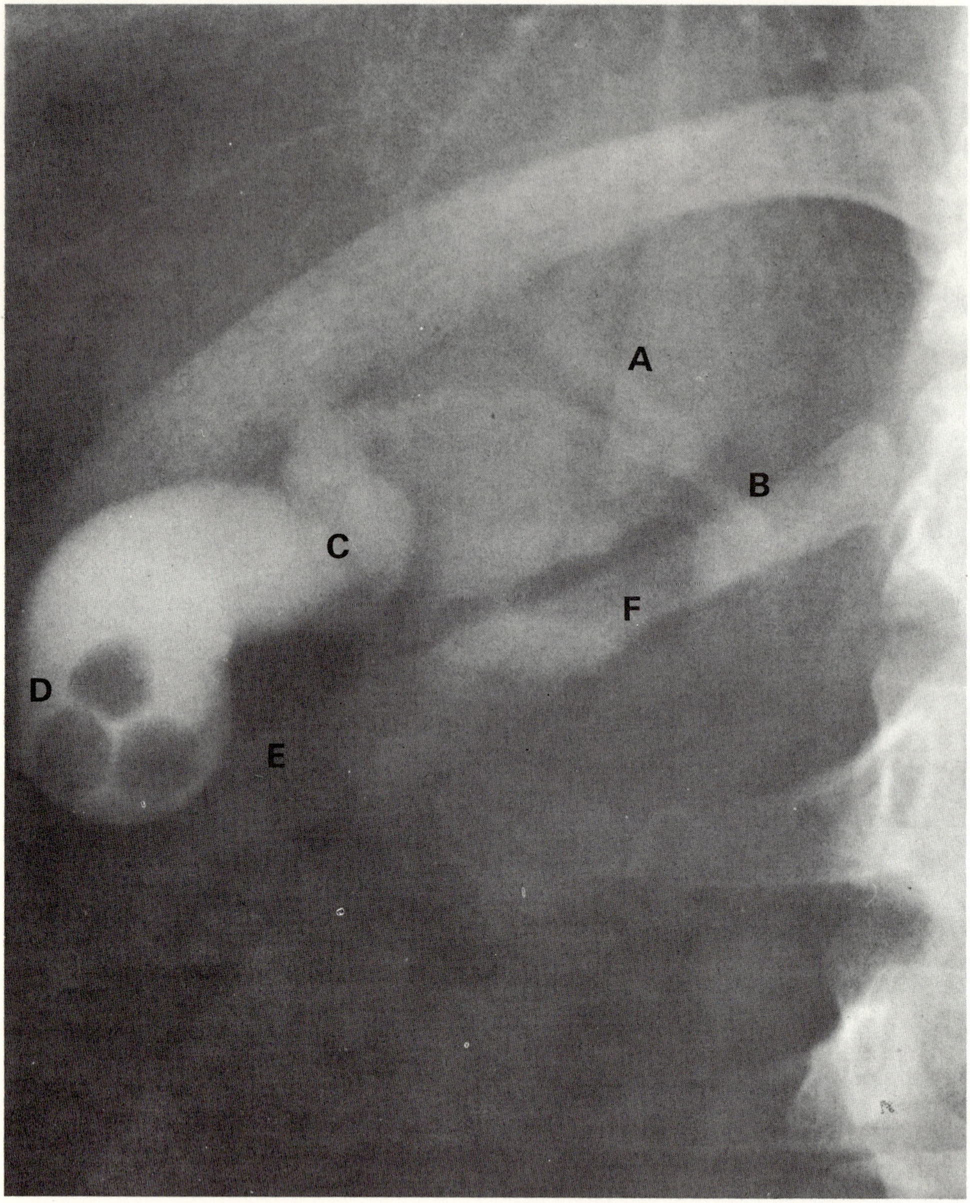

Fig. 9.4. An oral cholecystogram exposed after the patient has eaten fat.

A, B Hepatic ducts

C Neck of the gall bladder, continuous with the cystic duct above

D Three radioparent cholesterol gall stones (negative shadows)

E, F Radioparencies due to intestinal gas

small accumulations of intestinal gas. A radiograph exposed whilst the patient was standing erect (Fig. 9.5b) shows them floating in opacified bile and unmistakably identifies them.

ANATOMY OF THE GALL BLADDER

Anatomically the gall bladder is considered as having a fundus, a body and a neck. These features are visualised on Figs. 9.1a and 9.2a.

The term fundus is applied to the widened end of the gall bladder and its direction in the abdomen is downwards and forwards. Sometimes an anomalous fold occurs in the fundus (or the body) of the gall bladder: this is known as a Phrygian cap (see Fig. 9.1c) because it gives the fundus of the gall bladder an appearance on the radiograph similar in shape to the so-called cap of liberty or pirate's conical bonnet.

Posteriorly the fundus is close to the transverse colon and this relationship may be easily recognised from Fig. 9.1a. Here, a radiopaque residue from the contrast agent has well demarcated part of the transverse colon on the radiograph.

The body of the gall bladder is its central portion and the neck the narrowed end. The cystic duct becomes continuous with the neck at a point where there is a constriction and an abrupt change of direction from upwards and forwards to downwards and backwards. This change may be appreciated from the appearances on Fig. 9.4 but to a limited extent as the region is necessarily seen in two dimensions only.

Within the neck of the gall bladder and in the proximal half of the cystic duct, the mucous membrane is deeply folded and projects into the lumen in a number of oblique ridges, which are called the valves of Heister or the spiral valves because—when the neck or duct is distended—they give the exterior surface a twisted appearance. The term valve may be misleading. The function of these ridges appears rather to be that of a splint to prevent kinking and promote a free flow of bile whilst pressure varies in the gall bladder and common bile duct. Heister's valves are visualised radiologically in the gall bladder neck on Fig. 9.2a and the crenellated appearance of the cystic duct on Fig. 9.7a and b is due to them.

Sometimes there is a pouch demonstrated on the right wall

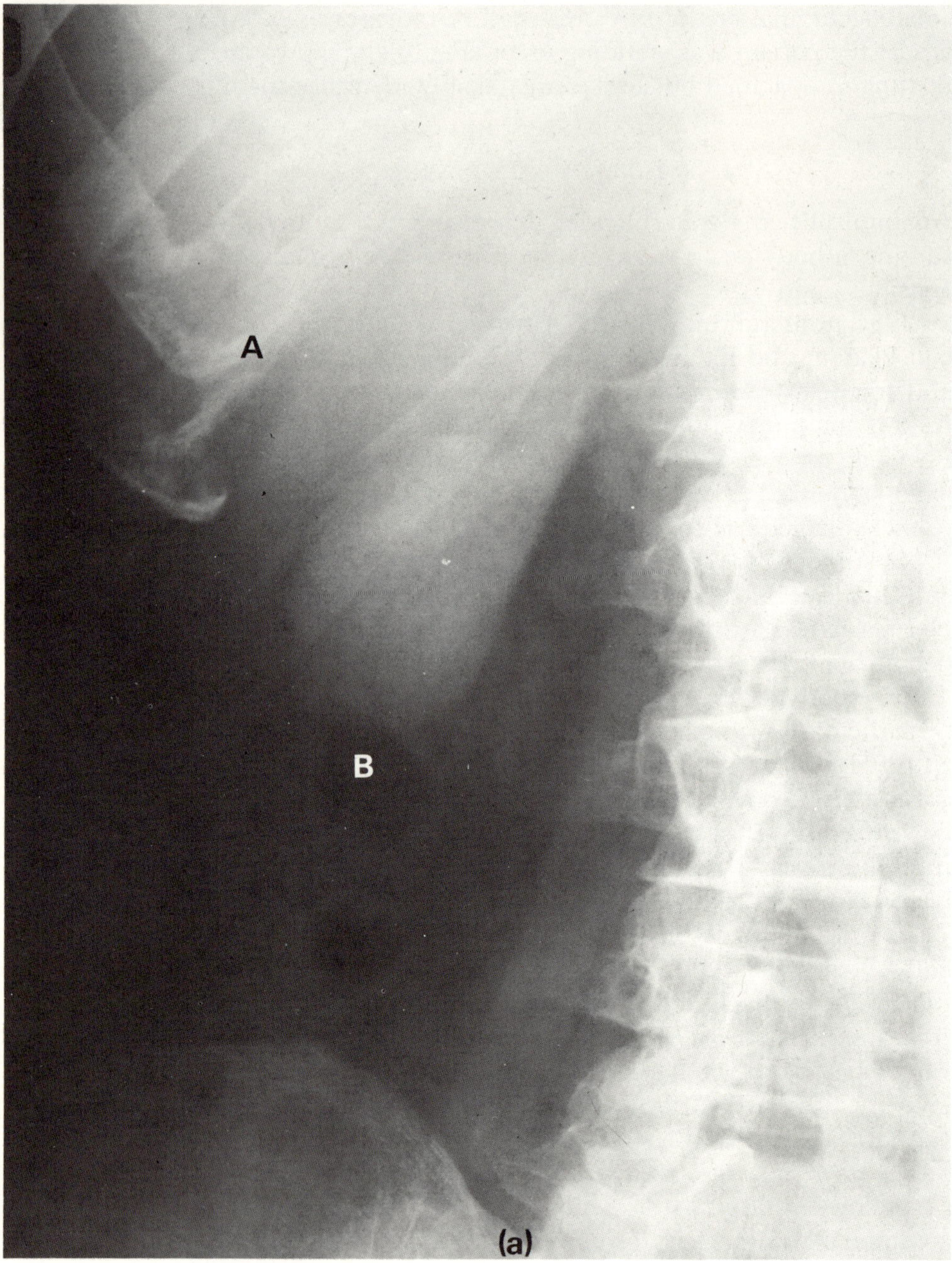

Fig. 9.5a. An oral cholecystogram exposed while the patient lay prone. The gall bladder contains many small cholesterol stones which are difficult to perceive.

A Calcification in rib cartilages

B Radioparency due to intestinal gas

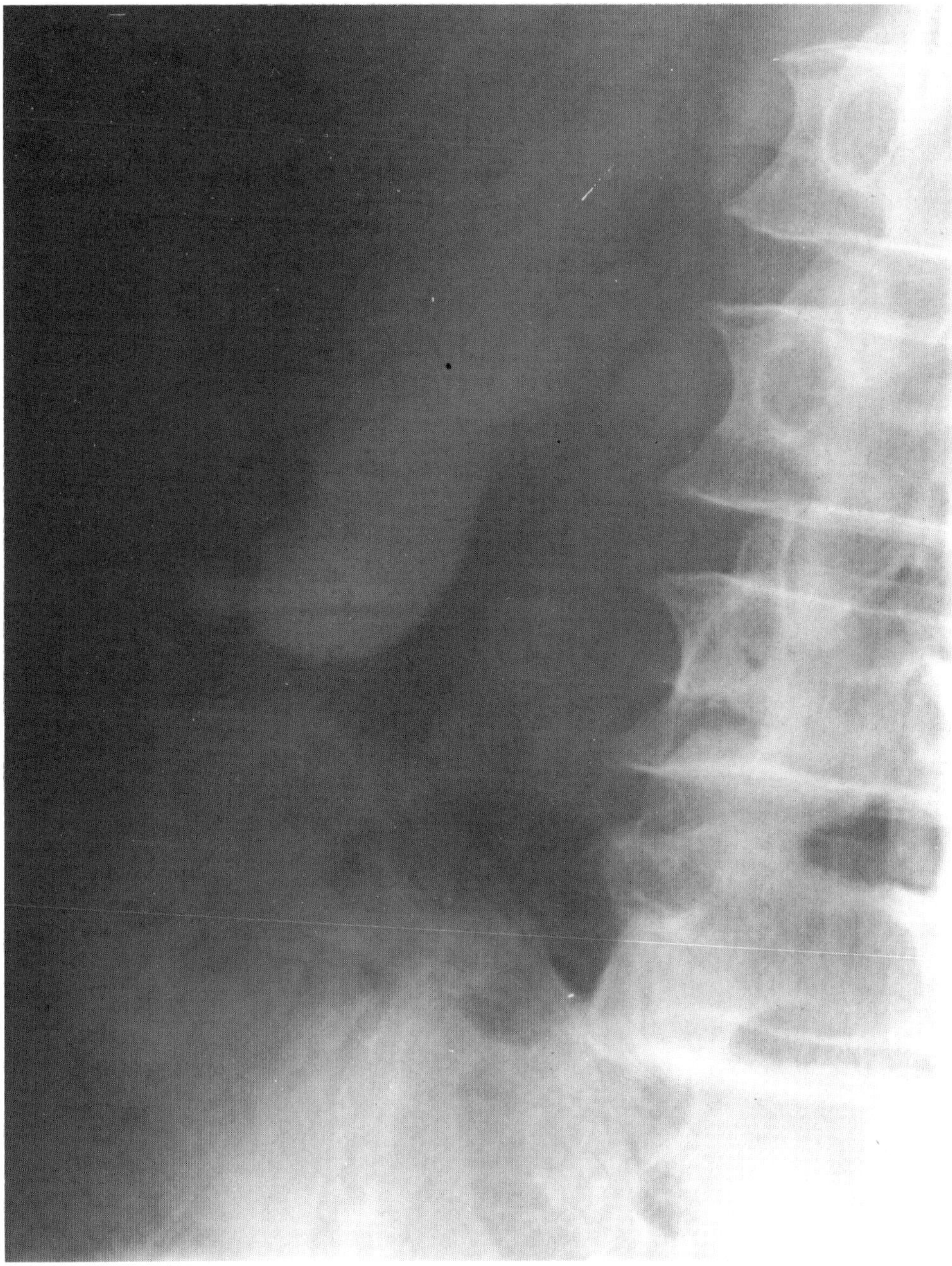

Fig. 9.5b. The same patient as in Fig. 9.5a but this radiograph was exposed while the patient stood upright. The cholesterol stones are floating on a layer of opacified bile and the diagnosis is unmistakable. The gall bladder has dropped considerably with the patient's change of position.

of the neck of the gall bladder, projecting downwards and backwards towards the duodenum. This is seen on Fig. 9.6 and is called Hartmann's pouch. The nature of Hartmann's pouch is open to question: by some surgeons it is regarded as a normal, constant anatomical feature of the gall bladder; others have shown it to be associated with pathology. Sometimes a gall stone becomes lodged in Hartmann's pouch, as might happen in the case of the single, large, transradiant stone which is seen in the body of the gall bladder on Fig. 9.6. There is evidence to suggest that patients in whom a Hartmann's pouch has been demonstrated may develop mucoceles of the gall bladder (a mucocele is a cyst or abnormal, dilated cavity containing accumulated mucus).

THE EXTRAHEPATIC DUCTS

The function of the bile ducts is to pass bile from the liver to the gall bladder, for storage and concentration, and from the gall bladder to the lumen of the duodenum at appropriate times to assist in the process of digestion. The normal physiology of the extrahepatic biliary system and of the mechanism whereby the gall bladder empties is not fully understood; but it is recognised that the liver secretes bile continuously (at a pressure of 150–250 mm of water) and forms about 16 litres of bile in 24 hours. The gall bladder is able to concentrate this up to tenfold and delivers 30–50 ml per day.

During oral cholecystography the bile ducts are not consistently well demonstrated. When visualised, they appear usually on radiographs exposed during the gall bladder's emptying phase, after the patient has taken food which includes some fat. Anatomical variants in the biliary tree occur with a frequency which is notorious to surgeons who must operate on it. In the so-called normal anatomy, two main ducts are described which leave the liver at the porta hepatis, a deep fissure on the liver's inferior surface. These are the right and left hepatic ducts which almost immediately join together to form the common hepatic duct, the junction occurring about 1·5 cm from the liver. The left hepatic duct is more oblique and therefore often a little longer than the

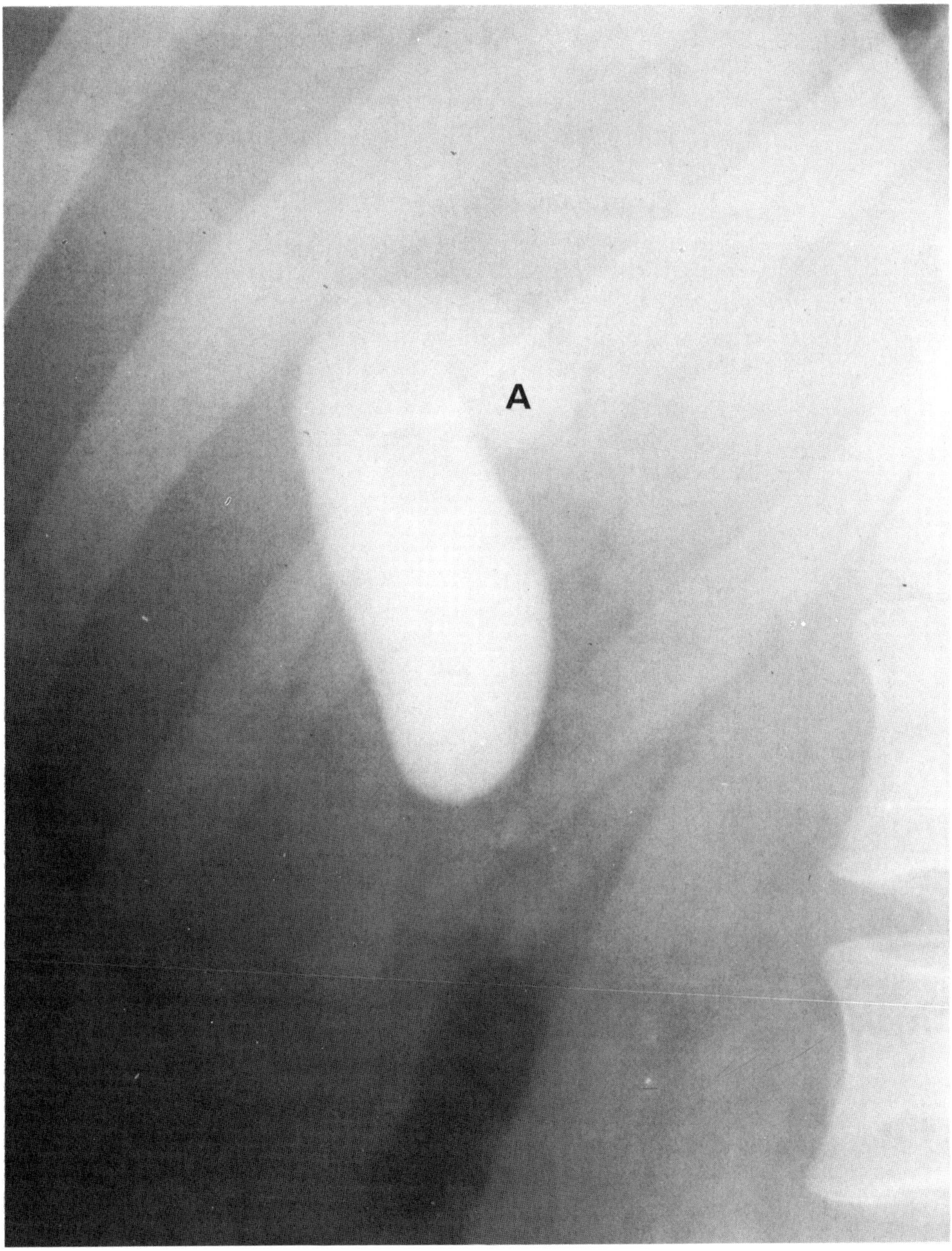

Fig. 9.6. An oral cholecystogram showing a gall bladder which has concentrated the contrast agent but contains a single, fairly large, radio-parent stone.
A Hartmann's pouch

right, although—depending on the course of the ducts and their content of contrast agent—this feature is not necessarily discernible from a radiograph: either duct may appear the longer.

The common hepatic duct passes downwards and is variable in length (1 to 5 cm), depending largely on the point at which it is joined by the cystic duct from the gall bladder. The cystic duct enters on the right wall of the hepatic duct at an acute angle and these ducts together form the common bile duct.

The course of the cystic duct from the neck of the gall bladder pursues a series of S-shaped bends, downwards, backwards and to the left. Typically the duct is about 2–3 cm long but its exact length, the course which it follows and the details of its termination with the common hepatic duct are all extremely variable between different individuals.

The common bile duct, which averages a length of 5 cm, continues in the same general direction, behind the head of the pancreas and the first part of the duodenum. At this point several features of the duct may be noticed:

(a) it may curve or even bend quite sharply to the right;
(b) its lumen may become a little narrower;
(c) it becomes embedded to a variable extent—sometimes totally embedded—in a deep groove on the posterior surface of the pancreas.

Aspects (a) and (b) are appreciated radiologically, although oral cholecystography is not the best way of doing so: the course of the ducts may be visualised during the procedure but their images are often faint and incomplete. Because of this, the anatomy of the common bile duct is further considered on p. 235.

The lumen of the common bile duct tapers to the appearance of a filament near the entry of the duct to the duodenum (see Fig. 9.11). It and the pancreatic duct approach and accompany each other through the posteromedial wall of the second part of the duodenum. The ducts are here (about 5 mm from the duodenal wall) surrounded by a common sheath of muscular and connective tissue, although their lumina are separate. They may remain separate and enter the duodenum separately; or they may fuse in a common channel (traditionally called the ampulla of Vater, although it is not an ampulla) and open into the duodenum on the apex of a papilla, the duodenal papilla.

A circular muscle (often called the sphincter of Oddi) surrounds the lower part of the bile duct and the termination of the pancreatic duct. It prevents reflux of duodenal contents and—when contracted—permits the gall bladder to fill. The admission of bile to the small bowel depends upon relaxation of this sphincter.

Figs. 9.7a and b and 9.8a and b illustrate the contraction and emptying of the gall bladder which occur when fat is ingested: compare the size of the gall bladder between Figs. 9.8a and 9.8b. Fig. 9.7a is a left anterior oblique view of a thin subject in whom the gall bladder is seen lying very close to the median line; the cystic duct (in which Heister's valves are demonstrated) passes upwards and then turns sharply downwards. The serpentine course of the duct is again indicated on Fig. 9.7b, together with the presence of Heister's valves. In both these radiographs, the appearance of a calcific 'calculus' in the neck of the gall bladder is illusory. It is caused by the end-on projection of part of the neck, where its route more or less coincides in direction with the central X-ray beam; that is, the appearance represents a turn or kink in the lumen, such that the observer is looking 'along' or through a greater depth of contrast agent, the opacity of which is thus increased at this point. The same effect may be seen sometimes in the ureter (see p. 192) and these illusions are among the proofs that a two-dimensional radiographic image of three-dimensional anatomy is not wholly satisfactory and may readily mislead an unpractised observer.

Fig. 9.8b further shows the cystic duct and its junction with the common hepatic duct; the upper part of the common bile duct is incompletely delineated below the junction.

Similar anatomy is demonstrated on Fig. 9.4, which is another oral cholecystogram exposed after the patient has ingested some fat. The anatomy of the extrahepatic ducts is further visualised on Figs. 9.9, 9.10 and 9.11, which are discussed in the following sections.

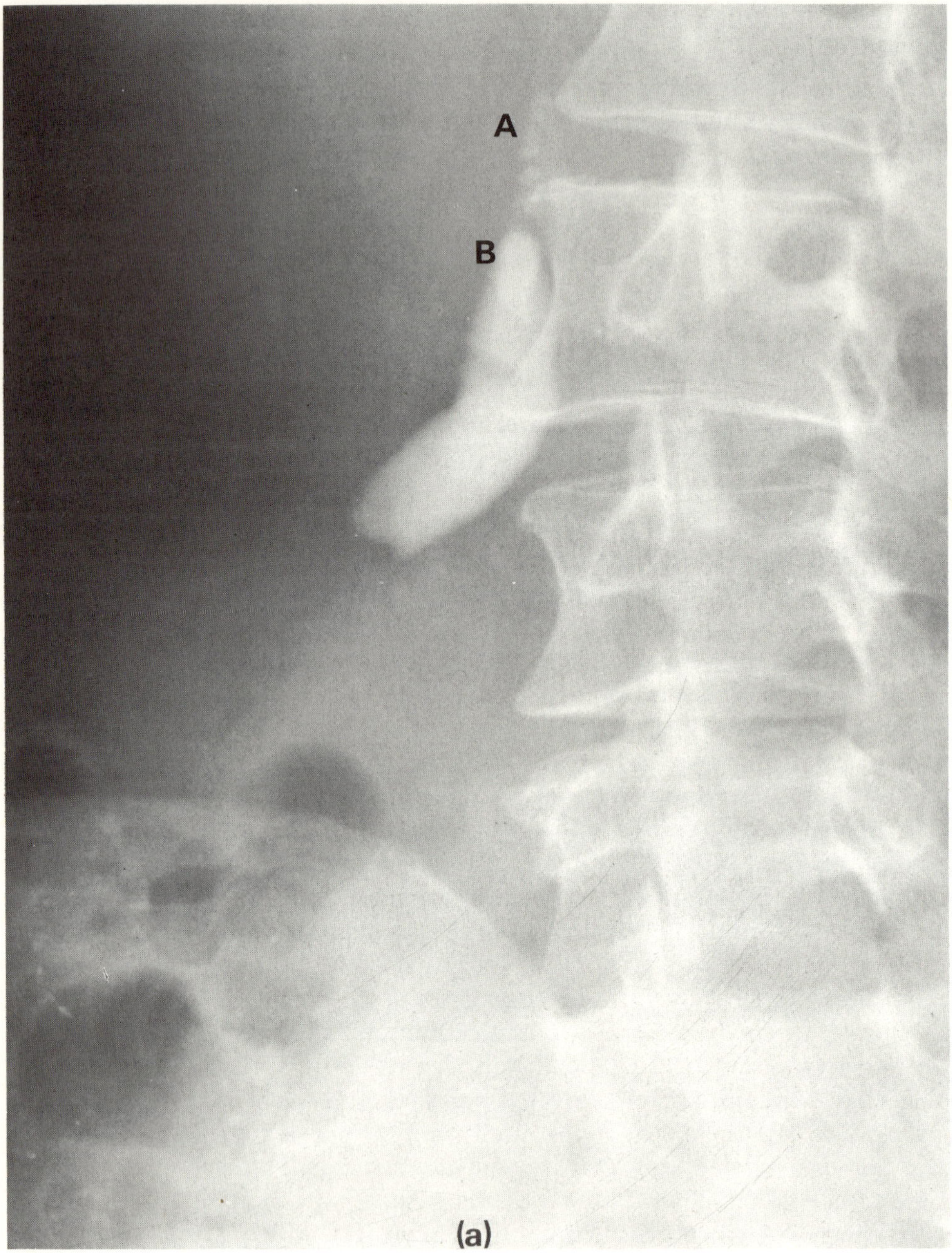

Fig. 9.7a. A left anterior oblique radiograph of a thin subject in whom an oral cholecystogram shows the gall bladder to be close to the midline. This radiograph was exposed an hour after the administration of fat and demonstrates the cystic duct, in which Heister's valves are present.

A Heister's valves B Neck of the gall bladder

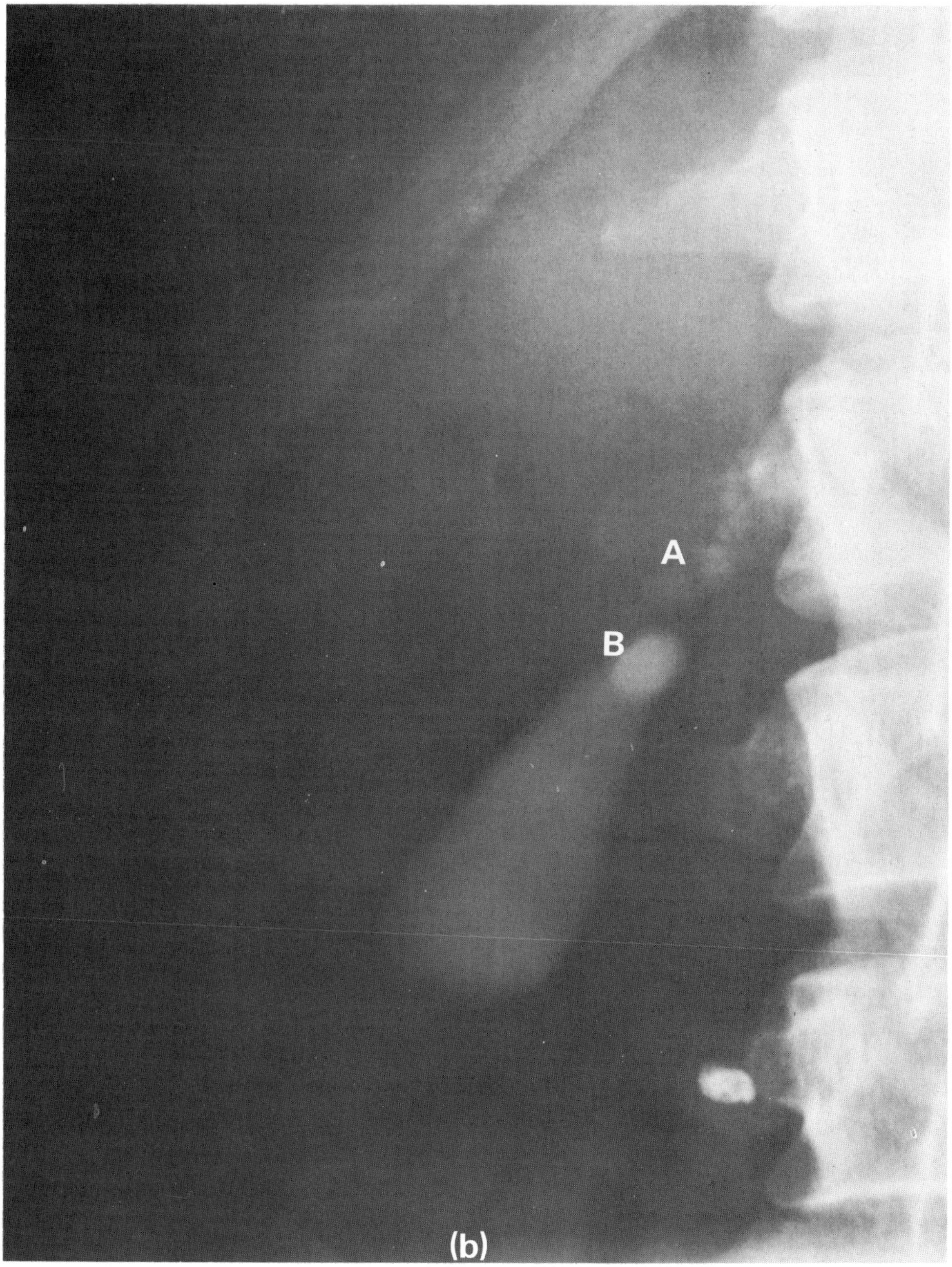

Fig. 9.7b. Another oral cholecystogram exposed after the administration of fat; this projection is posteroanterior.

A Heister's valves in the cystic duct

B Neck of the gall bladder

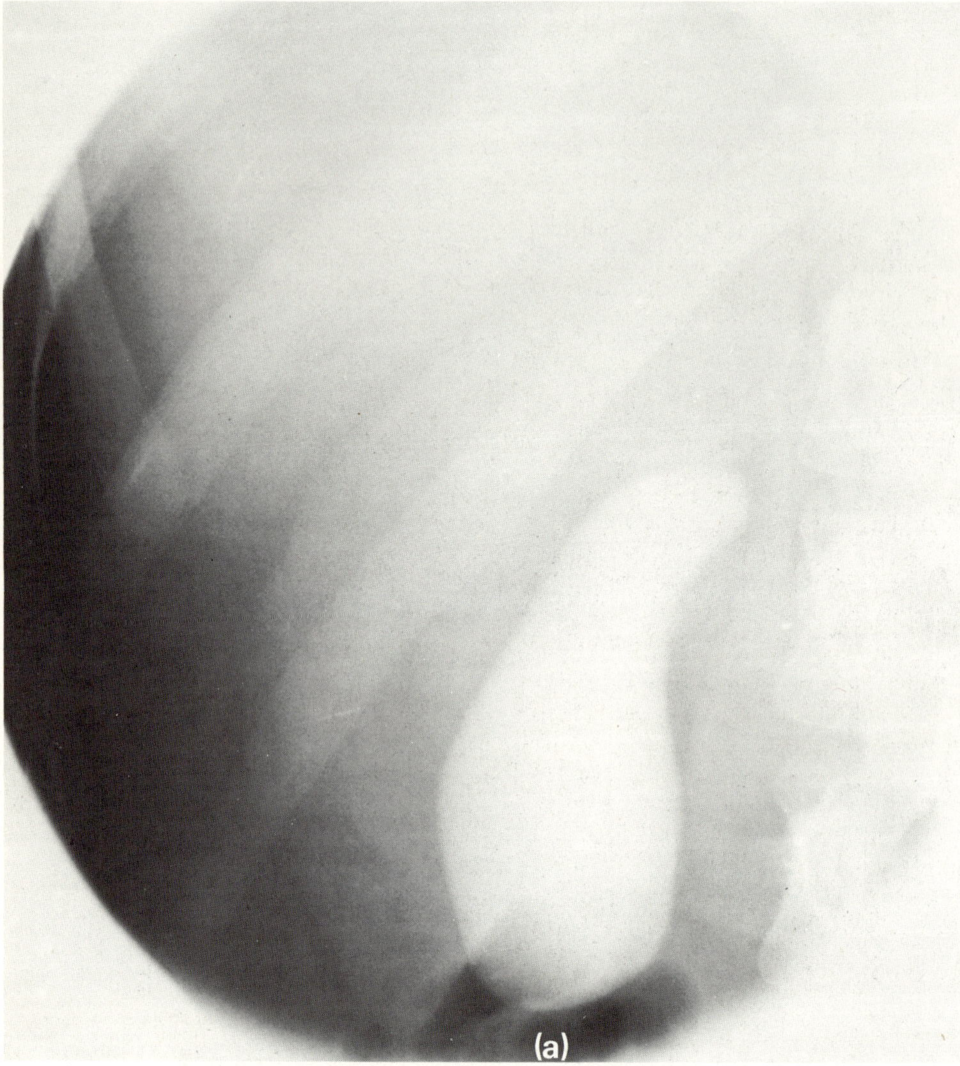

Fig. 9.8a. Radiographs of the same patient, exposed during oral cholecystography; **a** about 12 hours after taking the contrast agent and **b** (facing page) after the administration of fat.

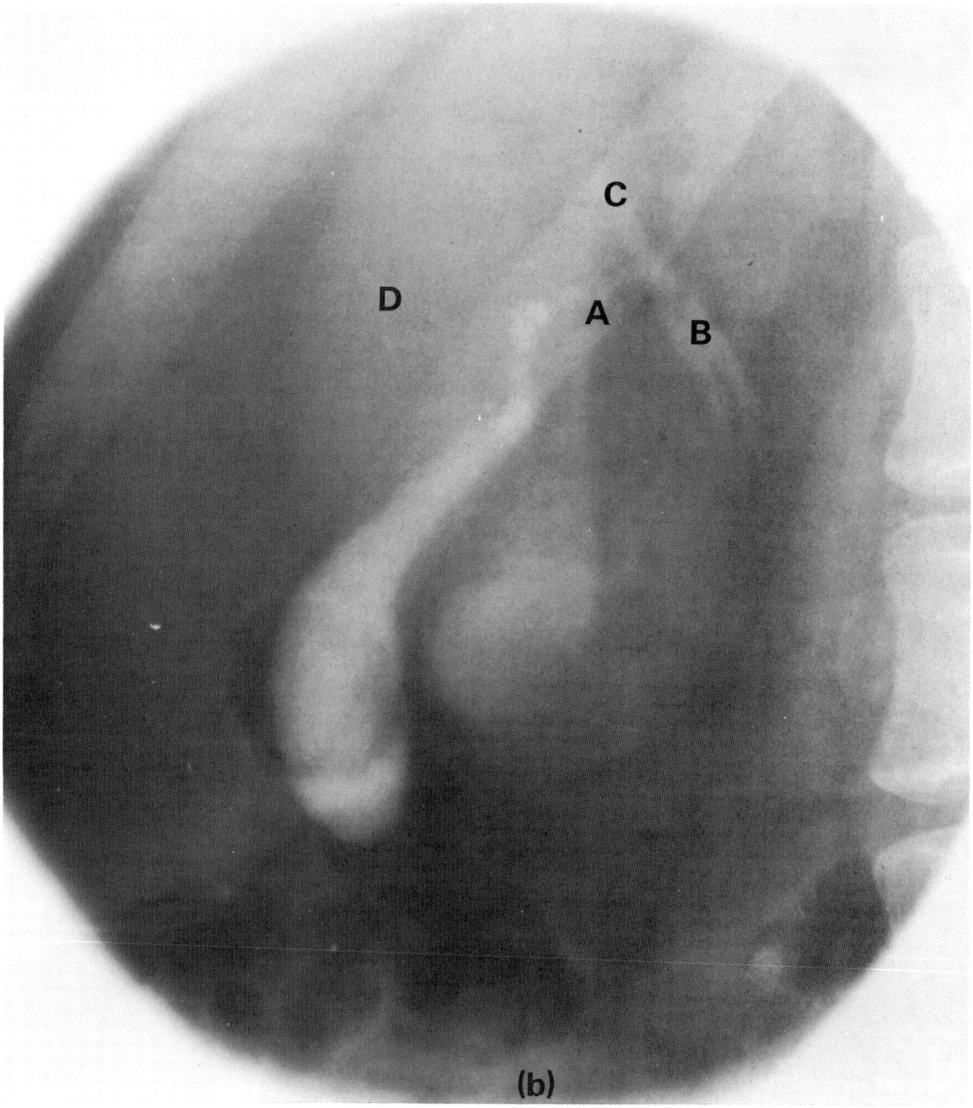

Fig. 9.8b. Contraction of the gall bladder and filling of the ducts are demonstrated.

A Cystic duct
B Common bile duct
C Common hepatic duct
D Right kidney

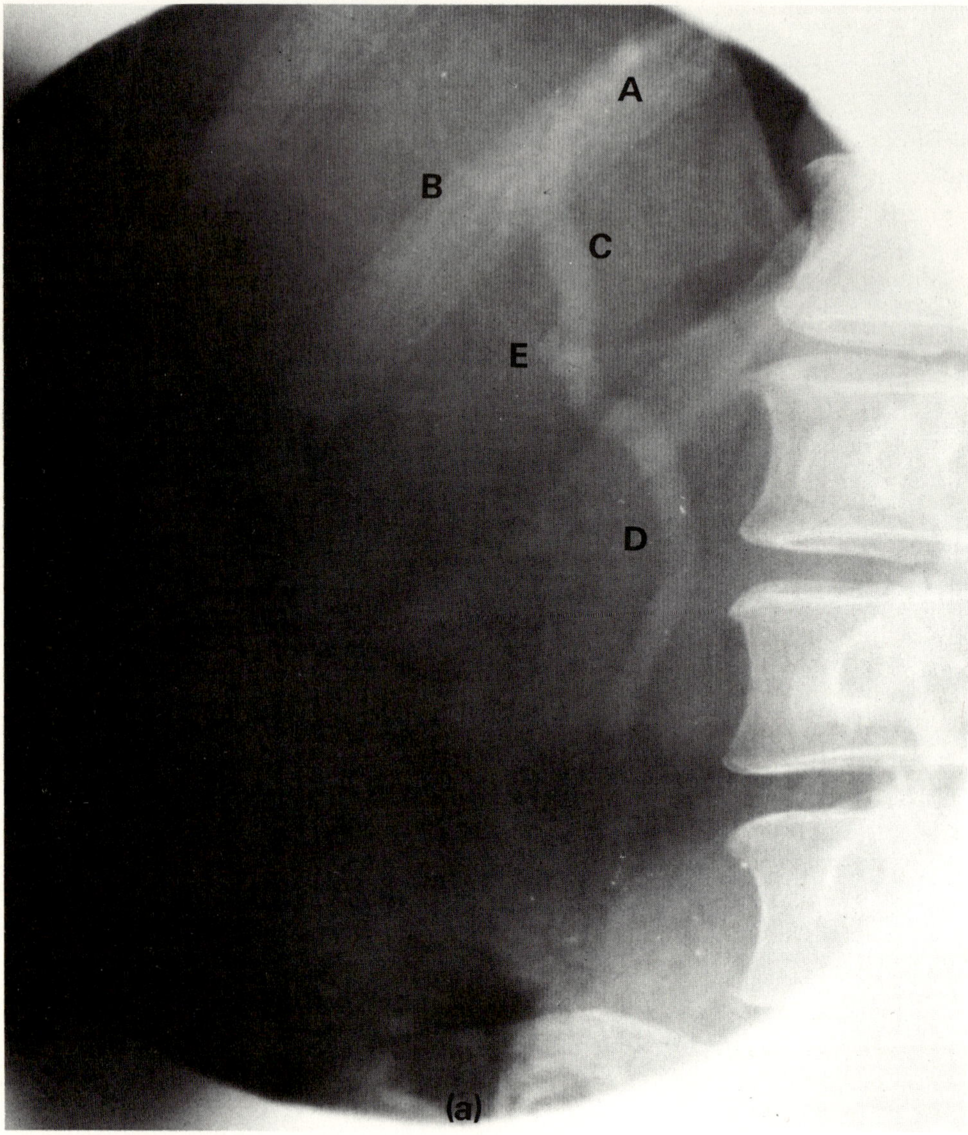

Fig. 9.9a. An intravenous cholangiogram (left anterior oblique projection) of a patient whose gall bladder has been removed.

A Left hepatic duct
B Right hepatic duct
C Common hepatic duct
D Common bile duct
E Stump of the cystic duct

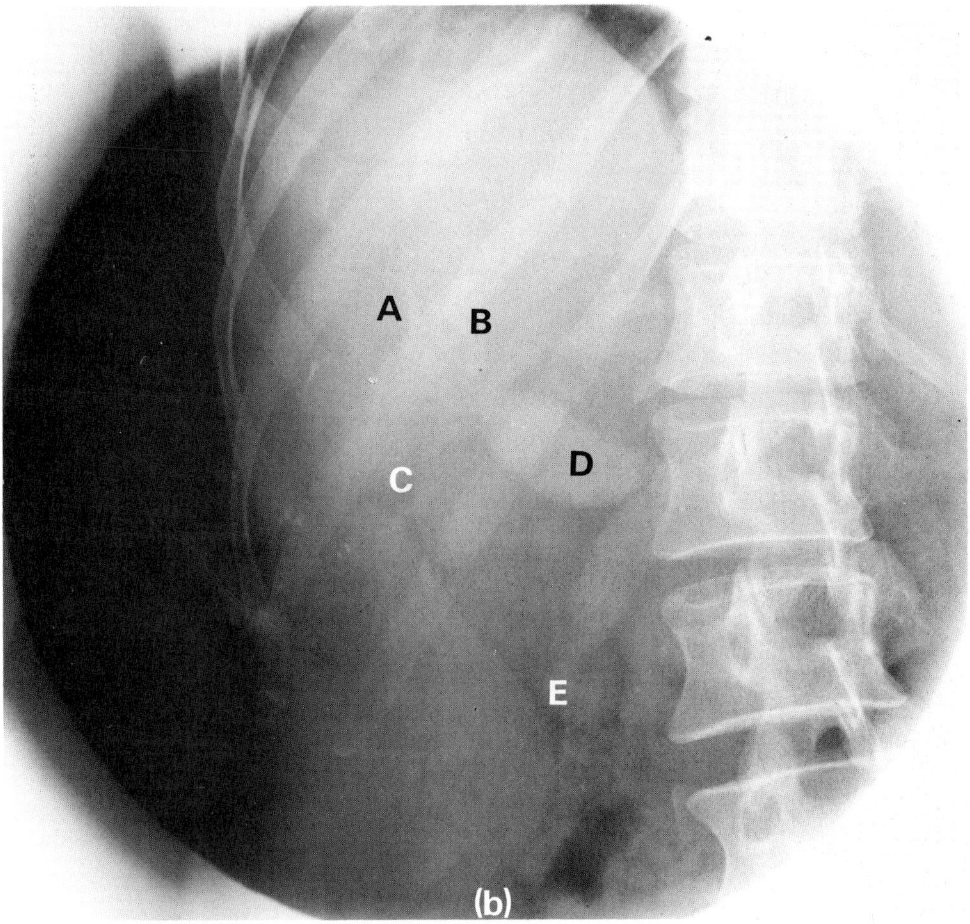

Fig. 9.9b. A similar intravenous cholangiogram of another patient after cholecystectomy. The ducts in this case have a much greater calibre. Some of the contrast agent has entered the duodenum.

A, B, C Hepatic ducts
D Common bile duct
E Contrast agent in the duodenum

Intravenous cholangiography

The need to demonstrate the common bile duct—more specifically the need to determine whether or not it contains stones—is the most frequent reason for submitting patients to intravenous cholangiography. The gall bladder may have been removed or it may be present and demonstrable in later stages of the cholangiogram.

Fig. 9.9a visualises much of the anatomy of the extra-hepatic biliary ducts in a patient who has had an earlier cholecystectomy. Contrast is faint in the right and left hepatic ducts and a few of their tributaries. The common hepatic duct is well outlined and the stump of the cystic duct where it enters the wall of the common bile duct is delineated.

The upper 7 to 8 cm of the common bile duct are filled with contrast agent. It illustrates the deviation of the duct to the right after an initial left-hand traverse behind the first part of the duodenum; and some reduction in its lumen as it proceeds; (see p. 226). The length of the duct varies in different subjects, from 1·5 cm to 9 cm.

Of greater radiological interest is the normal width of the common bile duct, as the diagnosis of an obstruction of the duct may depend upon the demonstration that it is dilated. X-ray examinations of the biliary tree have enabled many radiological measurements of the common bile duct to be made; it is recognised that, as the duct lies generally half-way between the anterior and posterior abdominal walls, some magnification (estimated as 10 per cent) is necessarily present in its X-ray image. Measured on a radiograph, the diameter of a normal duct has been stated to lie anywhere between values as small as 3 mm and as much as 15 mm. The average finding for the normal seems to be 3–6 mm and it is now generally accepted that a duct greater in diameter than 10 mm should be suspected of obstruction.

Fig. 9.9b is the intravenous cholangiogram of another patient whose gall bladder has been removed. Again, some contrast is present in hepatic ducts and the course of the common bile duct is delineated. Its appearance may be compared with its fellow on Fig. 9.9a. The overall greater width of the duct on Fig. 9.9b is a notable feature. It turns to the right much more sharply than in the case demonstrated on Fig. 9.9a and, beyond this point, its lumen is reduced in greater proportion. From the common bile duct, some of the contrast agent has entered the duodenum, which is faintly visualised in the vicinity.

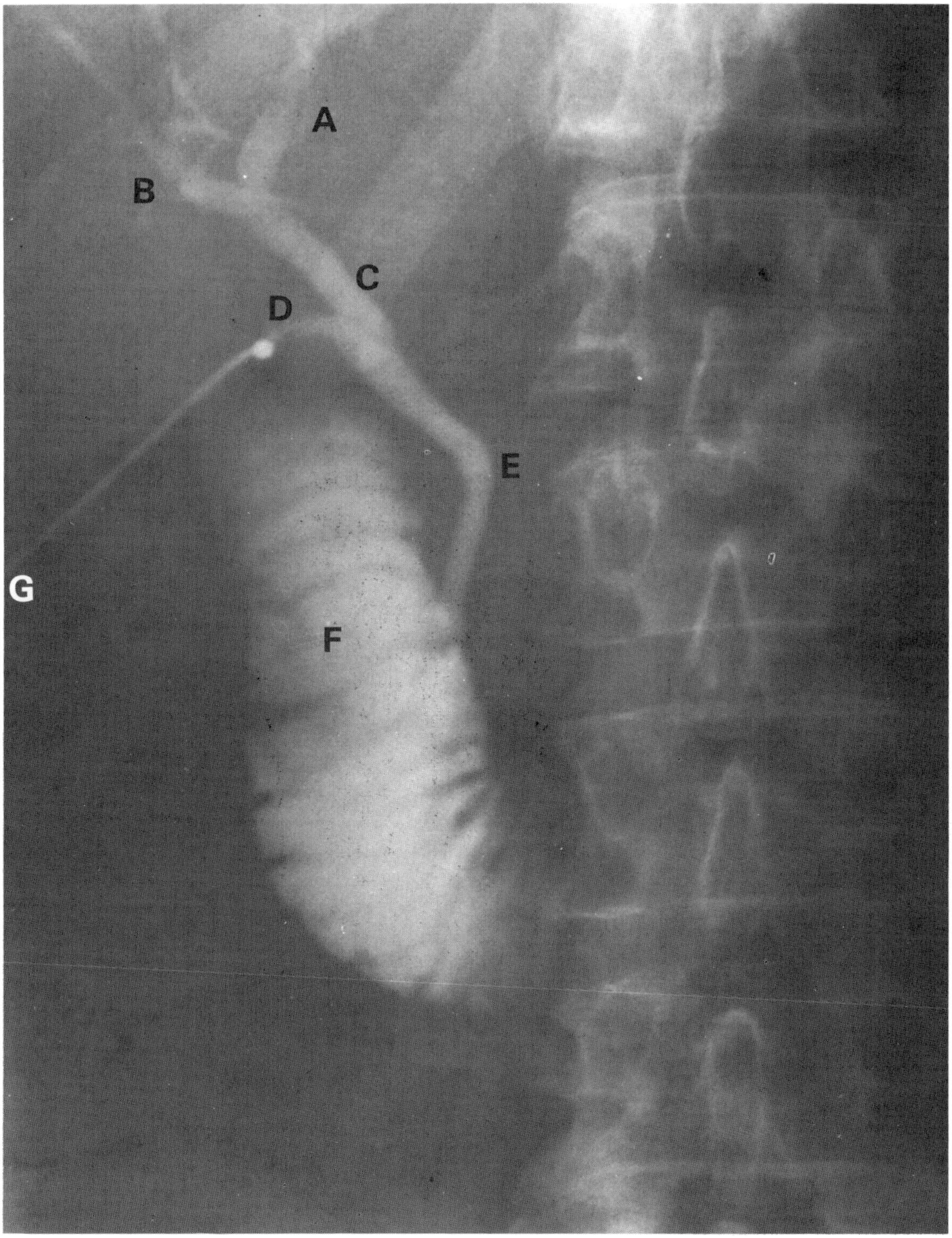

Fig. 9.10. An operative cholangiogram obtained during cholecystectomy for the purpose of determining if any stone is contained in the common bile duct.

A, B Hepatic ducts
C Common hepatic duct
D Cystic duct
E Common bile duct
F 2nd part of the duodenum filled with contrast agent
G Needle used for injection of the contrast agent

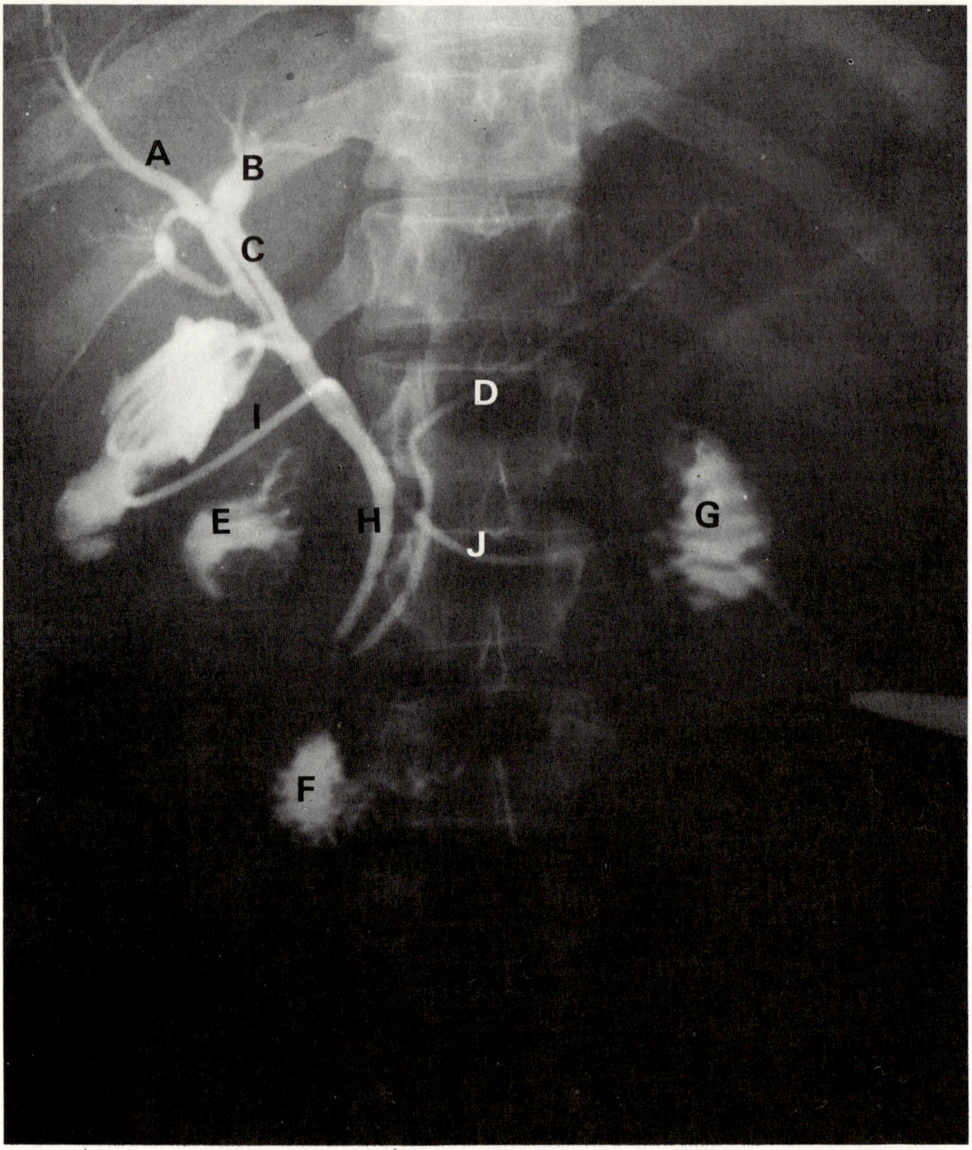

Fig. 9.11. A T-tube cholangiogram obtained after cholecystectomy, the contrast agent being introduced through a T-tube inserted at operation in the common bile duct for drainage purposes. Some of the contrast agent has refluxed along the pancreatic duct and some has entered the duodenum from the common bile duct.

A, B Hepatic ducts
C Common hepatic duct
D Pancreatic duct
E 2nd part of the duodenum
F 3rd part of the duodenum
G Contrast agent in the small bowel (duodeno-jejunal flexure)
H Common bile duct
I, J Tubing employed for the injection and lying across the anterior abdominal wall

Operative and post-operative cholangiography

During operative or post-operative cholangiography the extrahepatic biliary system is injected directly with a radiological contrast agent and the main anatomy of the ducts is normally well displayed on the resultant radiographs.

Fig. 9.10 is an example of operative cholangiography. The right and left hepatic ducts and a few tributaries are visualised; so also are the common hepatic duct and the common bile duct. The diameter of the common bile duct may normally appear greater during operative cholangiography than when filling of the duct has resulted from functional processes (as after oral or intravenous administration of a contrast agent). This is because the mechanical pressure of retrograde injection almost always is higher than the physiological normal and the duct temporarily distends to accommodate the increase.

The cystic duct is delineated on Fig. 9.10 proximal to the point of insertion of the needle used to give the contrast agent. Much of the contrast material has entered the duodenum and is obscuring the distal few millimetres of the common bile duct where it is behind the duodenum at its entry point on the posteromedial wall of the second part.

Fig. 9.11 shows post-operative cholangiography; the contrast agent has been injected through a T-shaped drainage tube inserted in the common hepatic and bile ducts at cholecystectomy. The left limb of the T is incompletely filled on this radiograph and is responsible for the deluding duplex appearance of the common hepatic duct. Above this are seen the right and left hepatic ducts, together with one major and some minor tributaries.

Fig. 9.11 offers a particularly effective display of regional anatomy as a quantity of contrast agent has refluxed along the pancreatic duct throughout its length, illustrating its relationship to the common bile duct. The reduction in the lumina of the ducts as they approach and traverse the duodenal wall is indicated. This is due to the presence of circular and longitudinal muscle fibres which appear in the walls of both the common bile duct and the pancreatic duct a few millimetres from the duodenum. Some contrast medium has entered the duodenum on Fig. 9.11 and is seen at three sites in the small bowel.

Chapter 10
Contrast Examinations: Liver, Spleen and Adrenal Glands

In textbooks of anatomy it is not customary to find the liver and spleen in adjacent sections of the same chapter. Usually, even in a short book, many pages separate these organs. Although both are glands by title, the liver participates in the digestive process, while the spleen is a ductless gland and a member of the reticulo-endothelial system.

Radiologically, however, there is a strong link between the two: by means of the procedure known as splenoportography the portal venous network of the liver may be demonstrated with a water-soluble contrast agent introduced through a percutaneous injection of the spleen. It is for this reason that the liver and spleen figure in a radiographic text as close neighbours.

In this chapter we shall consider, too, the adrenal glands, which are endocrine organs within the abdomen, capable of radiographic visualisation.

The liver

Only limited information about the liver is to be obtained from a plain radiograph (see Chapter 5, p. 123). While the right lateral border and the inferior margin of the right lobe may usually be determined with certainty, the left lobe of the liver cannot be located. Even if it is enlarged, no abnormal

X-ray appearance may result; enlargement of the right lobe elevates and may immobilise or restrict the movements of the diaphragm.

The diagnosis of hepatic disorder depends as a rule on methods other than radiology. In some conditions, however, an X-ray examination is helpful and we shall describe below the appearances associated with the liver during each of three procedures which are applicable. These are:

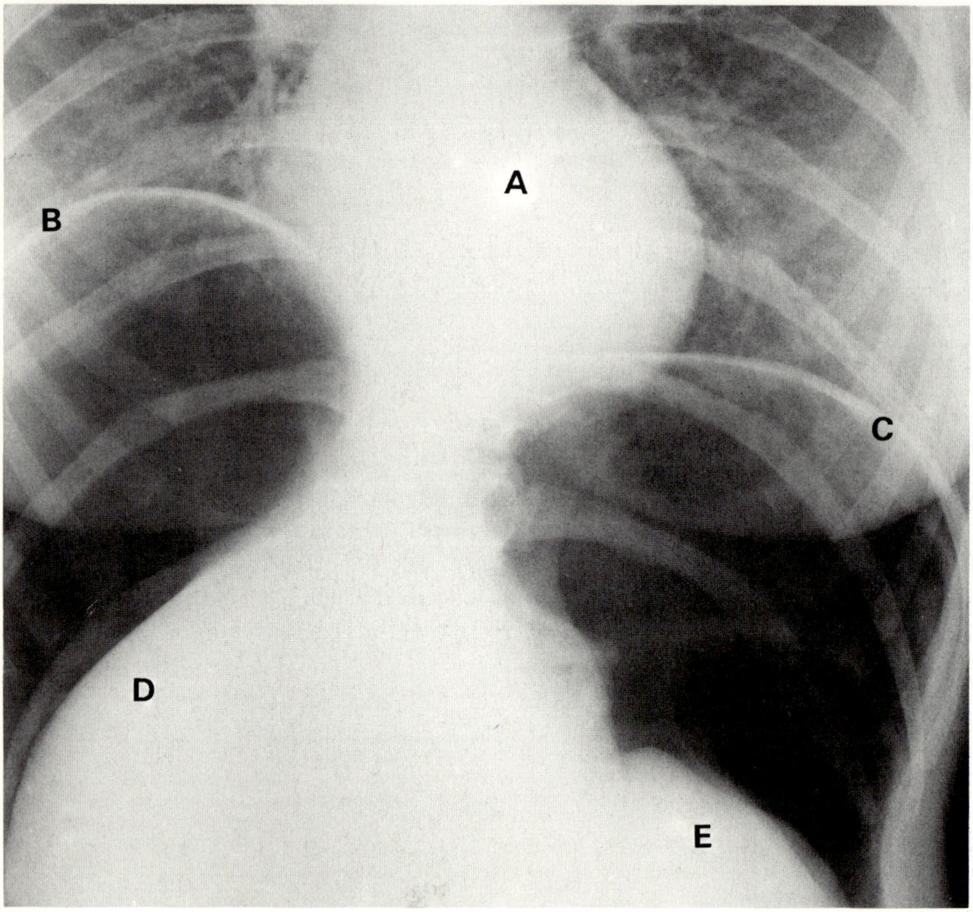

Fig. 10.1. A diagnostic pneumoperitoneum (posteroanterior radiograph).

A The heart

B Right dome of the diaphragm

C Left dome of the diaphragm

D The liver

E The spleen

(i) diagnostic pneumoperitoneum (the introduction of an appropriate gas to the peritoneal cavity);
(ii) splenoportography (puncture of the spleen and the introduction of an organic iodine compound to the splenoportal venous system);
(iii) selective hepatic arteriography by means of a catheter inserted in the coeliac axis or the superior mesenteric artery.

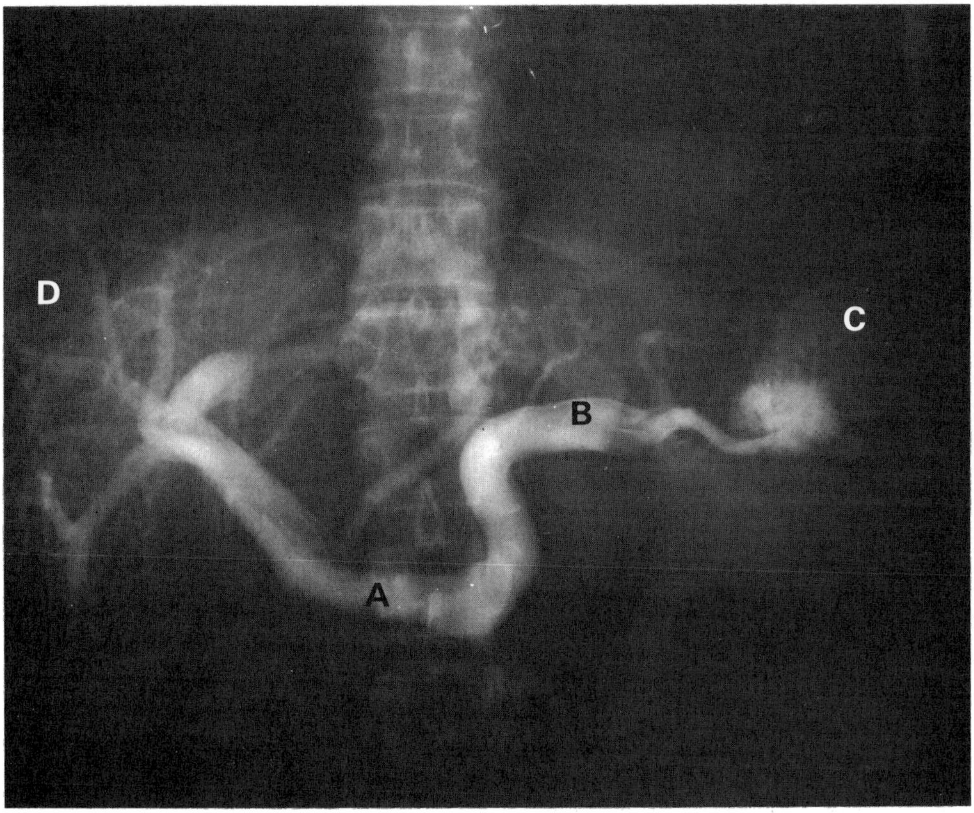

Fig. 10.2. Splenoportography (anteroposterior projection).
A The portal vein
B The splenic vein
C The spleen opacified by an injected contrast agent
D The liver, in which are seen ramifications of the opacified portal vein

DIAGNOSTIC PNEUMOPERITONEUM

The appearances of a diagnostic pneumoperitoneum are seen in Fig. 10.1. Its effect is to separate the superior surface of the liver from the right dome of the diaphragm, with the undersurface of which the liver is normally contiguous (see Chapter 5, p. 123). On Fig. 10.1 the rounded superior margin of the liver is clearly visualised within the radioparent region produced by the introduction of a volume of air (or other appropriate gas) to the abdominal cavity. From this procedure an opinion may be given on the size of the liver and its surface smoothness or irregularity, which are significant diagnostic features.

SPLENOPORTOGRAPHY

Fig. 10.2 shows typical appearances which result from the introduction of a radiological contrast agent to the pulp of the spleen. The contrast agent—flowing towards the liver—has filled the splenoportal venous axis. The union of the splenic vein with the superior mesenteric vein forms the portal vein at the level of lumbar vertebra 2.

The portal vein passes upwards and to the right, reaching the liver at the porta hepatis (see Chapter 9, p. 224). It divides into a right branch, which enters the right lobe of the liver; and a left branch, longer and reduced in calibre, which gives off branches to the caudate and quadrate lobes before entering the left lobe of the liver. Within the liver the portal vein ramifies after the manner of an artery.

The portal vein receives blood from the spleen, the pancreas, the gall bladder and all the abdominal part of the alimentary tube, except for the lower rectum and the anal canal. Radiologically, however, only those vessels are demonstrated which are situated between the liver and the site of injection of the contrast agent. When this is the spleen—as in splenoportography—only the splenoportal axis is seen.

SELECTIVE ARTERIOGRAPHY

Fig. 10.3a shows early arterial appearances resulting from the injection of a radiological contrast agent into the abdominal aorta; it may be compared with Fig. 8.10a to which it is similar. Figs. 10.3b and 10.3c illustrate respectively the different effects of selective arteriography through a catheter introduced to the coeliac axis and the superior mesenteric artery.

Coeliac axial injection

A radiological contrast agent injected in the coeliac axis may visualise (a) the arterial systems of the liver and spleen; and (b) the splenoportal venous trunk during the subsequent venous phase of the angiogram. Fig. 10.3b is an early arterial radiograph.

Superior mesenteric arterial injection

Contrast injection of the superior mesenteric artery should show the arterial supply to (a) the small intestine and (b) the proximal part of the large intestine. Radiographs exposed later than Fig. 10.3c in the series would reflect the venous return and demonstrate the superior mesenteric vein, which is not visualised during splenoportography.

This vessel returns blood from the small bowel, from the caecum and from the ascending and transverse parts of the colon. Beginning in the right iliac fossa from the union of veins draining the terminal ileum and caecum, the superior mesenteric vein passes upwards in front of the right ureter and the third part of the duodenum. Behind the neck of the pancreas, it unites with the splenic vein to form the portal vein.

Certain of the major blood vessels depicted on Fig. 10.3a, b and c have been described in an earlier chapter (Chapter 8) of this book: these are the hepatic artery (see p. 204), the splenic artery (see p. 205), the superior mesenteric artery (see p. 205) and the renal arteries (see p. 205). Many variations of the coeliac trunk and the superior mesenteric artery have been recognised and classified.

Other vessels shown on Fig. 10.3a, b and c are described in the paragraphs which follow.

The gastro-jejunal artery is a short large branch of the hepatic artery descending between the first part of the duodenum

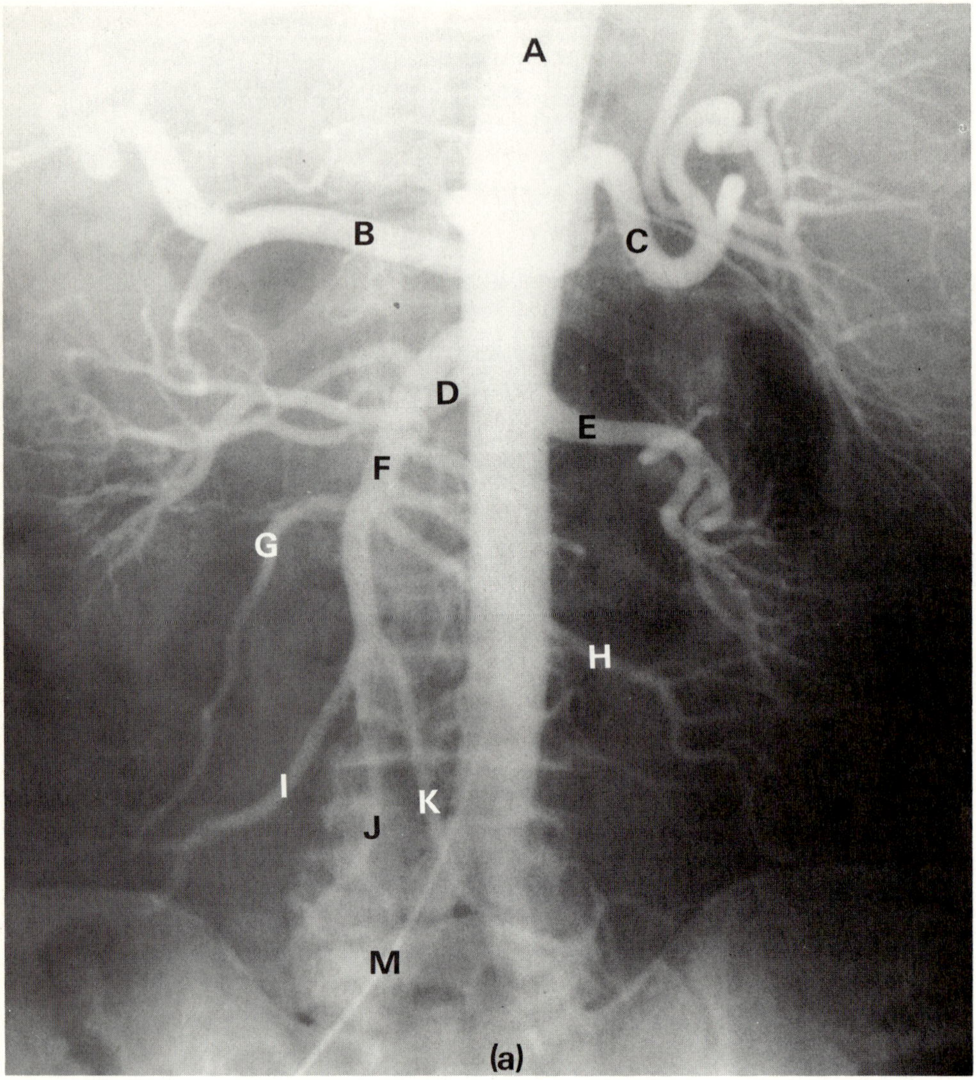

Fig. 10.3a. An abdominal aortogram exposed during injection of a contrast agent.

A The abdominal aorta
B Hepatic artery
C Splenic artery
D Right renal artery
E Left renal artery
F Superior mesenteric artery
G Right colic artery
H Jejunal branches of the superior mesenteric artery
I Ileocolic artery
J, K Ileal branches of the superior mesenteric artery
M Intra-arterial catheter

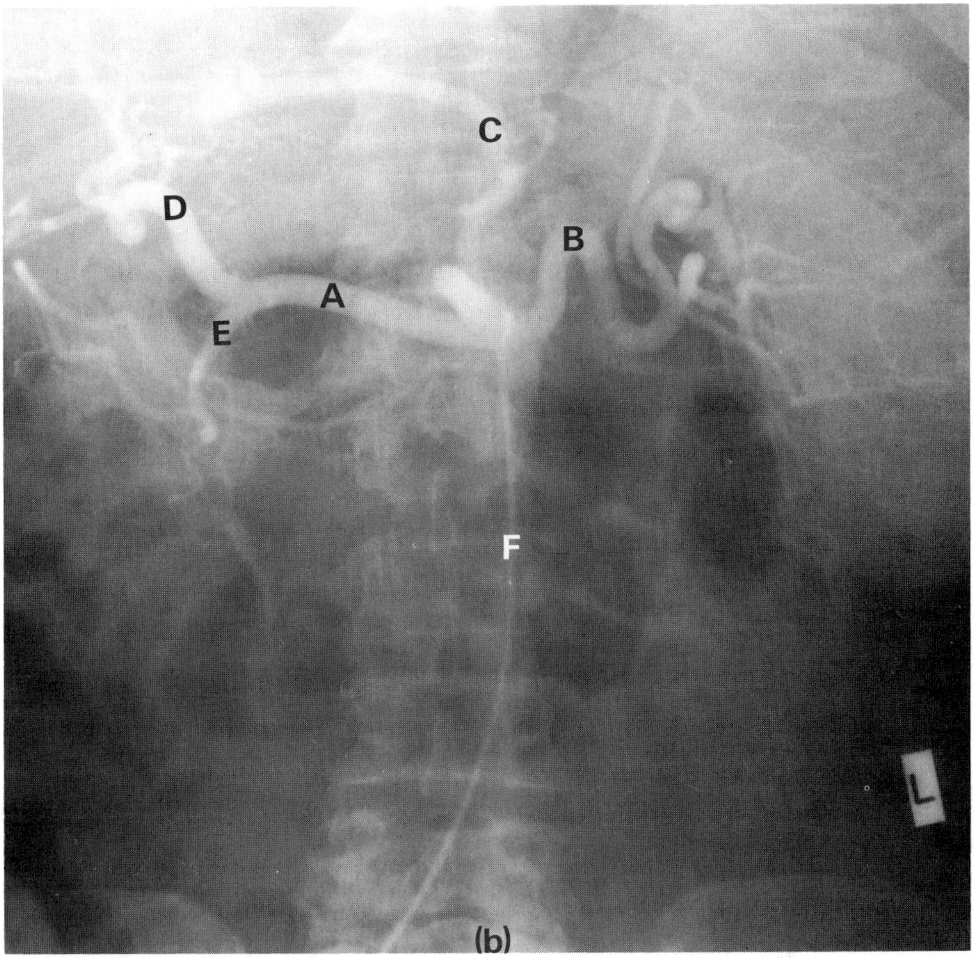

Fig. 10.3b. Selective arteriography. An intra-arterial catheter has been introduced to the coeliac axis and this radiograph was exposed during injection of a contrast agent.

A Hepatic artery
B Splenic artery
C Left hepatic artery
D Right hepatic artery
E Gastroduodenal artery
F Intra-arterial catheter

and the neck of the pancreas. Its branches supply the stomach, the duodenum and the pancreas.

The jejunal and ileal branches arise from the left side of the superior mesenteric artery and altogether are about 12–15 in number. Their courses are parallel to each other between

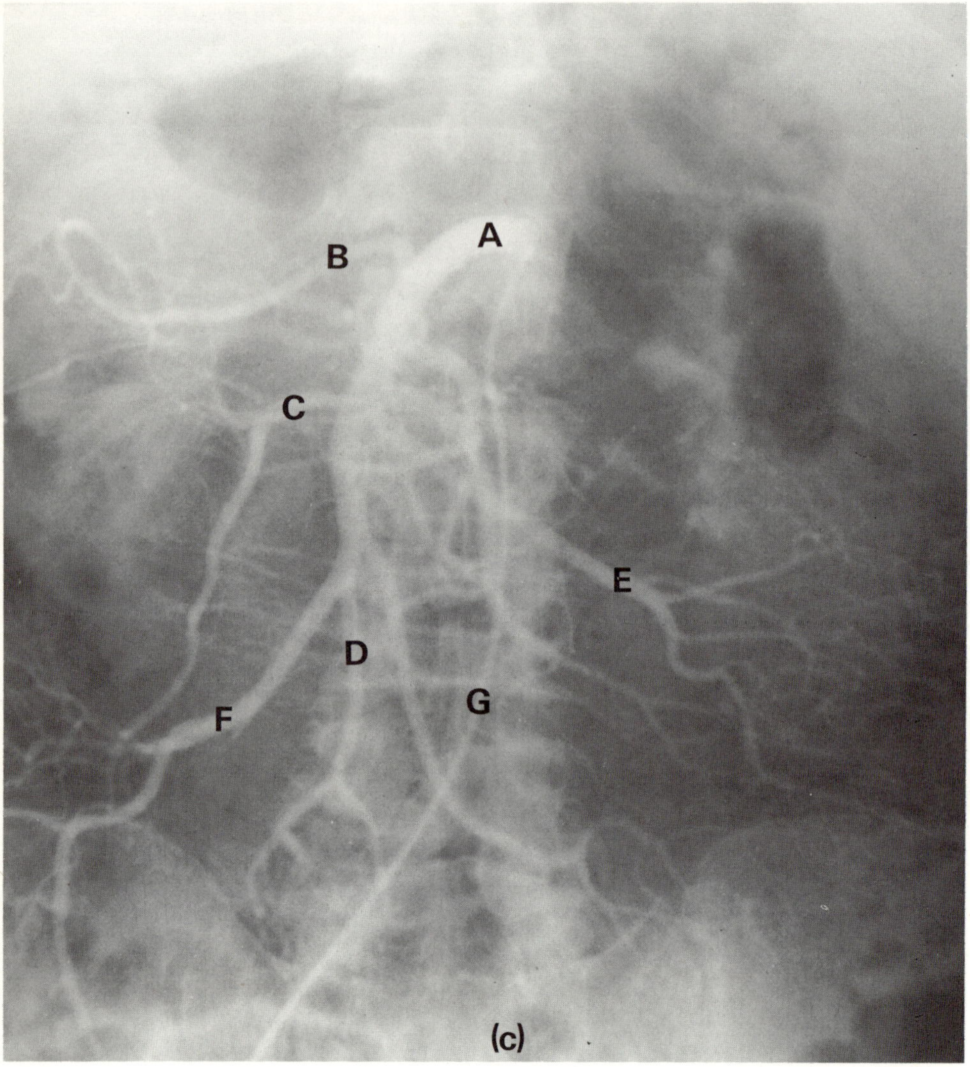

Fig. 10.3c. Selective arteriography. An intra-arterial catheter has been introduced to the superior mesenteric artery and a contrast agent injected directly in this vessel. This radiograph was exposed during the early phase of arterial filling. Later exposures would demonstrate the venous return.

A Superior mesenteric artery
B Middle colic artery
C Right colic artery
D Ileal branches
E Jejunal branches
F Ileocolic artery
G Intra-arterial catheter

layers of the mesentery. Each divides initially in two, forming branches which unite with other branches; several repetitions of this process result in a series of arterial arches, from the terminal group of which a number of straight vessels supply —more or less alternately—the right and left sides of the intestinal tube. Generally speaking the jejunal arteries are longer and fewer than the ileal vessels.

The right colic artery may arise from either the superior mesenteric artery or a stem which is common to it and the ileocolic artery. The right colic artery is directed to the right, behind the peritoneum and in front of the psoas major, towards the ascending colon.

The ileocolic artery is the lowest branch leaving the concavity of the superior mesenteric artery. Crossing in front of the right ureter and psoas major, it passes downwards and to the right towards the right iliac fossa.

The spleen

Some account of the spleen and its radiographic appearances has been given in Chapter 5 of this book (see p. 126). Visualisation of the spleen on a plain radiograph is relatively unlikely and partly a matter of chance but it may be demonstrated with the use of contrast agents.

On Fig. 10.1 the induction of a diagnostic pneumoperitoneum has resulted in the appearance of the spleen in outline against the air underlying the left dome of the diaphragm (as it has shown the liver similarly on the right). The rounded medial end of the spleen and its diaphragmatic surface, which faces backwards, upwards and to the left, have been demonstrated.

On Fig. 10.2 part of the spleen is delineated above the needle through which the contrast agent has been injected and of which the tip has penetrated the splenic pulp.

The spleen is highly vascular in structure. It has a red pulp, which gives the organ its dark red-brown colour and consists of a fine network of fibres; the meshes of this network are filled with blood from the splenic artery (see Chapter 8, p. 205). There is no real capillary system in the spleen.

The white pulp of the spleen is formed of lymphatic

tissue which surrounds many small branches of the splenic artery. In places in this network, the sheath is expanded to provide a lymphatic nodule (Malpighian body) in which lymphocytes are produced and through which the artery passes usually eccentrically.

The splenic vein, which is seen on Fig. 10.2, is a large vessel; but—unlike the splenic artery (see Figs. 10.3a and 8.10)—it is not tortuous. The splenic vein is formed from five or six branches which return blood from the spleen. It passes to the right across the posterior abdominal wall, a little below the splenic artery and so close to the pancreas that it grooves the upper part of the posterior surface of this gland. The splenic vein is connected to the pancreas by many small venous tributaries. Behind the neck of the pancreas, the union of the splenic vein with the superior mesenteric vein, at virtually a right angle, forms the portal vein.

The adrenal glands

The adrenal glands are seen radiographically by means of a contrast agent. Air (or oxygen or carbon dioxide or nitrous oxide), introduced behind the peritoneum may be used to demonstrate the adrenal glands, particularly when tomographs can be taken. Fig. 10.4 is an example of such a tomograph.

The adrenals are part of the endocrine system of glands which pass their secretions (hormones) directly to the blood stream and for this reason are sometimes called ductless glands. A hormone is a chemical substance which is produced in one part of the body, is conveyed by the blood stream and exerts an effect on distant organs and tissues, modifying their structure and function.

The adrenal glands are paired, each being a small flattened body which is surrounded by areolar tissue and situated to either side of the median plane in the renal fascia, above and in front of the upper end of either kidney.

Although a couple, the two glands are not exactly alike in shape: the right one is triangular, with its base directed downwards towards the upper part of the medial border of the kidney; the left gland is half-moon shaped, the concavity

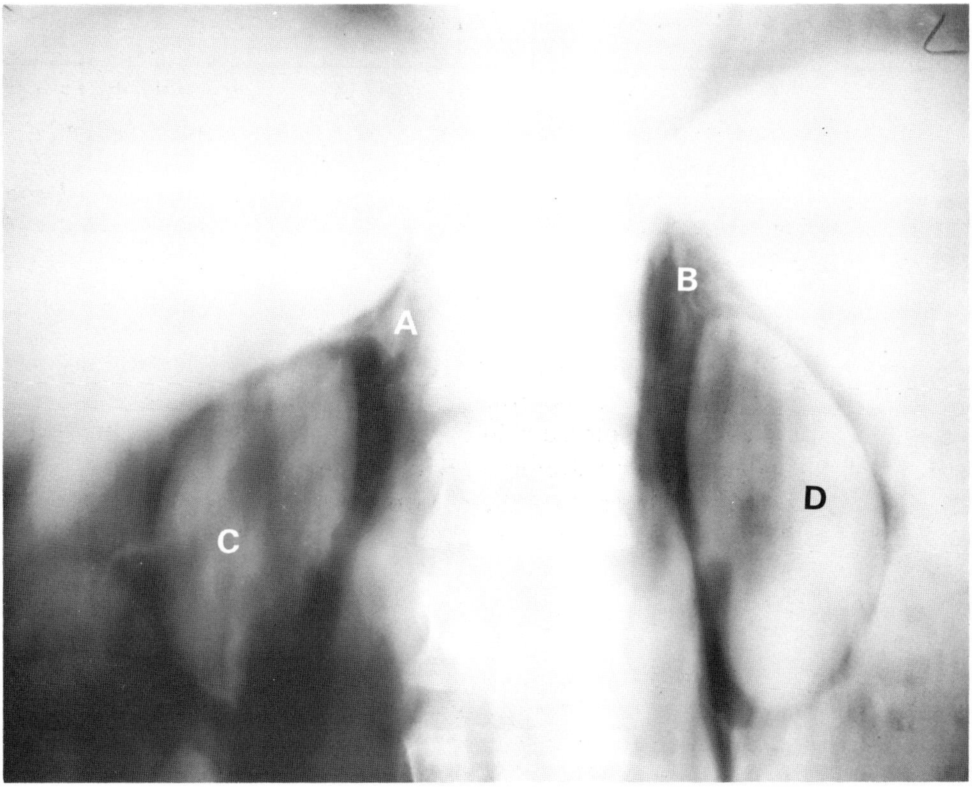

Fig. 10.4. A tomograph of the upper abdomen taken after the introduction of a negative contrast agent behind the peritoneum (pre-sacral air insufflation).

A	Right adrenal gland	C	Right kidney
B	Left adrenal gland	D	Left kidney

of the crescent being adapted to the medial border of the upper part of the left kidney. These differences cannot be fully appreciated from the appearances of the glands on Fig. 10.4.

STRUCTURE OF THE ADRENAL GLANDS

Each adrenal gland is composed of two functionally separate parts. The outer or cortical portion forms most of the gland. Its substance consists of a fine network of tissue containing epithelial cells which are arranged in different groupings at different levels. In the most superficial stratum the cell masses are rounded; in the next and largest zone the cell groups are arranged in radial columns; in the deepest layer the cellular patterns are irregular and branching.

The medullary part of the gland is very vascular, as it contains large thin-walled capillaries through which must pass all the blood of the organ. The fibrous framework of tissue in the medulla is continuous with that of the cortex but the spaces are filled with cells which are asymmetrical in shape. These are called chromaffin cells and are found elsewhere in the body in plexuses of the sympathetic nervous system.

Each adrenal gland is enclosed in a thin capsule of connective tissue.

FUNCTION OF THE ADRENAL GLANDS

The cortex and medulla of the adrenal glands operate independently in the production of hormones.

The cortex

The adrenal cortex secretes a great number of hormones, collectively called corticosteroids, which are classified in the following groups.

(i) *Glucocorticoids* (hydrocortisone and cortisone), which affect the metabolism of sugar in a way opposed to that of insulin and have also some anti-inflammatory action.

(ii) *Mineralocorticoids* (the major member is aldosterone) which control the balance of electrolytes in the body; that is, they are concerned with salt metabolism and levels of potassium, sodium and chloride in circulation.

(iii) *Sex hormones* (androgens and oestrogens) which are concerned with the development of normal secondary sexual characteristics.

The medulla

The medulla of the adrenal glands produces two hormones which are necessary in preparing the body either to fight or to flee at a time of emergency and alarm. The hormones are adrenalin, which stimulates the sympathetic nerve endings,

and noradrenalin, a powerful vasoconstrictor. There must be few of us who—at some or other time—have not experienced and recognised the uncomfortable release of these hormones which accompanies a start of fear. The hormonal effects are:
(i) a rise in blood pressure by constriction of vessels supplying the skin;
(ii) an increase in the circulating volume of the blood;
(iii) dilatation of the coronary arteries which supply the heart;
(iv) increased conversion of glycogen to glucose to maintain animal energy;
(v) dilatation of the bronchi;
(vi) dilatation of the pupil of the eye;
(vii) decreased peristalsis in the gut;
(viii) increased activity of sweat glands and contraction of the muscles which effect that condition of the skin which we describe as goose-flesh.

Chapter 11
Contrast Examinations: The Uterus and Uterine Tubes

The anatomy of the female reproductive organs usually is described in terms of their division in two groups: these groups respectively are (a) the internal organs, (b) the external organs. The internal structures lie within the pelvis and comprise the ovaries, the uterine tubes, the uterus and the vagina. The external group, which are situated below and anterior to the pubic arch, are known collectively as the vulva or pudendum; they include the mons pubis, the labia, the clitoris and the vaginal vestibule.

Students of radiographic anatomy may expect to find that virtually only two structures of the female reproductive system are often subject to radiological examination: these are the uterus and uterine tubes.

Plain radiography

Plain radiography of the pelvic cavity cannot usually demonstrate any of the female reproductive organs. From time to time, however, there may be indirect radiographic evidence of the topography of some part of the tract: such examples are seen on Figs. 5.17, 5.18 and 5.20. In all of these, material artificially introduced—for another purpose—to the vagina and uterus has provided some general indication of the location of the structure concerned.

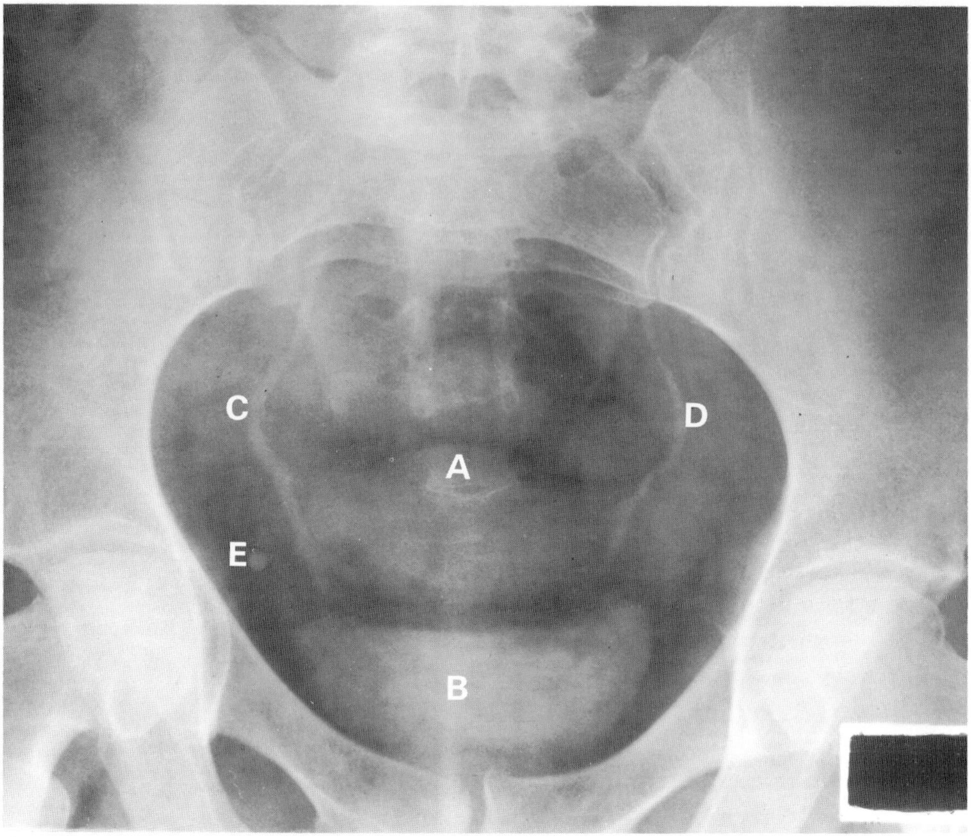

Fig. 11.1. A radiograph of the partially filled bladder and lower ureters taken during intravenous urography. Soft tissue outlines of the uterus are demonstrated and the uterus is seen to depress slightly the superior surface of the bladder.

A The uterus
B The bladder
C The right ureter
D The left ureter
E Pelvic phleboliths (see also Fig. 5.14).

A rather different instance occurs on Fig. 8.6. Here we see a depression of the upper surface of the bladder for which the uterus is probably responsible (see p. 194).

Fig. 11.1 is another example of an intravenous urogram. There is contrast agent in the lower part of each ureter and in the bladder. Above the bladder the soft tissue outline of the uterus has been demonstrated, possibly because of its physiological condition at the time of exposure, which may have been made just before or during menstruation (see p. 198).

Hysterosalpingography

Hysterosalpingography (uterosalpingography) is a procedure during which a radiological contrast agent is introduced to the uterus from the vagina, usually for the primary purpose of determining patency of the uterine tubes during investigations of infertility. Filling of the uterine tubes normally occurs from the uterus; and delineation of both the tubal and uterine lumina may be thus obtained.

No examination of the ovaries (the female reproductive glands) may be made by this means, although it is possible to visualise these—as well as the uterine silhouette and other pelvic organs—by the insufflation of a radioparent contrast agent, nitrous oxide or carbon dioxide, into the peritoneal cavity. This radiological process is known as gynaecography or pelvic pneumography. It is performed comparatively infrequently.

Figs. 11.2a and 11.2b show two examples of hysterosalpingography. The size, shape and situation of the uterus are each subject to variation between individuals and to alteration at different times and in different circumstances of life. For the purpose of anatomical description, it is usual to consider the uterus of an adult woman who has not experienced pregnancy. Since hysterosalpingography commonly is performed on patients who seek medical help because of an infertile marriage, the uterus of the anatomy book is also the one which tends to appear on radiographs in many X-ray departments.

THE UTERUS

The uterus is a thick-walled, muscular viscus, situated in the pelvic cavity below the plane of the pelvic inlet (an oblique plane passing through the sacral promontory posteriorly and the arcuate line of the hip bone on each side, anterolaterally). The uterus is globular or pear-shaped. Its narrow end is directed downwards and its long axis downwards and

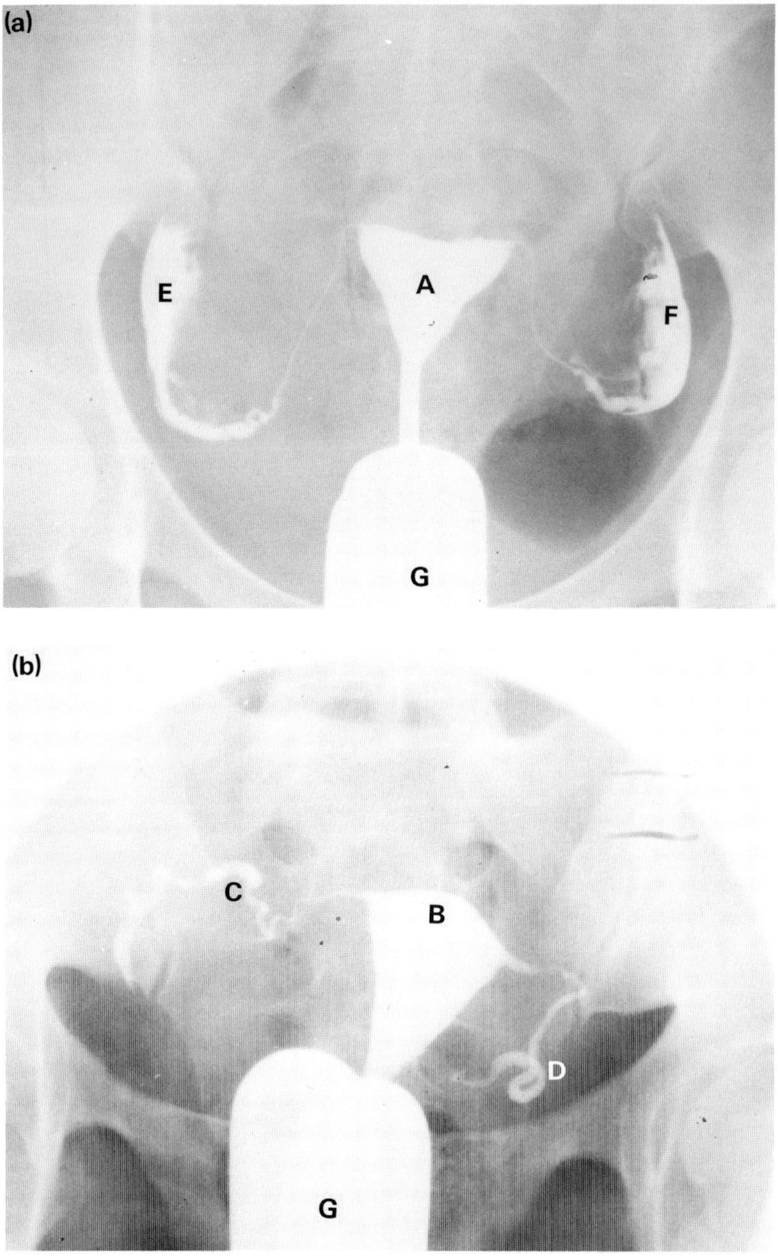

Fig. 11.2. Two examples of hysterosalpingography, showing the uterus and uterine tubes filled with a radiological contrast agent.

A The body of the uterus
B The fundus of the uterus
C The right uterine tube
D The left uterine tube
E Peritoneal spill from the right uterine tube
F Peritoneal spill from the left uterine tube
G Vaginal speculum

backwards, approximately following the axis of the pelvic inlet (a line at right angles to the plane of the inlet).

The bladder is below and in front of the uterus and the pelvic colon above and behind it. As the uterus is freely mobile, the degree of distension of either of these other organs influences the situation of the uterus.

The uterine tubes open into the upper part of the uterine cavity on either side. Fig. 11.2 illustrates:

(i) typical positions of the uterus within the true pelvis;

(ii) the size and shape of the uterine cavity which—because of the thickness of its walls—is very much smaller than the size of the whole organ;

(iii) the relationship of the uterus to the uterine tubes.

The uterus is constricted a little below its middle. The narrow portion of the uterine cavity is termed the internal os. The part above the internal os is the body of the uterus; the part below is the cervix. The fundus is the region of the body lying above a line joining the points of entrance of the uterine tubes.

The cavity of the body is triangular from side to side, as seen on Figs. 11.2a and 11.2b, but from before back it is

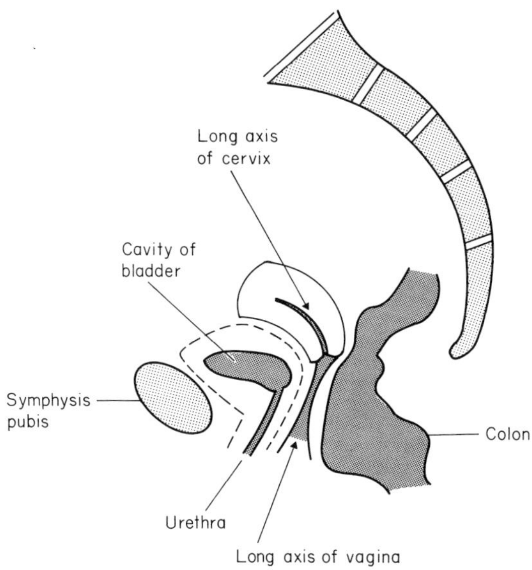

Fig. 11.3. A sagittal section of the female pelvis.

merely a slit, the anterior and posterior uterine walls being in contact with each other.

The cavity of the cervical canal is similarly flattened from before backwards. Coronally it is narrower and more cylindrical than the body and is wider at the middle than at either end. The cervix projects through the anterior wall of the vagina. Its rounded extremity bears a small, circular opening, the external os, which provides communication between the cervical and vaginal cavities. In sagittal section, the long axis of the cervix meets the long axis of the vagina at an angle which is open forwards and downwards, the uterus being anteverted on the vagina (see Fig. 11.3). When the bladder is full, the uterus is pushed upwards and the angle of anteversion becomes more obtuse.

On the evidence of a hysterosalpingogram, conclusions regarding the anatomy of the cervix and vagina should be avoided as both structures may be distorted—and on the radiograph are usually largely obliterated—by instruments, present for the introduction of the contrast agent.

THE UTERINE TUBES

The uterine tubes are seen filled with a radiological contrast agent in the two cases shown on Fig. 11.2. The tubes are paired structures situated in the free upper margins of the broad ligaments (folds of peritoneum which help to support the uterus). One tube opens on each side into the cavity of the uterus at each superior angle. The other end of the tube communicates with the peritoneal cavity, close to the ovary on the side in question. This communication is unique as it is the only opening which the peritoneal sac possesses; in the male the cavity is entirely closed.

The purpose of the uterine tubes is to provide a pathway to the uterus and a system of transport for an ovum as one is discharged from the ovary (occasionally more than one may be involved): this occurs once every month, usually approximately halfway through the menstrual cycle. However, it is not unknown for ovulation to occur at other times, even during menstruation.

Each uterine tube is about 10 cm long. Its opening into

the uterus is extremely small. The other end of the tube, close to the ovary, is characterised by a trumpet-shaped expansion (an infundibulum) and may be up to 3 mm in diameter. Here the circumference of the tube is prolonged in a number of irregular processes called fimbriae.

The uterine tube has serous, muscular and mucous coats.

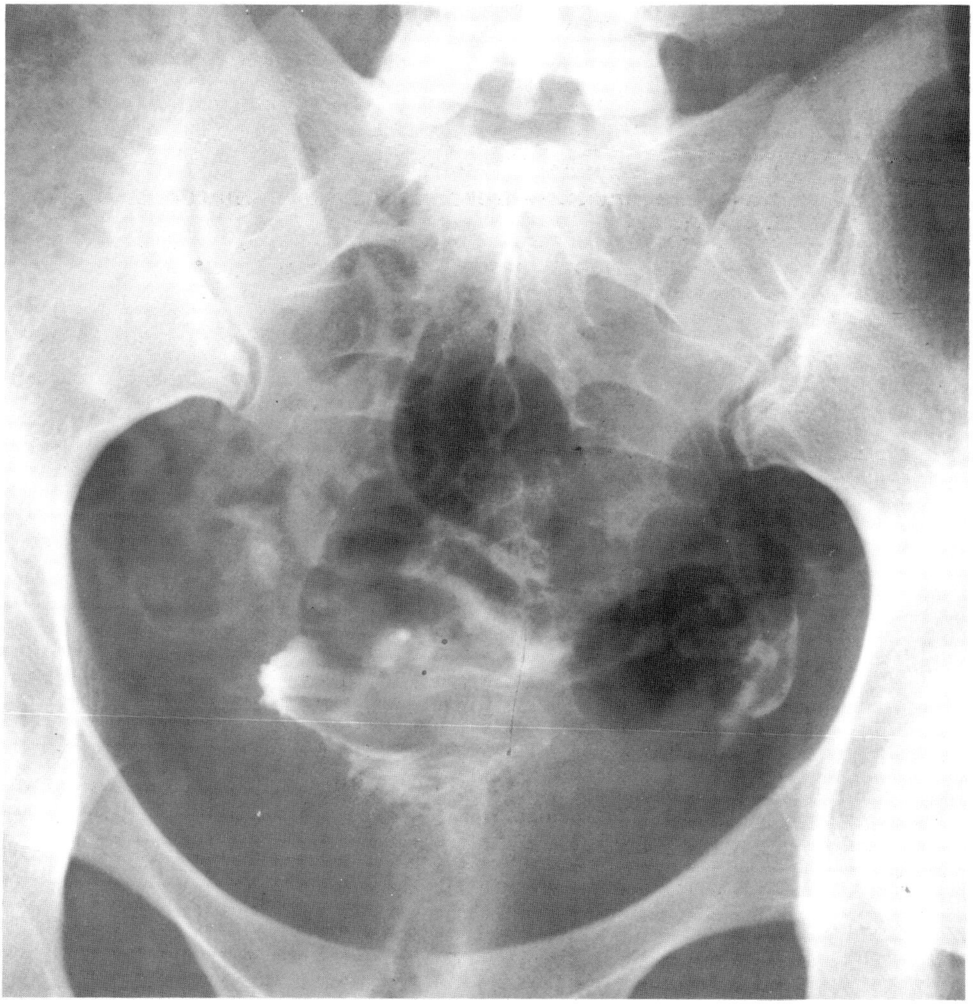

Fig. 11.4. A radiograph of the pelvis exposed some time (perhaps 20–30 minutes) after the completion of hysterosalpingography. Some contrast agent is seen free in the peritoneal cavity, which it has entered from the uterus by way of the uterine tubes.

The outer, serous coat is peritoneal, The middle, muscular coat—consisting of an external, longitudinal layer and an internal circular layer—is continuous with the corresponding muscular fibres of the uterus. Similarly, the innermost, mucous coat is continuous with the mucous lining of the uterus. The lining epithelium is columnar and ciliated; that is, it displays hair-like processes which are able to vibrate.

On its release from the ovary, movement of the ovum along the uterine tube is achieved as the result of three kinds of activity which occur in the tube:

(i) muscular contractions of the walls;
(ii) sweeping movements of the infundibulum over the ovary;
(iii) vibrations of the cilia of the epithelial lining, which actually become taller at the time of ovulation.

The activity of the uterine tubes is influenced by the hormones normally secreted during each menstrual cycle. Their motility is increased by oestradiol and depressed by progesterone. At ovulation the oestrogen-level in the blood is high. Following ovulation, the natural changes, which in effect prepare the uterus for receiving a fertilised ovum, mean that the progesterone-level is high. A result of this subtle chemical balance is that the activity of the uterine tubes is maximum when they may have a cargo to shift and becomes diminished when the ovaries are not releasing ova and there is no work to do.

During hysterosalpingography, the radiological contrast agent should enter the uterine tubes from the cavity of the uterus—provided that the tubes are not occluded—and thence will flow into the peritoneum from the fimbriated end of each tube. This peritoneal spill has already occurred on Fig. 11.2a but is not present on Fig. 11.2b. Fig. 11.4 is a radiograph of the pelvis taken a short time (perhaps 20 minutes) after hysterosalpingography was performed. It shows a small amount of contrast agent lying within folds of the pelvic peritoneum and is proof of the patency of one or both uterine tubes.

Chapter 12
The Lymphatic System in the Pelvis and Abdomen

Apart from calcification which may be seen from time to time, particularly in the lymph nodes of the mesentery, the lymphatics of the pelvis and abdomen are not apparent on a plain radiograph. If the lymphatic courses are to be demonstrated, a radiological contrast agent must be introduced: the procedure by which this is done is called lymphangiography and it enables lymph vessels and lymph nodes to be studied.

Normally the contrast agent flows quite quickly through the lymph channels and is not retained there for longer than a few hours. Lymph nodes fill more slowly and may hold the contrast for several weeks, being visible on a radiograph taken a month or more later; abnormally, nodes have been seen to retain contrast for as long as two years. It is expected that only a portion of the lymphatic pathways in any given area will opacify during lymphangiography; furthermore, to be sure that each of the opacified vessels and nodes is fully delineated and its architecture identified, it is necessary to expose radiographs of the abdomen in anteroposterior, oblique and lateral projections. Because of the delay which occurs between filling of the lymphatic channels and filling of the nodes, it is usual to X-ray the patient both immediately at the time of injection of a contrast agent and 24 hours later.

The courses of lymph vessels correspond to those of arteries and veins. This proximity may sometimes be the agent of a misleading radiological appearance when pressure from adjacent blood vessels gives the impression that a defect indicative of pathology is present in the contour of a lymph node. Elucidation of such a problem is usually dependent on an adequate variety of radiographic projections being made.

The lymph vessels

Lymph is a normally colourless fluid, similar to blood plasma but containing a lower concentration of protein: it is concerned with tissue metabolism. Lymph vessels are found in almost every body tissue which contains blood vessels; they are absent from such avascular structures as cartilage and hair. These vessels are delicately formed and their coats so transparent that the contained lymph is easily visible to anyone who may have the opportunity to look.

The smallest lymph vessels are enmeshed with surrounding tissue elements and blood vessels of the region which they drain. From these networks small vessels arise which feed either a lymph node or a larger lymphatic trunk. In general, lymph vessels are arranged as:

(i) superficial vessels which run immediately beneath the skin and are plentiful where skin and mucous membrane meet at the body's orifices;

(ii) deep vessels which are associated with vascular or neurovascular groupings.

The walls of the larger lymph vessels have a treble construction as follows:

(i) an inner coat of endothelial cells supported on a thin, elastic membrane;

(ii) a middle coat of smooth muscle fibres arranged transversely;

(iii) an external coat of connective tissue, through which run some longitudinal and oblique muscle fibres. In the case of small lymph vessels the walls are composed only of connective tissue lined with epithelium.

Like the veins which they accompany, the lymph vessels have semilunar valves of which the function is to prevent a backflow of lymph. They are most numerous near lymph nodes and are at nearer intervals to each other than the valves of veins. Because the walls of the vessel are expanded at the sites of attachment, these valves give the lymphatic vessels a beaded appearance which may be demonstrated on a radiograph (see Fig. 12.1a). Unlike veins, lymph vessels do not increase in calibre as they approach their termini.

The lymph nodes

Lymph nodes, sometimes incorrectly called glands, are small bean-shaped structures which are situated along the course of lymph vessels and lacteals (the lymph vessels of the mesentery). Lymph and chyle (the name given to the milky-white combination of lymph and emulsified fat which drains from the small intestine) pass through at least one of these bodies *en route* for the blood stream; thus, associated with each node are lymph vessels which enter it (afferent vessels) and lymph vessels which leave it (efferent vessels). On one side of each lymph node there is a hilum or notch at which blood vessels enter and leave the node, together with the efferent vessels; the afferent vessels enter at different points along the periphery of the node.

The structure of a lymph node is recognised as having two layers: a pale, outer, cortical layer and an inner, dark, medullary layer; but this nature is not apparent from a radiograph.

The functions of a lymph node are:

(i) to produce lymphocytes which are collected by the lymph *en passant*;

(ii) to participate in the production of antibodies and antitoxins;

(iii) to remove and destroy bacteria which lymph may carry to the nodes from the tissues.

The cisterna chyli and the thoracic duct

The lymph from the abdominal organs—except for a small part of the liver—and from most of the abdominal wall is returned to the blood stream by way of the cisterna chyli and the thoracic duct.

The cisterna chyli is a dilated part (a few centimetres long) of the abdominal lymphatic pathway and is situated in front of the bodies of lumbar vertebrae 1 and 2, just to the right of the abdominal aorta. It receives major lymphatic tributaries from the abdomen and pelvis and the thorax, as follows:
(i) the intestinal trunk (see p. 269);
(ii) and (iii) right and left lumbar trunks (see p. 269);
(iv) the retro-aortic trunk (see p. 269);
(v) and (vi) right and left descending lymphatic trunks, which are formed by efferent vessels from the intercostal lymph nodes on either side and descend to the cisterna chyli through the aortic opening of the diaphragm.

The thoracic duct, which is the body's main lymph vessel, begins at the upper end of the cisterna chyli, near the lower border of thoracic vertebra 12. Passing in an upward direction, the thoracic duct enters the thorax through the aortic opening of the diaphragm. Its passage through the posterior mediastinum is described elsewhere in this book (see Chapter 4, p. 104). Anomalous variations in the normal distribution of the lymphatic pathways—particularly in the context of the thoracic duct—are encountered in some subjects.

The pelvic and abdominal lymphatics

The injection of a radiological contrast agent to the lower extremities normally fills in sequence vessels and nodes of the following groups:
(i) inguinal;
(ii) external iliac;
(iii) common iliac;
(iv) para-aortic.

THE INGUINAL LYMPH NODES

Except for the ischial and gluteal regions, all the lymph from the lower limbs passes through a group of lymph nodes in either groin. These terminal lymph nodes constitute the inguinal lymph nodes. They are arranged in two groups as:

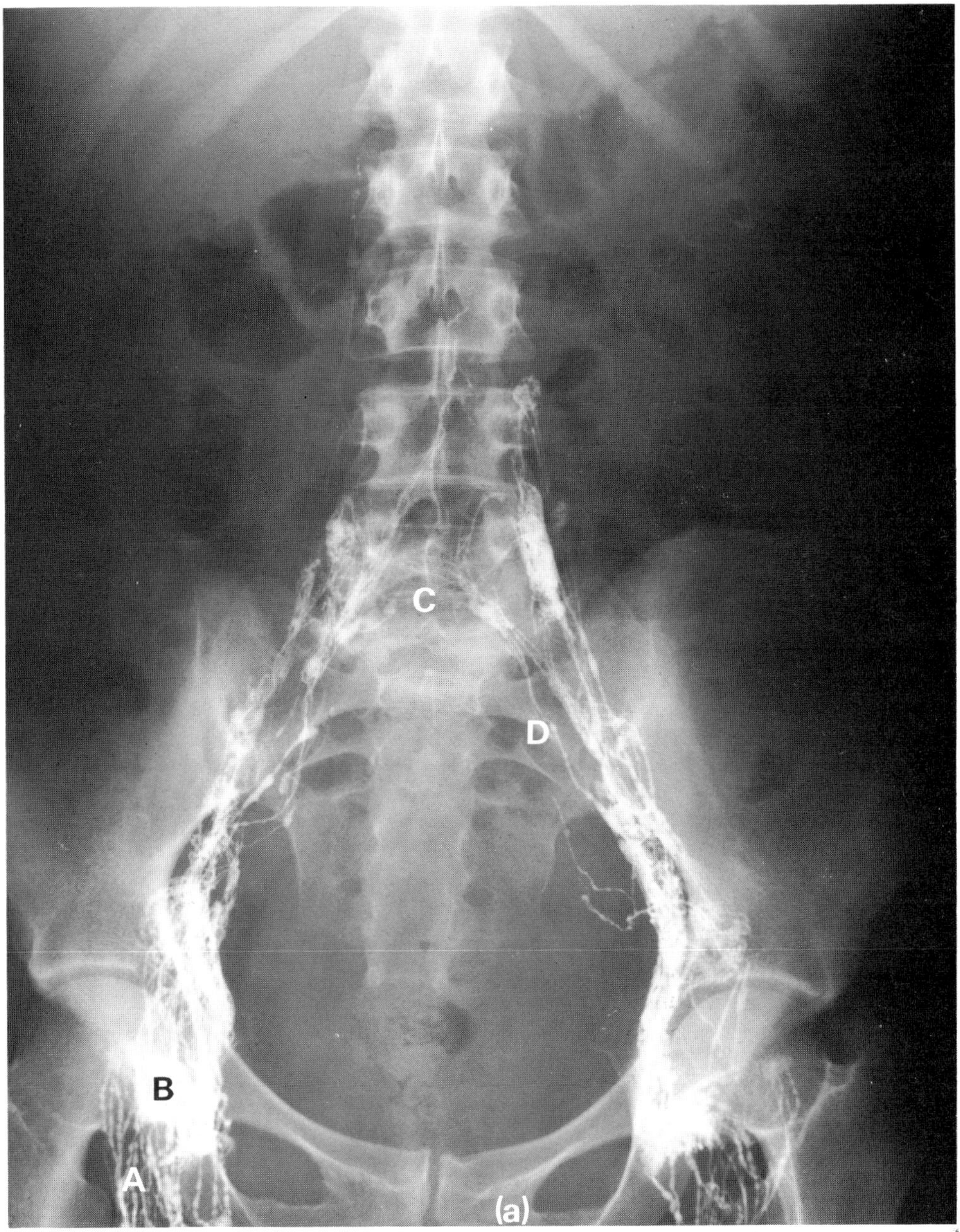

Fig. 12.1a. A radiograph of the abdomen which was obtained shortly after the injection of a contrast agent to a lymphatic channel of each lower extremity. Lymphatic channels and nodes in the pelvis and lower abdomen are demonstrated.

A Afferent lymph vessels to inguinal nodes
B First group of inguinal nodes
C Cross-over network of lymph vessels
D 'Beaded' appearance which is characteristic of a lymphatic valve

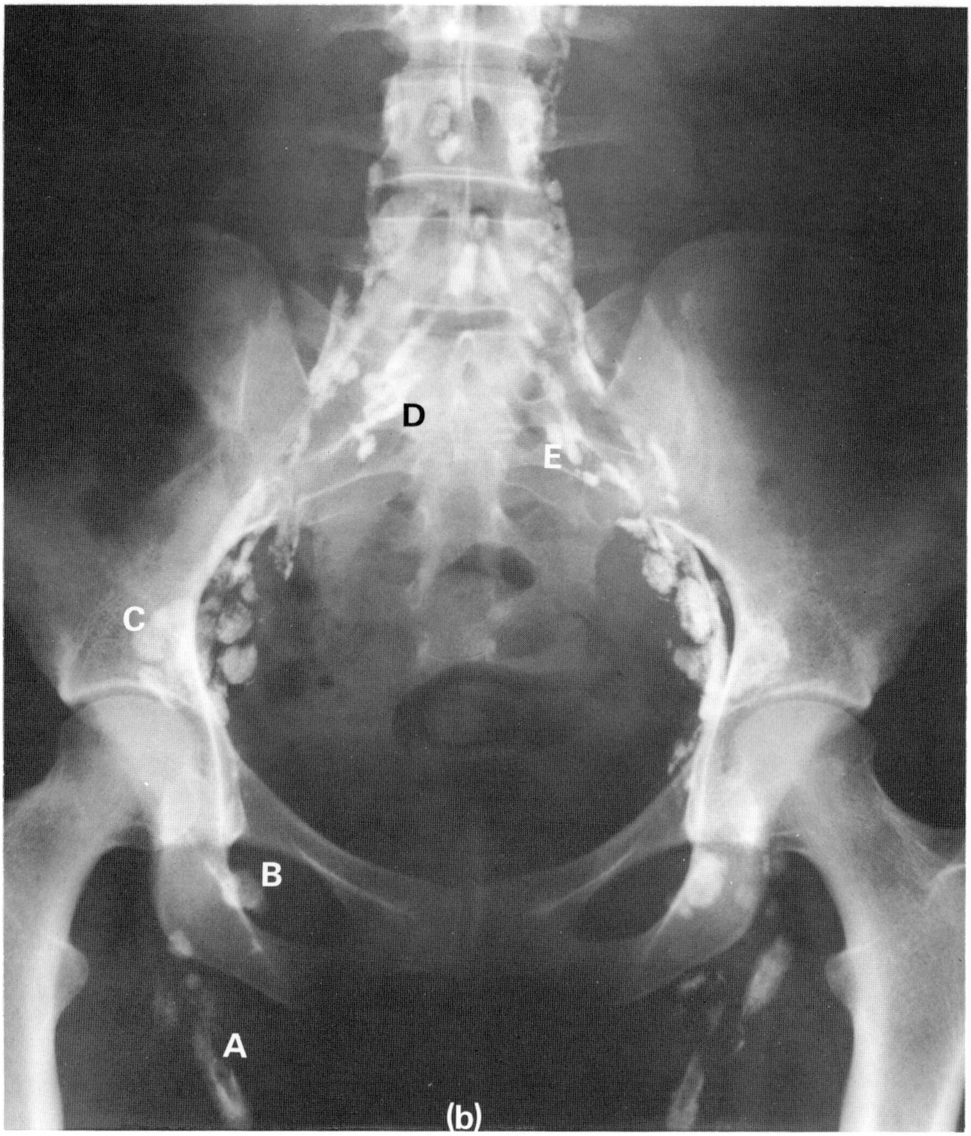

Fig. 12.1b. A lymphangiogram—not of the same patient as on Fig. 12.1a—which was exposed 24 hours after injection of a radiological contrast agent. The contrast agent has mainly dispersed from the pelvic and abdominal vessels but is retained in a number of lymph nodes.

A, B Inguinal lymph nodes
C External iliac nodes
D, E Common iliac nodes on each side

(i) superficial inguinal lymph nodes (an upper group of 5 or 6 and a lower group of 4 or 5);
(ii) deep inguinal lymph nodes, which vary in number from 1 to 3.

Inguinal lymph nodes are well seen in Fig. 12.1b. Fig. 12.1a demonstrates the numerous vessels which both enter the first inguinal lymph nodes and connect the nodes in the groin with each other. The efferent vessels from superficial and deep inguinal lymph nodes pass to the external iliac group.

THE EXTERNAL ILIAC AND THE COMMON ILIAC LYMPH NODES

The external iliac and the common iliac lymph nodes are two of the outlying groups which feed the para-aortic nodes and through which pass the lymph vessels of (a) the pelvis, (b) many of the pelvic viscera and (c) the anterior and lateral abdominal walls. These groups are associated with the iliac arteries and their branches.

External iliac nodes

The external lymph nodes (see Fig. 12.1b) number about 8 to 10 and are arranged in three groups along the external iliac arteries:
(i) a lateral group;
(ii) a medial group;
(iii) an inconstant anterior group.
The efferent vessels from these nodes pass to the common iliac lymph nodes.

The common iliac nodes

The common iliac nodes, which number from 4 to 6, are grouped on either side of and posterior to the common iliac artery. They are seen on Fig. 12.1b and in the oblique view which is Fig. 12.2.

One or two of these lymph nodes lie just below the bifurcation of the aorta, in front of the body of lumbar vertebra 5 or the sacral promontory. The efferent vessels from the common iliac nodes feed the para-aortic lymph nodes.

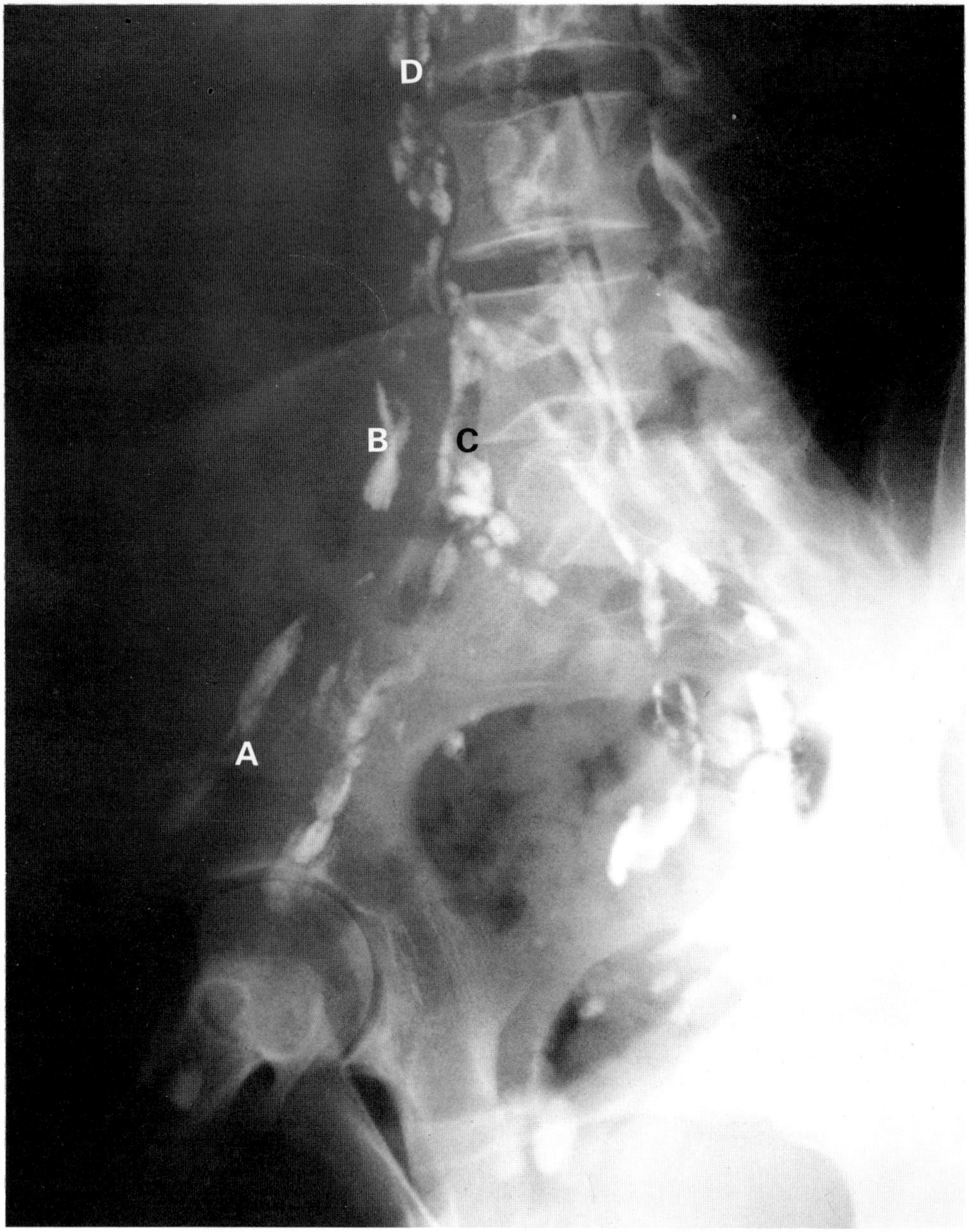

Fig. 12.2. A right posterior oblique projection obtained at the same time as the anteroposterior view depicted on Plate 12.1(b).

A External iliac nodes
D Para-aortic nodes
B, C Common iliac nodes

In Fig. 12.1a is seen the 'cross-over' network of lymph vessels which is usually found from the level of the sacrum upwards: otherwise the lymphatic drainage from each lower limb is separate and there is even only minor communication between the medial and lateral portions of either limb itself. The 'cross-over' system may extend along the whole area of the para-aortic lymph nodes.

THE PARA-AORTIC LYMPH NODES

The para-aortic lymph nodes, although they are not sharply separated from each other topographically, are arranged in groups which are associated with discrete drainage areas. The four groups are described in relation to the abdominal aorta as follows:

(i) pre-aortic or in front of the aorta;
(ii) and (iii) right and left lateral groups;
(iv) a retro-aortic group.

The first three are terminal lymph nodes; that is, the lymph vessels of the abdominal viscera all feed respectively to one or another of these groups.

The efferent vessels from the pre-aortic group unite to form an intestinal trunk which enters the cisterna chyli (see p. 263). Efferent vessels from the lateral aortic groups of lymph nodes form the lumbar trunks—one on either side—and these right and left lumbar trunks similarly enter the cisterna chyli.

The retro-aortic group is the individualistic member among the para-aortic lymph nodes. Unlike the others, its drainage area is unspecific. Only a few vessels directly feed retro-aortic nodes from adjacent muscles, bones and ligaments of the posterior abdominal wall: nearly all the retro-aortic afferents come from outlying members of the lateral aortic groups. The efferents of the retro-aortic group unite to form a fair-sized vessel which enters the cisterna chyli.

Para-aortic lymph nodes are seen in an anteroposterior view on Fig. 12.3a; and in oblique projection (not the same patient) on Fig. 12.3b. Fig. 12.4 shows para-aortic vessels from the lateral aspect.

It is to be emphasized that the lymphatics described in

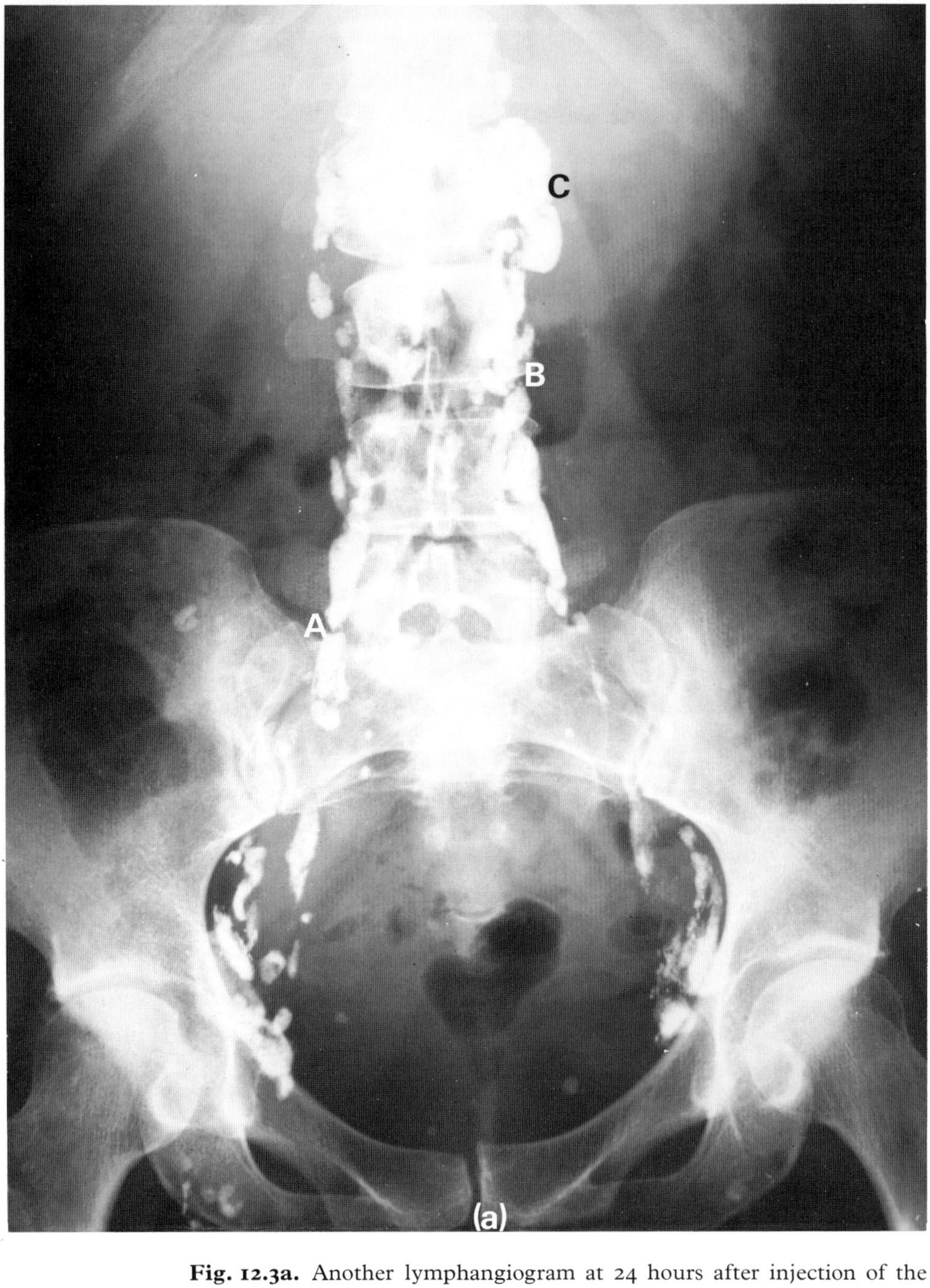

Fig. 12.3a. Another lymphangiogram at 24 hours after injection of the contrast agent, showing filling of the pelvic and abdominal lymph nodes.
A Common iliac lymph nodes B, C Para-aortic lymph nodes

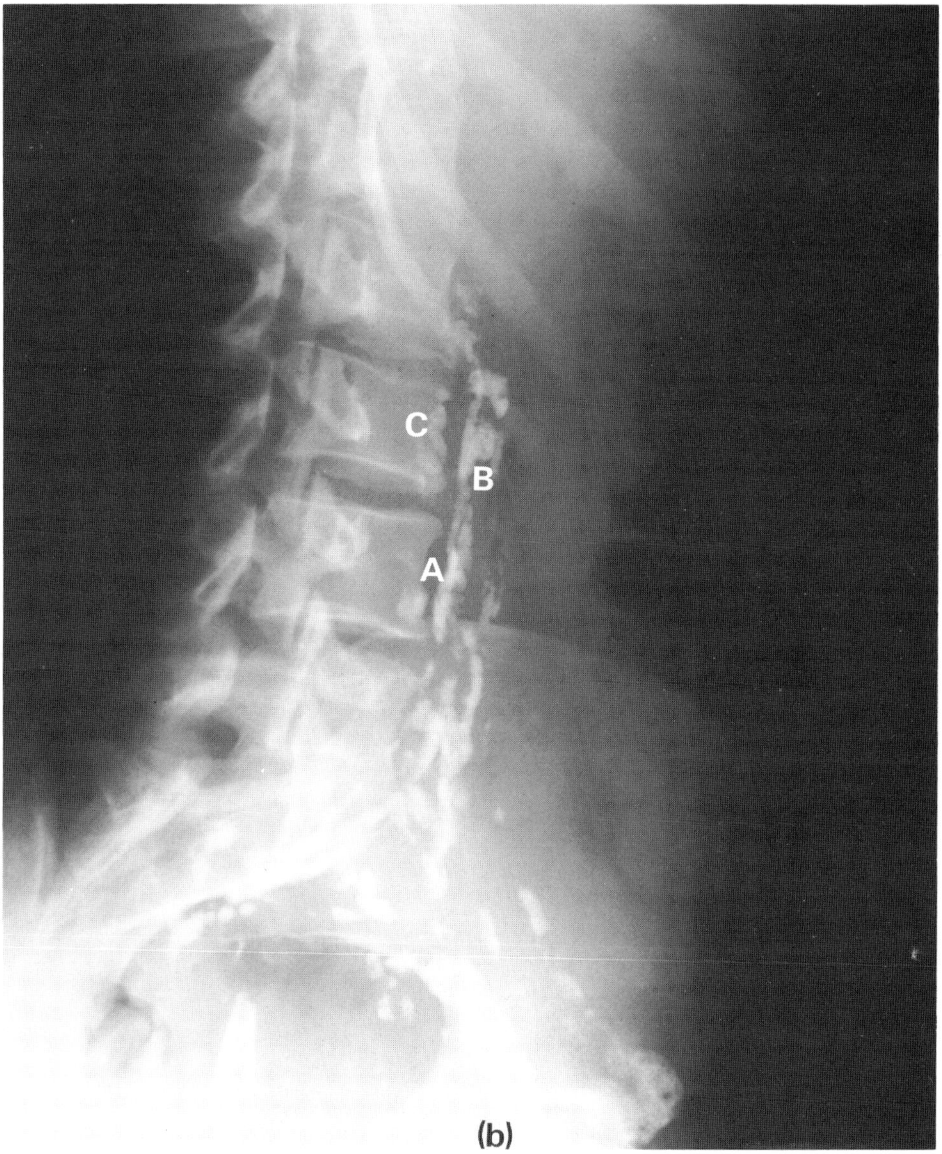

Fig. 12.3b. A left posterior oblique projection of the same patient as on Figs. 12.1b and 12.2.
A, B, C Para-aortic lymph nodes

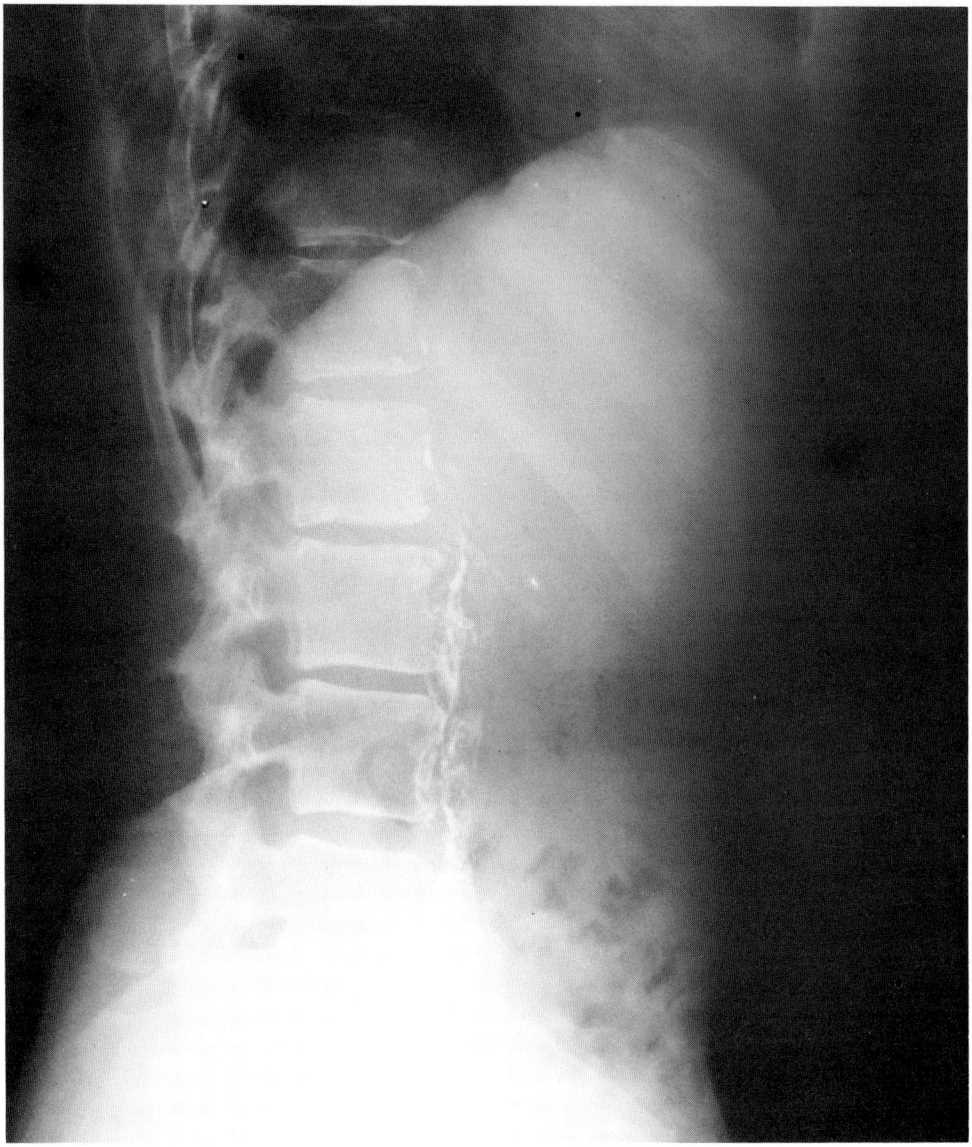

Fig. 12.4. A lymphangiogram in lateral projection, showing filling of para-aortic lymphatics.

this chapter consitute only a part of the complete system draining the pelvic and abdominal organs. There are many more visceral—and other—collecting vessels and nodes. The lymphatic groups, of which some account is given here, are simply those which usually are seen as the result of lymphangiography from the lower extremities. Even within such limits, there is no certainty that every vessel and node has been visualised at each examination. In effect this means that a normal lymphangiogram cannot justifiably be taken as proof that no pathology is present: it may exist in nodes which have not been demonstrated.

Index